Disorders of the Proximal Biceps Tendon: Evaluation and Treatment

Edited by
Samer S. Hasan, MD, PhD
Co-Director
Shoulder and Elbow Center
Cincinnati SportsMedicine and Orthopaedic Center
Cincinnati, Ohio

Augustus D. Mazzocca, MS, MD
Interim Director, New England Musculoskeletal Institute
Interim Chairman, Department of Orthopaedic Surgery
Department of Orthopaedic Surgery
University of Connecticut Health Center
Farmington, Connecticut

Series Editor
Adam J. Schwartz, MD
Assistant Professor
Department of Orthopaedic Surgery
Mayo Clinic
Phoenix, Arizona

AAOS
American Academy of Orthopaedic Surgeons

AAOS

AMERICAN ACADEMY OF ORTHOPAEDIC SURGEONS

STAFF

Hans Koelsch, PhD, *Director, Department of Publications*
Lisa Claxton Moore, *Managing Editor*
Steven Kellert, *Senior Editor*
Mary Steermann Bishop, *Senior Manager, Production and Content Management*
Courtney Astle, *Editorial Production Manager*
Abram Fassler, *Publishing Systems Manager*
Suzanne O'Reilly, *Graphic Designer*
Susan Morritz Baim, *Production Coordinator*
Karen Danca, *Permissions Coordinator*
Charlie Baldwin, *Production Database Associate*
Hollie Muir, *Production Database Associate*
Emily Nickel, *Page Production Assistant*
Michelle Wild, *Editorial Coordinator*

Published 2014 by the
American Academy of Orthopaedic Surgeons
6300 North River Road
Rosemont, IL 60018

The material presented in *Disorders of the Proximal Biceps Tendon: Evaluation and Treatment* has been made available by the American Academy of Orthopaedic Surgeons for educational purposes only. This material is not intended to present the only, or necessarily best, methods or procedures for the medical situations discussed, but rather is intended to represent an approach, view, statement, or opinion of the author(s) or producer(s), which may be helpful to others who face similar situations.

Some drugs or medical devices demonstrated in Academy courses or described in Academy print or electronic publications have not been cleared by the Food and Drug Administration (FDA) or have been cleared for specific uses only. The FDA has stated that it is the responsibility of the physician to determine the FDA clearance status of each drug or device he or she wishes to use in clinical practice.

Furthermore, any statements about commercial products are solely the opinion(s) of the author(s) and do not represent an Academy endorsement or evaluation of these products. These statements may not be used in advertising or for any commercial purpose.

ISSN
2328-272X

ISBN
978-0-89203-970-8
Printed in the USA

Bone and Joint Initiative USA

Contributors

Christopher S. Ahmad, MD
Associate Professor
Department of Orthopaedic Surgery
Columbia University
New York, New York

Stéphane Audebert, MD
Orthopaedic Surgeon
Clinique du Cambrésis
Cambrai, France

James R. Bailey, MD, LCDR, USN
Resident Physician
Department of Orthopaedic Surgery
Naval Medical Center San Diego
San Diego, California

Nikolas J. Baret
Research Coordinator
Orthopaedic Department
Hospital for Special Surgery
New York, New York

Knut Beitzel, MA, MD
Department of Orthopedic and Trauma Surgery
Trauma Center Murnau
Murnau, Germany

Hans C. Bengtson, MD
Clinical Fellow
Cincinnati SportsMedicine & Orthopaedic Center
Cincinnati, Ohio

Michael J. Bey, PhD
Director
Bone and Joint Center
Henry Ford Hospital
Detroit, Michigan

Sepp Braun, MD
Department of Orthopedic Sports Medicine
Technical University Munich
Munich, Germany

Benjamin Bruce, MD
Shoulder and Elbow Fellow
Department of Orthopaedic Surgery
Rush University Medical Center
Chicago, Illinois

Alissa J. Burge, MD
Assistant Attending Radiologist
Department of Radiology and Imaging
Hospital for Special Surgery
New York, New York

Matthew L. Busam, MD
Staff Orthopaedic Surgeon
Cincinnati SportsMedicine & Orthopaedic Center
Cincinnati, Ohio

Mark P. Cote, PT, DPT, MSCTR
Sports Medicine Clinical Outcomes Research Facilitator
Department of Orthopaedic Surgery
University of Connecticut Health Center
Farmington, Connecticut

Arash Dini, MD
Department of Orthopaedic Surgery
Tulane University School of Medicine
New Orleans, Louisiana

T. Bradley Edwards, MD
Attending Surgeon
Fondren Orthopedic Group
Texas Orthopedic Hospital
Houston, Texas

Contributors (cont.)

Eugene T.H. Ek, MBBS, PhD, FRACS
Fellow
Harvard Shoulder Service
Department of Orthopaedic Surgery
Massachusetts General Hospital
Boston, Massachusetts

Neal S. ElAttrache, MD
Chairman
Kerlan-Jobe Orthopaedic Foundation
Los Angeles, California

Elizabeth Gausden, MD
Orthopedic Resident
Department of Orthopedics
Hospital for Special Surgery
New York, New York

Lauren E. Geaney, MD
Resident
Department of Orthopaedics
University of Connecticut
Farmington, Connecticut

Arnaud Godenéche, MD
Orthopaedic Surgeon
Shoulder Unit – Shoulder Surgeon
Centre Orthopédique Santy
Lyon, France

Anil K. Gupta, MD, MBA
Sports Medicine Fellow
Department of Orthopaedic Surgery
Rush University Medical Center
Chicago, Illinois

Samer S. Hasan, MD, PhD
Co-Director
Shoulder and Elbow Center
Cincinnati SportsMedicine &
Orthopaedic Center
Cincinnati, Ohio

Wendell M.R. Heard, MD
Assistant Professor
Department of Orthopaedic Surgery
Tulane University School of Medicine
New Orleans, Louisiana

Andreas B. Imhoff, MD
Department Head
Department of Orthopedic Sports Medicine
Technical University Munich
Munich, Germany

Michael F. Joseph, PhD, PT
Assistant Professor
Kinesiology Department
University of Connecticut
Storrs, Connecticut

W. Ben Kibler, MD
Medical Director
Shoulder Center of Kentucky
Lexington Clinic
Lexington, Kentucky

Eric C. Makhni, MD
Resident
Department of Orthopaedic Surgery
Columbia Presbyterian Medical Center
New York, New York

CONTRIBUTORS (CONT.)

Augustus D. Mazzocca, MS, MD
Interim Director, New England Musculoskeletal Institute
Interim Chairman, Department of Orthopaedic Surgery
Department of Orthopaedic Surgery
University of Connecticut Health Center
Farmington, Connecticut

Frank McCormick, MD
Sports Medicine Fellow
Department of Orthopaedic Surgery
Rush University Medical Center
Chicago, Illinois

Lucas S. McDonald, MD, MPH, LCDR, USN
Clinical Instructor of Surgery
Resident Physician
Department of Orthopaedic Surgery
Naval Medical Center San Diego
San Diego, California

Edward G. McFarland, MD
The Wayne H. Lewis Professor of Orthopaedics and Shoulder Surgery
Co-Director, Division of Shoulder Surgery
Department of Orthopaedic Surgery
Johns Hopkins University
Baltimore, Maryland

John W. McNeil II, BA
Research Assistant
Department of Orthopaedics
Naval Medical Center San Diego
San Diego, California

Vasilios Moutzouros, MD
Orthopaedic Surgeon
Department of Orthopaedic Surgery
Henry Ford Hospital
Detroit, Michigan

Gregory P. Nicholson, MD
Associate Professor
Division of Sports Medicine and Elbow Surgery
Rush University Medical Center
Chicago, Illinois

Laurent Nové-Josserand, MD
Orthopaedic Surgeon
Shoulder Unit – Shoulder Surgeon
Centre Orthopédique Santy
Lyon, France

Michael J. O'Brien, MD
Assistant Professor of Clinical Orthopaedics
Department of Orthopaedic Surgery
Tulane University School of Medicine
New Orleans, Louisiana

Stephen J. O'Brien, MD, MBA
Attending Orthopaedic Surgeon
Department of Orthopaedics
Hospital for Special Surgery
New York, New York

Bradford O. Parsons, MD
Assistant Professor
Department of Orthopaedic Surgery
Mount Sinai School of Medicine
New York, New York

Contributors (Cont.)

Cathryn D. Peltz, PhD
Senior Research Engineer
Bone and Joint Center
Henry Ford Hospital
Detroit, Michigan

Hollis G. Potter, MD
Chief
Division of Magnetic Resonance Imaging
Department of Radiology and Imaging
Hospital for Special Surgery
New York, New York

Matthew T. Provencher, MD, CDR, USN
Professor of Surgery and Orthopaedics
Department of Orthopaedic Surgery
Naval Medical Center San Diego
San Diego, California

Clay Riley, MD
Orthopaedic Surgeon
Martin Knee and Sports Medicine Center
Little Rock, Arkansas

Anthony A. Romeo, MD
Professor, Department of Orthopaedic Surgery
Section Head, Shoulder and Elbow Surgery
Midwest Orthopaedics at Rush
Rush University Medical Center
Chicago, Illinois

Felix H. Savoie III, MD
Professor of Clinical Orthopaedics
Department of Orthopaedic Surgery
Tulane University School of Medicine
New Orleans, Louisiana

Lewis L. Shi, MD
Assistant Professor
Department of Orthopaedics
University of Chicago
Chicago, Illinois

Steven Slotkin, MS
Medical Student
Wayne State University
Detroit, Michigan

Eric W. Tan, MD
Resident
Department of Orthopaedic Surgery
Johns Hopkins University
Baltimore, Maryland

Samuel A. Taylor, MD
Fellow
Department of Orthopaedics
Hospital for Special Surgery
New York, New York

Bruno Toussaint, MD
Orthopaedic Surgeon
Clinique Generale
Annecy, France

Nikhil N. Verma, MD
Associate Professor
Midwest Orthopaedics at Rush
Rush University Medical Center
Chicago, Illinois

Brandon R. Vier, MD, LT, USN
Resident Physician
Department of Orthopaedic Surgery
Naval Medical Center San Diego
San Diego, California

Contributors (Cont.)

Mandeep S. Virk, MBBS
Orthopaedic Resident
Department of Orthopaedic Surgery
University of Connecticut
Farmington, Connecticut

Gilles Walch, MD
Orthopaedic Surgeon
Shoulder Unit – Shoulder Surgeon
Centre Orthopédique Santy
Lyon, France

Jon J.P. Warner, MD
Chief
Harvard Shoulder Service
Department of Orthopaedic Surgery
Massachusetts General Hospital
Boston, Massachusetts

Allan Young, MBBS, MSpMed, PhD, FRACS
Shoulder Surgeon
Sydney Shoulder Specialists
Sydney, New South Wales, Australia

Preface

The evaluation and treatment of injuries to the proximal or long head of the biceps tendon and the superior labrum have evolved greatly over the past few decades and are topics of great interest and considerable controversy. Superior labrum anterior to posterior (SLAP) injuries were not recognized until the advent of modern shoulder arthroscopy less than 30 years ago. Moreover, although open biceps tenodesis was first described more than 60 years ago, most current treatment methods, including open and arthroscopic repairs, are new and evolving.

Although the understanding of biceps and labral anatomy and pathoanatomy has increased immensely in recent years, much controversy persists regarding the accurate diagnosis of symptomatic proximal biceps tendon injuries and the optimal treatment of these lesions, including the precise indications for both SLAP repair and biceps tenotomy. In addition, no two patients with proximal biceps tendon injuries are exactly alike, and myriad factors related to patient health, habitus, activity level, expectations, and associated shoulder injuries influence the treatment algorithm.

To place attention on this controversial topic, we asked a group of international surgical leaders to share their insights and experiences related to the evaluation and treatment of proximal biceps tendon injuries. The authors have delivered magnificently, and the result is a monograph covering anatomy and biomechanics, clinical evaluation, and nonsurgical and surgical management of biceps and SLAP injuries, including the treatment of specific patient populations. This monograph represents the most comprehensive treatment of proximal biceps tendon injuries to date and fills a gap in the AAOS educational portfolio. Some redundancy between chapters has been deliberately retained to present multiple perspectives on a specific topic. We believe that this modest overlap is a strong point of this monograph rather than a shortcoming.

On a personal note, editing this monograph has been a rewarding experience for both of us. Throughout this process we have learned a great deal more about the proximal biceps tendon and superior labrum than we knew beforehand, and we hope that the reader experiences a similar effect. Finally, this monograph has been a team effort and acknowledgments are in order. We thank all of the authors for their timely and quality contributions, which greatly simplified our work as coeditors. We also thank the editorial staff at AAOS, who have guided this project from takeoff to landing, including Hans Koelsch, PhD, publications department director; Lisa Claxton Moore, managing editor; Steven Kellert, senior editor; and Michelle Wild, editorial coordinator. Finally, we acknowledge and appreciate the infinite patience of our two families who have put up with us as we took on this challenge. Thank you all.

Samer S. Hasan, MD, PhD
Augustus Mazzocca, MS, MD
Editors

Table of Contents

CHAPTER 1

Anatomy and Biomechanics: Normal Anatomy and Pathoanatomy of the Superior Labrum

Elizabeth Gausden, MD
Samuel A. Taylor, MD
Stephen J. O'Brien, MD, MBA

Introduction

The glenohumeral joint has tremendous mobility because of its osseous architecture and relatively unconstrained ligamentous support. The humeral head abuts the glenoid rather than articulating within it, and has been compared with a golf ball on a tee.[1] Although this relationship allows considerable mobility, it simultaneously makes the joint susceptible to instability.

Normal Anatomy, Morphology, and Function

The stability of the glenohumeral joint is maintained by a complex interaction of static and dynamic restraints. The labrum is an important component of that stability.

The shape of the glenoid fossa varies and may be pear-shaped, oval-shaped, or notched.[2] The pear-shaped variant is found in 55% of the population and has a notch on the anterior border of the glenoid that separates the superior third from the inferior two thirds of the glenoid.[3]

The glenoid labrum attaches circumferentially to the glenoid, which increases its surface area, facilitates weight bearing, and provides an attachment site for several tendoligamentous structures. The labrum consists mostly of collagenous tissue fibers and is approximately 4 to 6 mm wide and 4 mm thick.[3] The cross section of the labrum appears predominantly triangular, and it functions as a bumper at the boundary of the glenoid fossa.[4] A recess exists between the labral lip and the capsule that is normally deeper ventrally than dorsally.[3] The labrum deepens the fossa without altering its radius of curvature.[4] With an intact labrum, the glenoid can accommodate 50% to 75% of the humeral head in the coronal plane and two thirds of the humeral head in the sagittal plane.[5,6] The increased glenohumeral contact area improves stability. In a cadaver model, Lippitt and Matsen[7] demonstrated the contribution of the labrum to glenohumeral stability: full resection of the labrum produced a 20% decrease in resistance to humeral head translation.

None of the following authors nor any immediate family member has received anything of value from or has stock or stock options held in a commercial company or institution related directly or indirectly to the subject of this chapter: Dr. Gausden, Dr. Taylor, and Dr. O'Brien.

The labrum also helps distribute load within the shoulder joint. Greis et al[8] evaluated the effect of progressive labral resection on glenohumeral contact pressures in eight fresh-frozen cadaver shoulders. The authors reported that a loss of the anteroinferior labrum decreased contact surface area by 15% and simultaneously produced a mean increase of 8% to 20% in contact pressure. Furthermore, resection of the anteroinferior labrum also shifted the contact area—contact pressures were increased in the anteroinferior quadrant and decreased in the posterosuperior quadrant.

The labrum is also intimately associated with the capsular ligaments and glenohumeral ligaments and provides insertion points for the long head of the biceps (LHB) tendon and the long head of the triceps tendon.[9] The capsule is located on the periphery of the labrum and envelopes the glenohumeral joint, extending from the glenoid neck to the anatomic neck of the humeral head. Inferiorly, a 1-cm-deep reserve fold of capsule exists in the axilla, allowing the humeral head to translate inferiorly during abduction.[3] Superiorly, the capsule attaches to the coracoid process and extends inferiorly down the biceps tendon, covering the intertubercular groove of the humerus[10] The glenohumeral ligaments help provide strength and stability within this capsule.[11] The coracohumeral ligament often appears as two bands stretching from the coracoid process to the greater tuberosity and partially to the lesser tuberosity, and is an inferior stabilizer of the glenohumeral joint.[12] In a cadaver study, the coracohumeral ligament had two times the stiffness and three times the tensile load of the superior glenohumeral ligament (SGHL).[13] Overall, the capsule and its ligamentous contributions restrain against translation during active and passive motion.[12]

The SGHL originates with or just anterior to the origin of the LHB tendon.[14,15] The SGHL consists of oblique and direct fibers, which arise from the supraglenoid tubercle and labrum, respectively,[16] and proceed parallel to the LHB tendon, inserting into the fovea capitis and lying superior to the lesser tuberosity. Some fibers insert into the base of the bicipital groove; the rest contribute to the transverse humeral ligament. The SGHL may be thin, and is absent in approximately 10% of normal shoulders.[11,17]

The middle glenohumeral ligament (MGHL) can have a highly varied appearance that ranges from gossamer to thick and cord-like; however, it can be absent in up to 27% of patients.[17] The MGHL typically originates from the labrum just anterior to the SGHL or from the adjacent glenoid neck. Tuoheti et al[18] noted that the MGHL typically attaches between the 12 o'clock and 1 o'clock positions on the labrum. Although the MGHL has been noted to insert on the humerus medial to the lesser tuberosity, a variant that inserts solely onto the capsule has also been reported.[19]

The inferior glenohumeral ligament (IGHL) complex is composed of an anterior band, a posterior band, and an interposed axillary pouch. The IGHL originates from the glenoid labrum, or glenoid neck (the anterior band originates between the 2 o'clock and 4 o'clock positions and the posterior band originates between the 7 o'clock and 9 o'clock positions), and inserts on the anatomic neck of the humerus[10] (**Figure 1**). The IGHL complex is the most important stabilizer when the shoulder is in abduction, bearing forces up to 45 N at 60° and 90° of abduction, and is the most frequently injured capsular ligament.[12]

The advent of shoulder arthroscopy has increased interest in labral anatomy, as well as any associated pathology. Furthermore, advances in shoulder imaging, particularly with MRI, have resulted in better understanding of the anatomy and function of the glenoid labrum. Despite the capabilities of modern MRI, the anatomic variability of the labrum can make differentiating normal variants from pathologic lesions quite difficult. In a study of arthroscopically normal labra, approximately 50% demonstrated signal changes on MRI.[20]

The labrum is morphologically heterogeneous, particularly regarding its association with the glenoid. Anatomic studies indicate that the superior and anterosuperior parts of the labrum attach loosely to the glenoid.[4] Cooper et al[9] studied 42 shoulder specimens and reported that attachments from the superior labrum to the glenoid fossa were present in less than 11%; in those cases, the labrum attached to the neck of the scapula rather than the glenoid fossa. Rispoli et al[21] identified an overlap of the labrum onto the bony surface of the glenoid of 2.6 mm to 7.3 mm. Inferiorly, the labrum's cross-section shape is round and it attaches firmly onto the glenoid.[4] The meniscoid-like superior labrum described in cadaver studies has been suggested as an artifact of the degenerative process of the labrum.[22]

FIGURE 1

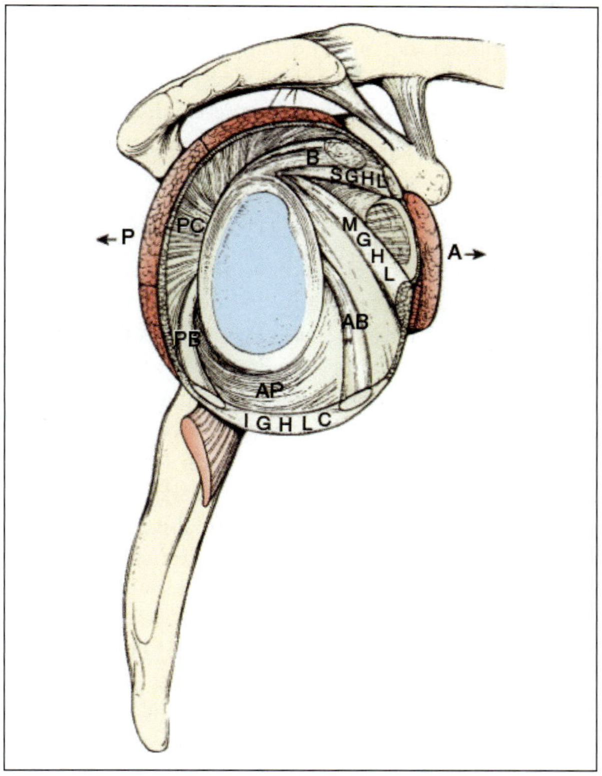

Illustration of the inferior glenohumeral ligament complex (IGHLC), composed of an anterior band, a posterior band, and an interposed axillary pouch. (AB = anterior band of the IGHL, AP = axillary pouch, B = biceps, MGHL = middle glenohumeral ligament, PB = posterior band of the IGHL, PC = posterior capsule, SGHL = superior glenohumeral ligament. (Reproduced with permission from Taylor SA, McCarthy MM, Newman AM, O'Brien SJ: Arthroscopy and the subdeltoid space and biceps tendon transfer, in Craig EV, ed: *Master Techniques in Orthopaedics: The Shoulder,* ed 3. Philadelphia, PA, Lippincott Williams & Wilkins, 2012, pp 205-221.)

Histology

Although the labrum has been described as fibrocartilaginous, the superior labrum consists entirely of collagen fibers without any interposed chondrocytes.[9] At the insertion of the glenohumeral ligaments and the LHB tendon superiorly, the labrum becomes indistinguishable from the tendon histologically.

The posterosuperior labrum closely resembles the collagen fibers of the LHB tendon, and the anterosuperior labrum contains more elastic fibers and semicircular fibers.[23] Furthermore, Tuoheti et al[18] described an all-posterior or posterior-dominated histologic origin of the LHB tendon from the labrum in 84 of 101 cadaver specimens (83.1%) examined. The elasticity of the anterosuperior labrum, particularly in the zone that connects the glenohumeral ligament to the LHB tendon, may be needed to accept tensile stress within the rotator interval in this region.[23]

In the lower quadrants, the labrum may be considered fibrocartilaginous where the collagen fibers of the inferior labrum at the periphery blend with the articular cartilage of the glenoid fossa, creating a transition zone.[4,9] The transition zone, which is histologically cartilaginous, explains the strong insertion of the labrum inferiorly.[9]

Because of the heterogeneous nature of the labrum and its insertions, Huber and Putz[9] proposed the term periarticular fiber system (PAFS) to include the labrum, the biceps and triceps tendons, and the insertions of the inferior humeral ligaments. The authors insisted that only the inferior quadrants of the PAFS should be referred to as the glenoid labrum because the superior region of the PAFS is merely a connection that exists between the SGHL and MGHL in the periphery of the glenoid fossa.

The LHB Tendon

The LHB tendon is intimately associated with the superior labrum—the combination is referred to as the biceps-labral complex. Historically, anatomy texts have described the supraglenoid tubercle as the origin of the LHB tendon.

The precise origin of the LHB tendon varies, but it most commonly arises from the superior labrum. In a landmark study, Vangsness et al[24] examined 100 cadaveric shoulders and found that in 50% of specimens, the LHB tendon originated from the supraglenoid tubercle. In the other 50%, the LHB tendon originated from and was virtually indistinguishable from the superior labrum. Four types of biceps attachments to the glenoid labrum were described. A type I biceps attaches solely to the posterior labrum, a type II biceps attaches predominantly posteriorly, a type III biceps attaches equally to the anterior and posterior labrum, and a type IV biceps attaches mostly to the anterior labrum.

Vangsness et al[24] and Pal et al[25] concluded that grossly, most LHB tendons originate from the superior labrum posterior to the supraglenoid tubercle (type I or type II).

The tissues of the superior labrum and the biceps tendon also blend histologically in this region.[4] One histologic study found that despite its macroscopic appearance, all of the LHB tendon fibers emanate from the posterior labrum.[18] Dierickx et al[26] reviewed 3,000 arthroscopic procedures and classified the anatomic variations of the intra-articular portion of the LHB tendon into four main types: the mesotenon type, which permits good movement between the LHB tendon and the rotator cuff; the adherent type, which has a stronger connection between the LHB tendon and the capsule; the split type; and the complete absence of the LHB tendon. The authors distinguished between two types of split LHB tendon origins: one in which the biceps originates partially from the inferior surface of the supraspinatus and partially from the glenoid, and one referred to as the "split biceps reversed type" in which a segment of the LHB tendon extends from the split and diverges laterally to the inferior surface of the capsule.

Great controversy exists over the biomechanical function of the LHB tendon. Many authors think that it functions as a humeral head depressor,[27] but most clinicians question whether this is clinically important for normal shoulder function.

Vascular Supply and Innervation

The branches of the suprascapular, the anterior humeral circumflex, and the posterior humeral circumflex arteries all contribute to the vascular supply of the labrum.[4] These three arteries create an anastomotic network that reaches the labrum from its peripheral glenoid attachment, mostly radially. Circumferential vessels have also been identified that unite with the radial branches, but no vessels reach the labrum from the underlying glenoid bone.[4] Penetration of the blood vessels from the periphery to the inner portions of the labrum is limited, particularly in the more meniscoid regions of the labrum. The superior and anterosuperior labrum have the lowest blood flow, possibly decreasing the likelihood of regeneration of these areas following a labral tear.[4]

The shoulder follows Hilton's law in that nerves that cross a joint also innervate the joint.[19] The axillary, suprascapular, and occasionally, the branches of the musculocutaneous nerves all contribute to the innervation of the shoulder capsule and labrum. Alpantaki et al[28] described the sensory and sympathetic elements of the LHB tendon and noted an asymmetric distribution of this neural network, primarily in the proximal portion of the tendon.

Normal Anatomic Variants

As the field of arthroscopy developed and MRI technology progressed, variations in the structure of the superior glenoid labrum have been identified and studied.[4,11,29-33] These variants were described as physiologic, not pathologic, suggesting that repairing variants such as a Buford complex would result in poor outcomes.[29] Imaging studies have reported incidences of the variants and remarked on the possibility of mistaking them for a detached labrum.[33] Despite the original descriptions of the variants as normal, more recent studies have questioned the physiologic nature of superior labral variants. Some anatomic variants have been associated with higher rates of labral injury.[34] Huber and Putz[9] studied 42 shoulders and reported that all had a gap between the labrum and the articular cartilage of the glenoid fossa superiorly; the authors argued that this gap is always present and should not be considered pathologic. Other authors reported that normal variants should be defined as not extending inferiorly to the anterior glenoid notch, which typically is between the 2 o'clock and 3 o'clock positions.[29,35]

Sublabral Recess

The supraglenoid tubercle is approximately 5 mm medial to the superior ridge of the glenoid rim.[32] The absence of a labral attachment inferior to the tubercle creates a synovial recess, often called a sublabral recess, and is generally located between the 11 o'clock and 1 o'clock positions.[4,32] This recess can be mistaken for a superior labrum anterior to posterior (SLAP) lesion on imaging,[11,33] but the two can be distinguished using magnetic resonance arthrography. With a physiologic sublabral recess, the injected contrast medium extravasates smoothly between the glenoid and the labrum; with a SLAP tear, the contrast extravasates irregularly and tracks posteriorly to the insertion of the biceps tendon.[32] No association is known to exist between a sub-

FIGURE 2

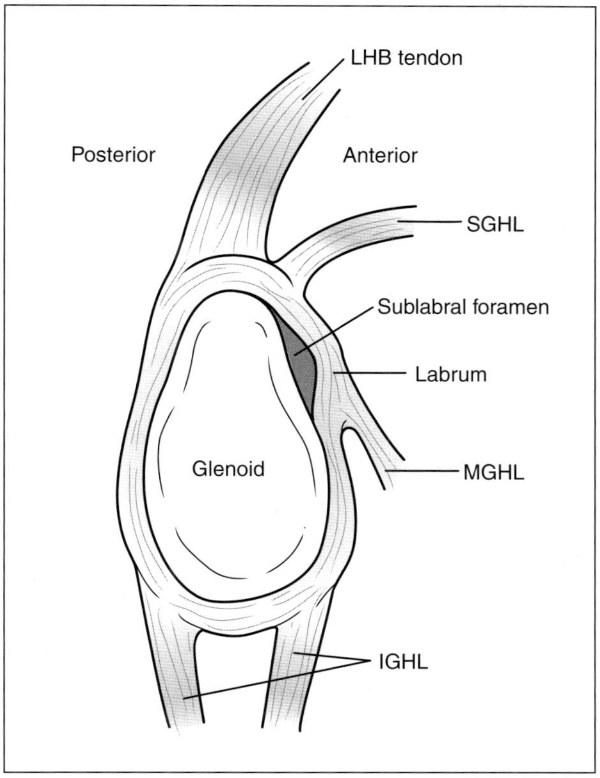

Illustration of a sublabral foramen variant. The sublabral foramen occurs at the 2 o'clock position, anterior to the origin of the biceps. LHB = long head of the biceps.

FIGURE 3

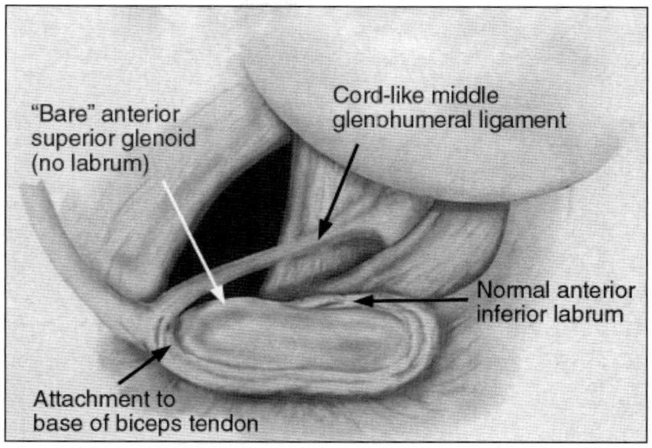

Illustration of the Buford complex shows the thickened MGHL in association with an absent anterosuperior labrum. (Adapted with permission from Williams MM, Snyder SJ, Buford D Jr: The Buford complex—the "cordlike" middle glenohumeral ligament and absent anterosuperior labrum complex: A normal anatomic capsulolabral variant. *Arthroscopy* 1994;10[3]:241-247.)

labral recess variant and the formation of pathologic lesions. The clinical significance of this variant may be limited to being confused with a pathologic labral lesion and used as a space for the entry of loose bodies.[36]

Sublabral Foramen

A sublabral foramen (**Figure 2**) occurs anterior to the biceps origin at approximately the 2 o'clock position, whereas a sublabral recess occurs at the 12 o'clock position at the attachment of the biceps tendon. A sublabral foramen is the gap between the glenoid cartilage and the labrum in this region, which creates a space that can be probed during arthroscopy.[4,37] The incidence of a sublabral foramen is between 8% and 18%.[29-31,33,38]

A notch in the anterosuperior osseous glenoid has been associated with this type of labral variability, and in the future may be used to radiographically distinguish an anatomic variant.[11] A sublabral foramen can potentially be confused for a Bankart lesion. An association between the presence of a sublabral foramen and SLAP lesions has been reported in one review of 713 arthroscopic procedures.[34]

Buford Complex

The Buford complex is the absence of the anterosuperior labrum occurring in conjunction with a thickened, cordlike MGHL. Williams et al[29] reviewed 200 shoulder arthroscopies and identified the Buford complex in three patients. In this variant, the cord-like MGHL attaches to the superior labrum inferior to the base of the biceps tendon and there is an absence of anterosuperior labrum between the MGHL and the biceps tendon superiorly. The incidence of a Buford complex has been reported between 1.5% and 6%[29,31] (**Figure 3**).

Some authors have suggested an association between the Buford complex and anterior shoulder instability.[39] A complete absence of the labrum resulted in reduced concavity depth and increased translation of the hu-

FIGURE 4

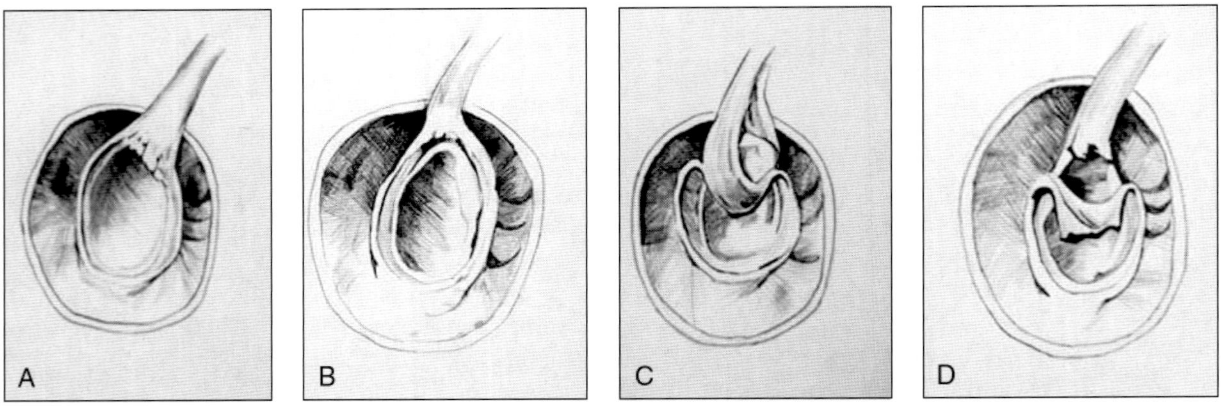

Snyder classification for types of SLAP lesions. **A,** type I; **B,** type II; **C,** type III; **D,** type IV. (Reproduced with permission from Snyder SJ, Karzel RP, Del Pizzo W, Ferkel RD, Friedman MJ: SLAP lesions of the shoulder. *Arthroscopy* 1990;6[4]:274-279.)

meral head.[7] In addition to instability, several studies have reported a significant relationship between the Buford complex and SLAP tears.[31,40] Ilahi et al[31] studied 108 arthroscopic procedures and identified 7 shoulders with a Buford complex, 5 of which had a significant SLAP tear.

Pathology and Biomechanical Dysfunction

SLAP Lesion

Lesions of the biceps anchor were first identified by Andrews et al.[41] The authors reported on 73 throwing athletes who had symptoms for a mean of 12 months and were found to have tears in the glenoid labrum. During arthroscopy, 10% of patients had a tear identified in the biceps tendon, and 83% had a tear identified near the biceps tendon insertion. The authors proposed that the biceps tendon decelerates the arm in the late phase of throwing and compresses the glenohumeral joint, and is therefore vulnerable to injury in overhead athletes. Furthermore, Burkhart and Morgan[12] described a forceful contraction of the biceps tendon during the abduction and external rotation phase of throwing, creating peel-back of the superior labrum.

Snyder et al[42] adeptly identified superior labral tears as a clinically significant entity and coined the term SLAP tears to classify these lesions (**Figure 4**). The authors reviewed 700 shoulder arthroscopic procedures and identified 27 posterior-to-anterior tears in the superior labrum. Two major mechanisms were identified to result in SLAP tears: a compressive force such as a fall onto an outstretched hand, or a traction force such as repetitive throwing and overuse.

According to the Snyder classification, a type I SLAP tear consists of a frayed superior labrum with limited degeneration and an intact biceps anchor. These lesions frequently represent a more chronic, repetitive mechanism. The clinical relevance of type I lesions is controversial. The treatment of type I lesions refractory to nonsurgical management is arthroscopic débridement of the tear. A type II (unstable) SLAP tear involves detachment of the superior labrum and biceps anchor from the superior glenoid. These lesions are the most common type of SLAP tear and are amenable to surgical repair. Morgan et al[43] conducted a study of 102 patients with type II SLAP tears and found that 30% had a rotator cuff tear. The authors suggested that a posterior SLAP tear predisposed the shoulder to chronic instability, which results in secondary cuff tears. Repair of type II lesions refractory to nonsurgical management depends on the size of the tear: generally, tears comprising more than 30% of the biceps-labral complex are treated with suture anchors and smaller tears are treated with débridement.[44] A type III (stable) SLAP tear is a bucket-handle labral detachment with an intact biceps anchor. A type IV (unstable) SLAP tear is a

FIGURE 5

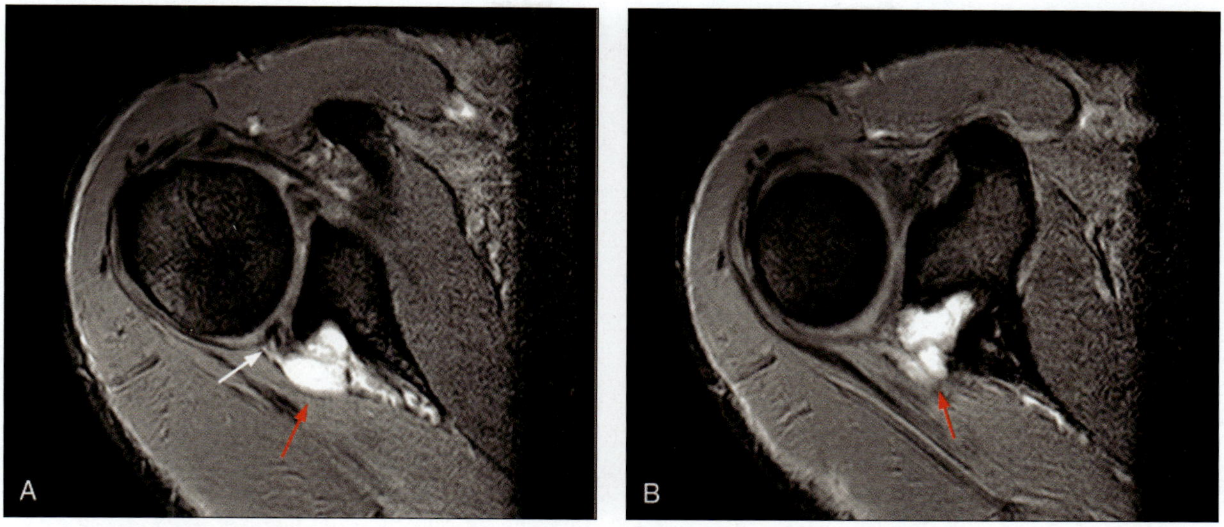

Axial T2-weighted fat-saturated MRIs of a right shoulder demonstrate a posterior labral tear (white arrow) with a large, multiloculated paralabral cyst (red arrows), which extended into the spinoglenoid (**A**) and suprascapular (**B**) notches, likely resulting in significant compression of the suprascapular nerve. (Adapted with permission from Westrick RB, Fogarty BT, Johnson MP: Posterior labral tear with a paralabral cyst causing suprascapular nerve compression. *J Orthop Sports Phys Ther* 2013;43[7]:511.)

bucket-handle labral detachment with involvement of the biceps attachment.

Other authors have provided additional subcategorizations; however, the most clinically relevant aspect of any classification scheme is whether the biceps anchor is stable or unstable.[45,46] Distinguishing between the normal anatomic variants described previously and pathologic labral tears can be difficult, both arthroscopically and on imaging. Misdiagnosis of a normal anatomic variant can result in unnecessary surgery and may ultimately limit glenohumeral range of motion. Williams et al[29] reported the misdiagnosis and surgical repair of a Buford complex that resulted in decreased external rotation in a patient and necessitated a subsequent procedure. On shoulder arthrography, contrast tracking in a smooth pattern between the labrum and the glenoid articular cartilage without extension to the biceps insertion is consistent with a sublabral sulcus.[32] An irregular contrast pattern tracking between the glenoid and the labrum as well as an increase in the area between the two is more consistent with a SLAP tear.[37] Some authors insist that normal variants do not extend inferior to the anterior glenoid notch, between the 2 o'clock and 3 o'clock positions on the glenoid, so extension of contrast past this point often indicates pathology.[29,35]

Paralabral Cyst With Suprascapular Nerve Compression

The sequelae of a labral tear may include the formation of a glenoid-labral cyst[47,48] (**Figure 5**). Tirman et al[33] hypothesized that the extrusion of intra-articular fluid into surrounding tissues after a labral tear may result in the formation of a cyst in a process similar to the formation of meniscal and popliteal cysts. Paralabral cysts, also referred to as spinoglenoid cysts or ganglion cysts, typically extend to the spinoglenoid notch, and sometimes to the suprascapular notch.[49] The suprascapular nerve lies approximately 1.8 cm medial to the posterior glenoid rim,[50] and may be compressed by a paralabral cyst. Posterior labral cysts larger than 1.0 cm in diameter are associated with nerve compression and muscle atrophy.[51-53] The sensory branch of the suprascapular nerve innervates the posterior capsule, and Fritz et al[53] postulated that irritation of this branch can result in poorly localized shoulder pain.

Various studies have investigated the results of both nonsurgical and surgical management of paralabral cysts.[49,52,54] Nonsurgical management usually begins with a course of rest and NSAIDs. Ultrasonographically guided aspiration of the cysts may also be successful. Cases that are refractory to nonsurgical treatment can be managed with open or arthroscopic procedures to eliminate nerve compression due to the paralabral cysts. Piatt et al[54] reported on 73 patients with spinoglenoid notch cysts: 19 underwent nonsurgical treatment, 11 underwent needle aspiration, 6 underwent isolated arthroscopic treatment of the labral defect with no treatment of the cyst itself, and 27 underwent cyst excision with labral repair using either an arthroscopic or open approach. Although only 53% of patients in the nonsurgical treatment group were satisfied with their outcome, 97% of the patients in the surgical treatment group were satisfied with their outcome at a mean follow-up of 20.5 months. Youm et al[49] described a case series of 10 patients with paralabral cysts who underwent arthroscopic labral repair without cyst aspiration, débridement, or excision. The authors found that the 4 patients with preoperative suprascapular neuropathies fully recovered and 8 patients in the study had MRIs that showed resolution of the cyst. Schroder et al[52] later reported on a larger series of 42 patients with paralabral cysts who all underwent arthroscopic labral repair but not direct management of the cyst: the cysts resolved in 37 patients (88%) and diminished in size in the other 5; all patients experienced improvement in symptoms.

Conclusion

The authors of this chapter prefer to start with a course of nonsurgical treatment of paralabral cysts that includes rest and NSAIDs. If refractory to nonsurgical management, the authors prefer arthroscopic excision of the cysts.

References

1. Tischer T, Vogt S, Kreuz PC, Imhoff AB: Arthroscopic anatomy, variants, and pathologic findings in shoulder instability. *Arthroscopy* 2011;27(10):1434-1443.
2. Anetzberger H, Putz R: The scapula: Principles of construction and stress. *Acta Anat (Basel)* 1996;156(1): 70-80.
3. Prescher A: Anatomical basics, variations, and degenerative changes of the shoulder joint and shoulder girdle. *Eur J Radiol* 2000;35(2):88-102.
4. Cooper DE, Arnoczky SP, O'Brien SJ, Warren RF, DiCarlo E, Allen AA: Anatomy, histology, and vascularity of the glenoid labrum: An anatomical study. *J Bone Joint Surg Am* 1992;74(1):46-52.
5. Perry J: Anatomy and biomechanics of the shoulder in throwing, swimming, gymnastics, and tennis. *Clin Sports Med* 1983;2(2):247-270.
6. Howell SM, Galinat BJ: The glenoid-labral socket: A constrained articular surface. *Clin Orthop Relat Res* 1989;(243):122-125.
7. Lippitt S, Matsen F: Mechanisms of glenohumeral joint stability. *Clin Orthop Relat Res* 1993;(291):20-28.
8. Greis PE, Scuderi MG, Mohr A, Bachus KN, Burks RT: Glenohumeral articular contact areas and pressures following labral and osseous injury to the anteroinferior quadrant of the glenoid. *J Shoulder Elbow Surg* 2002;11(5):442-451.
9. Huber WP, Putz RV: Periarticular fiber system of the shoulder joint. *Arthroscopy* 1997;13(6):680-691.
10. O'Brien SJ, Neves MC, Arnoczky SP, et al: The anatomy and histology of the inferior glenohumeral ligament complex of the shoulder. *Am J Sports Med* 1990;18(5):449-456.
11. Shortt CP, Morrison WB, Shah SH, Zoga AC, Carrino JA: Association of glenoid morphology and anterosuperior labral variation. *J Comput Assist Tomogr* 2009;33(4):584-586.
12. Burkhart SS, Morgan CD: The peel-back mechanism: Its role in producing and extending posterior type II SLAP lesions and its effect on SLAP repair rehabilitation. *Arthroscopy* 1998;14(6):637-640.
13. Boardman ND, Debski RE, Warner JJ, et al: Tensile properties of the superior glenohumeral and coracohumeral ligaments. *J Shoulder Elbow Surg* 1996;5(4): 249-254.
14. Yeh L, Kwak S, Kim YS, et al: Anterior labroligamentous structures of the glenohumeral joint: Correlation of MR arthrography and anatomic dissection in cadavers. *AJR Am J Roentgenol* 1998;171(5):1229-1236.
15. de Palma AF, Callery C, Bennett GA: Variational anatomy and degenerative lesions of the shoulder joint. *Instr Course Lect* 1949;6:255.

16. Kask K, Põldoja E, Lont T, et al: Anatomy of the superior glenohumeral ligament. *J Shoulder Elbow Surg* 2010;19(6):908-916.
17. O'Brien SJ, Warren RF, Schwartz E: Anterior shoulder instability. *Orthop Clin North Am* 1987;18(3):395-408.
18. Tuoheti Y, Itoi E, Minagawa H, et al: Attachment types of the long head of the biceps tendon to the glenoid labrum and their relationships with the glenohumeral ligaments. *Arthroscopy* 2005;21(10):1242-1249.
19. O'Brien SJ, Voos JE, Neviaser AS, Drakos MC: Developmental anatomy of the shoulder and anatomy of the glenohumeral joint, in Rockwood CA Jr, Matsen FA III, Wirth MA, Lippitt SM, eds: *The Shoulder,* ed 4. Philadelphia, PA, Saunders Elsevier, 2009, pp 1-32.
20. Zanetti M, Carstensen T, Weishaupt D, Jost B, Hodler J: MR arthrographic variability of the arthroscopically normal glenoid labrum: Qualitative and quantitative assessment. *Eur Radiol* 2001;11(4):559-566.
21. Rispoli DM, Athwal GS, Sperling JW, Cofield RH: The macroscopic delineation of the edge of the glenoid labrum: An anatomic evaluation of an open and arthroscopic visual reference. *Arthroscopy* 2009;25(6):603-607.
22. Pfahler M, Haraida S, Schulz C, et al: Age-related changes of the glenoid labrum in normal shoulders. *J Shoulder Elbow Surg* 2003;12(1):40-52.
23. Arai R, Kobayashi M, Toda Y, Nakamura S, Miura T, Nakamura T: Fiber components of the shoulder superior labrum. *Surg Radiol Anat* 2012;34(1):49-56.
24. Vangsness CT Jr, Jorgenson SS, Watson T, Johnson DL: The origin of the long head of the biceps from the scapula and glenoid labrum: An anatomical study of 100 shoulders. *J Bone Joint Surg Br* 1994;76(6):951-954.
25. Pal GP, Bhatt RH, Patel VS: Relationship between the tendon of the long head of biceps brachii and the glenoidal labrum in humans. *Anat Rec* 1991;229(2):278-280.
26. Dierickx C, Ceccarelli E, Conti M, Vanlommel J, Castagna A: Variations of the intra-articular portion of the long head of the biceps tendon: A classification of embryologically explained variations. *J Shoulder Elbow Surg* 2009;18(4):556-565.
27. Warner JJ, McMahon PJ: The role of the long head of the biceps brachii in superior stability of the glenohumeral joint. *J Bone Joint Surg Am* 1995;77(3):366-372.
28. Alpantaki K, McLaughlin D, Karagogeos D, Hadjipavlou A, Kontakis G: Sympathetic and sensory neural elements in the tendon of the long head of the biceps. *J Bone Joint Surg Am* 2005;87(7):1580-1583.
29. Williams MM, Snyder SJ, Buford D Jr: The Buford complex—the "cord-like" middle glenohumeral ligament and absent anterosuperior labrum complex: A normal anatomic capsulolabral variant. *Arthroscopy* 1994;10(3):241-247.
30. Rao AG, Kim TK, Chronopoulos E, McFarland EG: Anatomical variants in the anterosuperior aspect of the glenoid labrum: A statistical analysis of seventy-three cases. *J Bone Joint Surg Am* 2003;85-A(4):653-659.
31. Ilahi OA, Cosculluela PE, Ho DM: Classification of anterosuperior glenoid labrum variants and their association with shoulder pathology. *Orthopedics* 2008;31(3):226.
32. Rudez J, Zanetti M: Normal anatomy, variants and pitfalls on shoulder MRI. *Eur J Radiol* 2008;68(1):25-35.
33. Tirman PF, Feller JF, Palmer WE, Carroll KW, Steinbach LS, Cox I: The Buford complex—a variation of normal shoulder anatomy: MR arthrographic imaging features. *AJR Am J Roentgenol* 1996;166(4):869-873.
34. Kanatli U, Ozturk BY, Bolukbasi S: Anatomical variations of the anterosuperior labrum: Prevalence and association with type II superior labrum anterior-posterior (SLAP) lesions. *J Shoulder Elbow Surg* 2010;19(8):1199-1203.
35. Tuite MJ, Blankenbaker DG, Seifert M, Ziegert AJ, Orwin JF: Sublabral foramen and buford complex: Inferior extent of the unattached or absent labrum in 50 patients. *Radiology* 2002;223(1):137-142.
36. Kaplan K, Sahajpal DT, Jazrawi L: Loose bodies in a sublabral recess: Diagnosis and treatment. *Bull Hosp Jt Dis* 2006;63(3-4):161-165.
37. De Maeseneer M, Van Roy F, Lenchik L, et al: CT and MR arthrography of the normal and pathologic anterosuperior labrum and labral-bicipital complex. *Radiographics* 2000;20(Spec No):S67-S81.
38. Kwak SM, Brown RR, Resnick D, Trudell D, Applegate GR, Haghighi P: Anatomy, anatomic variations, and pathology of the 11- to 3-o'clock position of the glenoid labrum: Findings on MR arthrography and anatomic sections. *AJR Am J Roentgenol* 1998;171(1):235-238.

39. del Rey FC, Vázquez DG, López DN: Glenohumeral instability associated with Buford complex. *Knee Surg Sports Traumatol Arthrosc* 2009;17(12):1489-1492.
40. Bents RT, Skeete KD: The correlation of the Buford complex and SLAP lesions. *J Shoulder Elbow Surg* 2005;14(6):565-569.
41. Andrews JR, Carson WG Jr, McLeod WD: Glenoid labrum tears related to the long head of the biceps. *Am J Sports Med* 1985;13(5):337-341.
42. Snyder SJ, Karzel RP, Del Pizzo W, Ferkel RD, Friedman MJ: SLAP lesions of the shoulder. *Arthroscopy* 1990;6(4):274-279.
43. Morgan CD, Burkhart SS, Palmeri M, Gillespie M: Type II SLAP lesions: Three subtypes and their relationships to superior instability and rotator cuff tears. *Arthroscopy* 1998;14(6):553-565.
44. Gregush RV, Snyder SJ: Superior labral repair. *Sports Med Arthrosc* 2007;15(4):222-229.
45. Shankman S, Bencardino J, Beltran J: Glenohumeral instability: Evaluation using MR arthrography of the shoulder. *Skeletal Radiol* 1999;28(7):365-382.
46. Maffet MW, Gartsman GM, Moseley B: Superior labrum-biceps tendon complex lesions of the shoulder. *Am J Sports Med* 1995;23(1):93-98.
47. Moore TP, Fritts HM, Quick DC, Buss DD: Suprascapular nerve entrapment caused by supraglenoid cyst compression. *J Shoulder Elbow Surg* 1997;6(5):455-462.
48. Chochole MH, Senker W, Meznik C, Breitenseher MJ: Glenoid-labral cyst entrapping the suprascapular nerve: Dissolution after arthroscopic debridement of an extended SLAP lesion. *Arthroscopy* 1997;13(6):753-755.
49. Youm T, Matthews PV, El Attrache NS: Treatment of patients with spinoglenoid cysts associated with superior labral tears without cyst aspiration, debridement, or excision. *Arthroscopy* 2006;22(5):548-552.
50. Bigliani LU, Dalsey RM, McCann PD, April EW: An anatomical study of the suprascapular nerve. *Arthroscopy* 1990;6(4):301-305.
51. Ogino T, Minami A, Kato H, Hara R, Suzuki K: Entrapment neuropathy of the suprascapular nerve by a ganglion: A report of three cases. *J Bone Joint Surg Am* 1991;73(1):141-147.
52. Schroder CP, Skare O, Stiris M, Gjengedal E, Uppheim G, Brox JI: Treatment of labral tears with associated spinoglenoid cysts without cyst decompression. *J Bone Joint Surg Am* 2008;90(3):523-530.
53. Fritz RC, Helms CA, Steinbach LS, Genant HK: Suprascapular nerve entrapment: Evaluation with MR imaging. *Radiology* 1992;182(2):437-444.
54. Piatt BE, Hawkins RJ, Fritz RC, Ho CP, Wolf E, Schickendantz M: Clinical evaluation and treatment of spinoglenoid notch ganglion cysts. *J Shoulder Elbow Surg* 2002;11(6):600-604.

CHAPTER 2

Anatomy and Biomechanics: Normal Anatomy and Pathoanatomy of the Proximal Biceps Tendon

Bradford O. Parsons, MD

Introduction

The long head of the biceps (LHB) tendon is intra-articular and traverses from the glenohumeral joint into the proximal brachium. Often recognized as a potential source of shoulder pain and dysfunction, tremendous controversy exists regarding the normal anatomy and pathoanatomy of the LHB tendon, its function in the shoulder, its role as a potential source of shoulder pathology, and ultimately, the best treatment of LHB pathology. Some authors consider the biceps to be vestigial, or the "appendix" of the shoulder, whereas others think that it plays an important role in the biomechanics, function, and pathology of the shoulder.[1] This chapter summarizes LHB anatomy, reviews the current biomechanics of the LHB tendon related to the role the biceps plays in shoulder motion and function, and discusses LHB tendon pathonanatomy.

Anatomy

The LHB originates from the supraglenoid tubercle of the scapula and traverses across the humeral head, exiting the glenohumeral joint into the intertubercular groove of the proximal humerus. The anatomy, and its variants, can be divided into three distinct aspects, the origin (in association with the superior labrum), the soft-tissue sling or pulley that envelopes the LHB tendon and stabilizes it on reaching the bicipital groove, and the more distal intertubercular groove aspect of the tendon that ends at the musculotendinous junction.

The origin of the biceps is at the top of the glenoid rim on the supraglenoid tubercle and is most often contiguous with the superior labrum along the glenoid rim.[2,3] Although most often originating from the superior labrum, various origins have been described, including directly off of the supraglenoid tubercle and separate from the labrum,[2] an extra-articular origin,[4] a bifurcate intra-articular origin from the labrum/capsule and the rotator cuff,[5,6] and congenital absence of the tendon.[7] When the origin is contiguous with the superior labrum, it is most often at the top of the glenoid, just posterior to the base of the coracoid, although variations of the attachment to the labrum have been observed.[3] The intra-articular section of the LHB tendon has been found to be approximately 25 mm in length from its origin to its exit into the bicipital groove and has a mean diameter of 5 to 6 mm.[8,9]

Dr. Parsons or an immediate family member is a member of a speakers' bureau or has made paid presentations on behalf of Zimmer and Arthrex; and serves as a paid consultant to or is an employee of Zimmer and Arthrex.

FIGURE 1

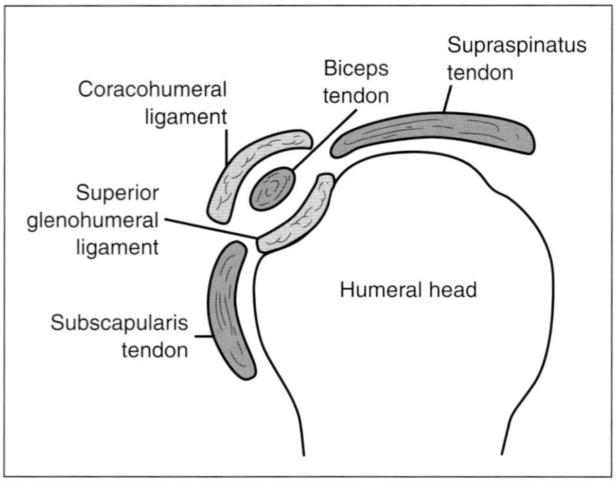

Illustration of the biceps sling or pulley shows four components: the coracohumeral ligament, the superior glenohumeral ligament, the subscapularis tendon, and the supraspinatous tendon.

As the LHB tendon exits the glenohumeral joint, it turns at a 35° to 40° angle and enters into the biceps sling at the top of the groove.[10] This pulley system, or sling, is composed of four components: the coracohumeral ligament (CHL), superior glenohumeral ligament (SGHL), the subscapularis tendon, and the supraspinatus tendon[10,11] (**Figure 1**). The floor of the pulley consists of the SGHL, which forms a U-shaped sling, and is reinforced by the upper border of the subscapularis insertion. The roof of the pulley, composed of the CHL, is posteriorly bordered by the supraspinatus insertion. These components of the pulley are integral aspects of the rotator interval and therefore have additional implications on glenohumeral stability and motion, particularly rotation.

The intertubercular component of the LHB tendon is distal to the biceps pulley, residing within the bicipital groove. Variations of bony groove shape and dimensions have been described in the literature; some patients have a very deep, conforming bicipital groove, and others have a very shallow groove.[12,13] In the groove, the LHB tendon is stabilized by the transverse humeral ligament (THL), which is a continuation of the confluence of the superior pulley and the CHL, the subscapularis reflection anteriorly, and the supraspinatus posteriorly. Interestingly, the THL fibers do not have a transverse orientation, but a vertical striation instead, which can be an important distinction when attempting to localize the distal biceps groove and tendon at arthroscopy or during biceps tenodesis procedures. Within the biceps groove, the LHB tendon is surrounded by vascular synovial tissue that has a network of sympathetic sensory fibers.[14] Some surgeons consider this synovial tissue and its innervation to be a source of pain in patients who have persistent anterior shoulder pain following intra-articular LHB tenotomy (without bicipital groove débridement) or following in-groove localized biceps tenodesis.[15,16]

The LHB tendon's blood is supplied from a combination of the attachment to the superior labrum proximally and from terminal branches of the anterior humeral circumflex artery, which are consistently observed along the posterior aspect of the bicipital groove[17] (**Figure 2**). The length of the LHB tendon is fairly consistent and can be referenced using landmarks such as the lower border of the subscapularis insertion and lesser tuberosity (which often also marks the end of the biceps groove), the crossing vessels of the anterior circumflex humeral artery (which lie midway between the inferior aspect of the lesser tuberosity and the superior border of the pectoralis insertion), and the upper border of the pectoralis major insertion. The biceps tendon extends a mean of 5.6 cm to the lower border of the subscapularis and the lesser tuberosity, a mean of approximately 8.0 cm to the upper border of the pectoralis major, and a mean of 12.0 cm to the musculotendinous junction, which is often found deep to the pectoralis insertion.[8,17] Knowledge of the biceps tendon length at the previously listed landmarks can help the surgeon appropriately tension the LHB tendon when performing arthroscopic or open tenodesis techniques.

Biomechanics of the LHB Tendon

The function of the LHB is controversial and few conclusions can be made from clinical and basic science data. Isolating the biceps when assessing its role in shoulder function is challenging, including immobilization of the elbow to remove any effect of flexion or supination on biceps shoulder function, as well as translating cadaver test results to clinical function. Most early

FIGURE 2

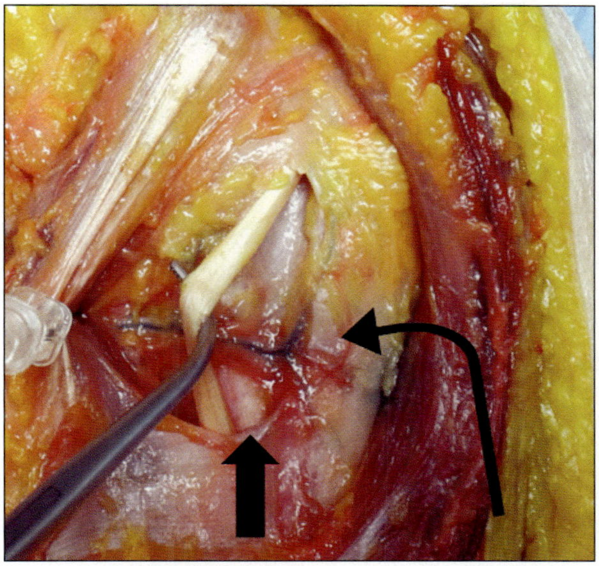

Photograph shows the terminal branch of the anterior circumflex artery (curved arrow) and courses across the bicipital groove at a consistent point midway between the top of the pectoralis major and bottom of the lesser tuberosity subscapularis insertion. In a cadaver study, these vessels were consistently observed 1.5 cm ± 2.4 mm proximal to the pectoralis major tendon (arrow) and may be a landmark for the distal aspect of the bicipital groove. (Adapted with permission from Neviaser AS, Glashow JL, Parsons BO, Gladstone JN, Flatow EL: Paper #17: Landmarks for placement and tensioning during arthroscopic suprapectoral biceps tenodesis. *Closed Meeting Proceedings.* White Sulphur Springs, WV, American Shoulder and Elbow Surgeons, October 12-15, 2011, p 5.)

investigators considered the biceps to be a humeral head depressor and stabilizer during elbow flexion and supination, based on early biomechanical work by Kumar et al.[18] More recent studies have used cadaver models to analyze the role of the biceps in humeral head stability and have concluded that the LHB tendon contributes to that stability by decreasing joint translation.[19-21] Rodosky et al[22] examined the role of the biceps in abduction and external rotation and found that the LHB tendon contributes to the anterior stability of the shoulder. Although most cadaver and biomechanical series demonstrated a stabilizing effect of the LHB tendon on the glenohumeral joint, a precise model for ideal testing of the LHB tendon's functional role in the shoulder is controversial and not well delineated. Current series[18-21] have substantial heterogeneity in loading parameters, elbow position, magnitude of LHB tendon loading and other variables, which make extrapolating clinical reality from biomechanical data very difficult.

To better assess the role of the LHB tendon in vivo, many investigators have conducted electromyographic (EMG) analysis of the biceps for shoulder function and the effects of glenohumeral joint kinematics. Levy et al[23] and Yamaguchi et al[24] conducted EMG analyses of the shoulder and documented minimal biceps activity of the biceps during shoulder motion, and therefore considered the biceps to be a passive contributor to shoulder function. Conversely, Sakurai et al[25] documented increased levels of biceps activity during shoulder function. The need to negate or remove elbow motion or its effect on EMG is inherent in the challenge ascertaining LHB tendon function in shoulder kinematics. Jobe et al[26] identified this challenge by analyzing pitching mechanics and demonstrated biceps activity during the cocking phase of throwing to elbow flexion and again when the arm decelerates during follow-through. Importantly, during functional shoulder motion, concomitant elbow motion (flexion, extension, and pronation-supination) often occurs, limiting the ability of EMG to isolate the role of the LHB tendon on shoulder kinematics. Based on current data, it is difficult to clearly define the role of the LHB tendon in shoulder kinematics and stability. The controversy surrounding the biceps does not end there. Further challenges await, specifically, what constitutes a diseased biceps, and how is the pathologic biceps best treated?

LHB Pathoanatomy

The diseased LHB is commonly addressed in combination with other shoulder pathology because of its potential as a pain generator. Although the exact role of the LHB in shoulder pain is controversial, the biceps as well as the surrounding tenosynovium and the THL contain neural elements, which may help explain how the diseased biceps hurts. Soifer et al[27] performed a cadaver study of 14 shoulders and identified free nerve fibers in the biceps tendon, tendon sheath, and THL. The presence of these neural elements may help explain the role of the pathologic LHB and its surrounding sheath in shoulder pain, although what constitutes a pathologic biceps is controversial.

FIGURE 3

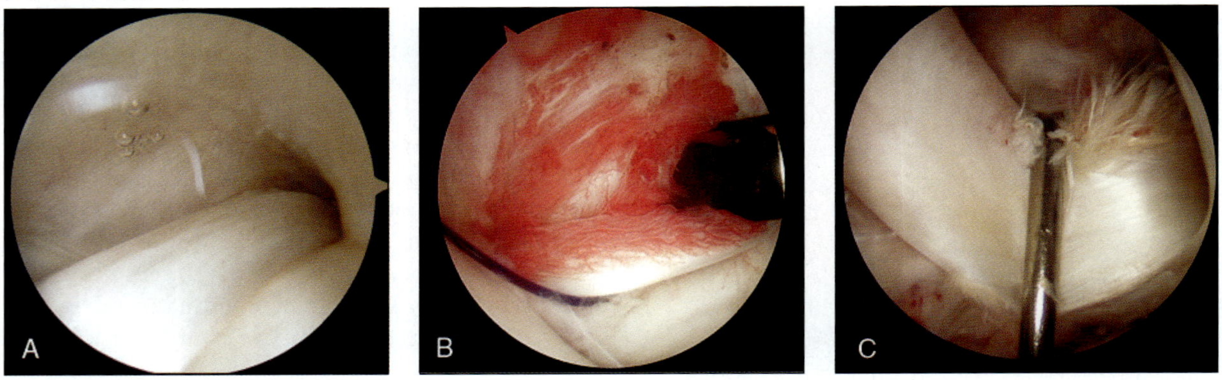

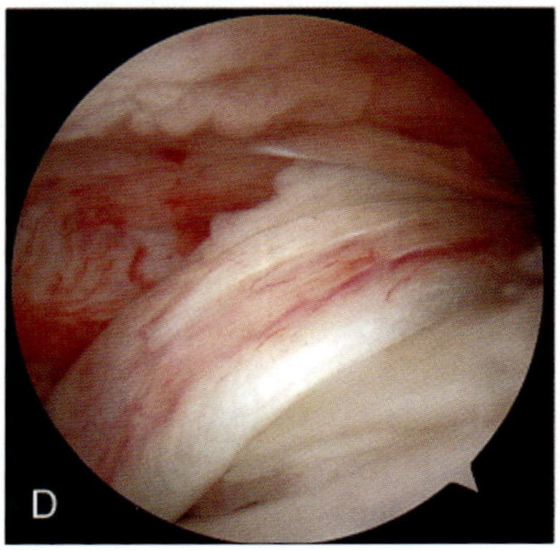

Arthroscopic views show a normal long head of the biceps (LHB) tendon (**A**) and one with severe synovitis (**B**). **C,** Degeneration and fraying are seen in a patholosic LHB tendon. **D,** A "lipstick" lesion is shown.

LHB pathology can be classified by its locale and its etiology. Pathologic locations include the biceps origin and the intra-articular portion of the tendon, pulley lesions, and the tendon pathology within the biceps groove. Lesions can include tendinitis, rupture, and instability. The spectrum of pathology can range from subtle pathology such as bicipital pulley lesions or hidden tendinitis in the bicipital groove, to more obvious pathology such as frank dislocation of the LHB tendon from the groove or complete tendon rupture. This section discusses the spectrum of LHB tendon pathology, its etiology, and its location along the course of the tendon, with the exception of pathology at the origin, which is discussed in a separate chapter.

LHB tendon pathology can occur as a result of trauma, repetitive microtrauma and overuse, inflammatory conditions, or from instability. The most common pathology is inflammatory, which most commonly occurs with other shoulder pathology, such as a rotator cuff tear or impingement, or more rarely, in isolation, and is termed primary bicipital tenosynovitis.[28,29] Biceps tendinitis is inflammation of the LHB tendon and is often characterized by synovitis and erythema of the tendon as it exits the joint and enters the bicipital groove. However, LHB tendinosis (for example, regarding the extent of erythematous streaking, synovitis, or "lipstick" lesions) is not well delineated in the literature, and no consensus on the definition exists (**Figure 3**). Often, the diagnosis of biceps tendinosis is not based on surgical inspection alone, and should include data from the patient's history of symptoms, physical examination findings, and imaging evidence including MRI or ultrasonographic findings.

As the pathology progresses, the tendon can degenerate, and become delaminated and frayed, and may lose its normal gliding excursion. The tendon shape can also alter because of bicipital tendinitis, forming an hourglass deformity, much like an inflamed tendon in the hand in patients with trigger finger.[30] Some authors have cited altered anatomy, such as a narrow bicipital groove that entraps the tendon, as a predisposing factor for bicipital tendinitis.[31] The sequelae of arthritis or fractures involving the bicipital groove area also can produce friction on the tendon, resulting in degeneration of the LHB tendon.[32]

Traumatic rupture of the LHB tendon has been observed, most commonly in patients older than 50 years, and typically occurs at its origin or as the tendon angles to enter the bicipital groove.[9,33] Rupture can occur with minimal trauma, and is often associated with preexisting biceps tendinitis. In thin patients with developed biceps muscles, rupture can result in a deformity of the contour of the proximal aspect of the biceps muscle (a Popeye deformity). Most commonly, pain is associated with the acute rupture, but often resolves quickly, and although some series have reported subjective biceps cramping with repetitive use in patients following LHB tendon rupture, most symptoms resolve by 6 months.[34]

The other common source of biceps pathology is instability of the LHB tendon in the proximal bicipital groove. Injury to the biceps reflection pulley can result in subluxation of the LHB tendon, or, as the pulley integrity progressively deteriorates, the LHB tendon can fully dislocate from the upper groove, which is commonly observed in upper subscapularis tendon tears (**Figure 4**). The spectrum of pulley lesions observed at arthroscopy have been classified by Habermeyer et al:[34] type I lesions are isolated lesions of the SGHL (the floor of the pulley); type II, combined SGHL lesions and leading-edge partial-thickness articular supraspinatous tears; type III, combined SGHL lesions and upper subscapularis tears; and type IV, combined lesions of the SGHL, supraspinatous, and subscapularis. Types I and III are the most common, with anteroinferior instability of the LHB tendon. When observed either on MRI or at arthroscopy, the tears require careful examination to ensure the subscapularis insertion is not torn. Anterosuperior or posterior instability is rare but can occur; this may be seen in type II or IV pulley lesions, involving the roof of the pulley (coracohumeral ligament) and the anterior supraspinatous tendon.

Anterior shoulder pain provoked by internal rotation and adduction, which can result in impingement of the pulley and upper subscapularis onto the anterior glenoid rim or the undersurface of the coracoid, has also been described. This has been termed anterosuperior impingement syndrome or coracoid impingement, and with repetitive trauma, may result in pulley lesions and subscapularis pathology.[10,35,36] Reducion of the coracohumeral distance between the coracoid and the lesser tuberosity may predispose the shoulder to coracoid impingement and lesions of the pulley or the subscapularis.[37] Sistermann[38] has also observed chondromalacia of the humeral head at the entrance of the bicipital groove at arthroplasty in 16% of patients. This finding was termed the "biceps footprint" and was most often associated with secondary sources of bicipital pathology such as rotator cuff tearing or glenohumeral instability, and may be another sign of bicipital pathology.

FIGURE 4

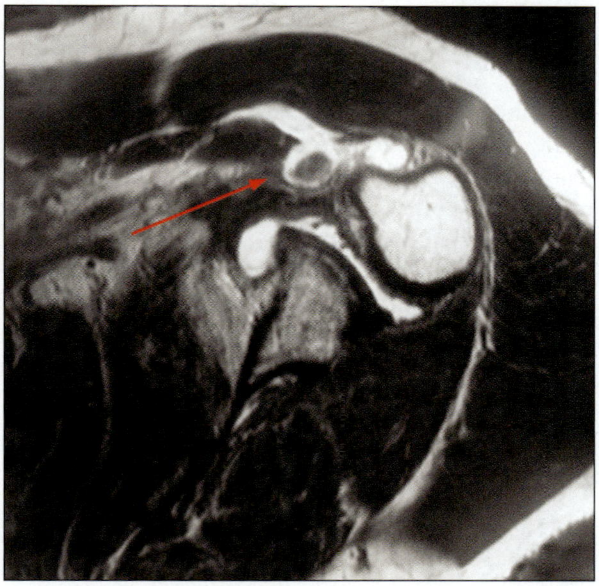

MRI showing long head of the biceps tendon subluxation. This condition is often a sign of an upper subscapularis tendon tear, but isolated pulley lesions (arrow) can also be a source of biceps instability and may be more subtle and therefore missed on MRI.

Conclusion

LHB tendon pathology has been recognized as a source of shoulder pain and is often observed at arthroscopy in association with other shoulder problems including impingement and rotator cuff tears, or may be primary to the LHB tendon or its anatomy. Although the anatomy of the LHB tendon has been well described, anatomic variation still makes identification of a subtle tendon or associated pathologic lesion difficult. An LHB tendon may appear to have signs of tendinopathy to one surgeon, but may seem relatively normal to another surgeon. Additionally, the lack of clear understanding of the functional role of the LHB tendon in the shoulder and arm makes determining the best course of management of biceps pathology more controversial. Clearly, more scientific investigation into the anatomy, biomechanics, and kinematics of the LHB tendon is required to answer definitively these questions.

References

1. Lippmann R: Bicipital tenosynovitis. *N Y State J Med* 1944;44:2235-2240.
2. Vangsness CT Jr, Jorgenson SS, Watson T, Johnson DL: The origin of the long head of the biceps from the scapula and glenoid labrum: An anatomical study of 100 shoulders. *J Bone Joint Surg Br* 1994;76(6):951-954.
3. Tuoheti Y, Itoi E, Minagawa H, et al: Attachment types of the long head of the biceps tendon to the glenoid labrum and their relationships with the glenohumeral ligaments. *Arthroscopy* 2005;21(10):1242-1249.
4. Hyman JL, Warren RF: Extra-articular origin of biceps brachii. *Arthroscopy* 2001;17(7):E29.
5. Enad JG: Bifurcate origin of the long head of the biceps tendon. *Arthroscopy* 2004;20(10):1081-1083.
6. Wittstein J, Lassiter T Jr, Taylor D: Aberrant origin of the long head of the biceps: A case series. *J Shoulder Elbow Surg* 2012;21(3):356-360.
7. Franco JC, Knapp TP, Mandelbaum BR: Congenital absence of the long head of the biceps tendon: A case report. *J Bone Joint Surg Am* 2005;87(7):1584-1586.
8. Denard PJ, Dai X, Hanypsiak BT, Burkhart SS: Anatomy of the biceps tendon: Implications for restoring physiological length-tension relation during biceps tenodesis with interference screw fixation. *Arthroscopy* 2012;28(10):1352-1358.
9. Elser F, Braun S, Dewing CB, Giphart JE, Millett PJ: Anatomy, function, injuries, and treatment of the long head of the biceps brachii tendon. *Arthroscopy* 2011;27(4):581-592.
10. Habermeyer P, Magosch P, Pritsch M, Scheibel MT, Lichtenberg S: Anterosuperior impingement of the shoulder as a result of pulley lesions: A prospective arthroscopic study. *J Shoulder Elbow Surg* 2004;13(1):5-12.
11. Werner A, Mueller T, Boehm D, Gohlke F: The stabilizing sling for the long head of the biceps tendon in the rotator cuff interval: A histoanatomic study. *Am J Sports Med* 2000;28(1):28-31.
12. Hitchcock HH, Bechtol CO: Painful shoulder; observations on the role of the tendon of the long head of the biceps brachii in its causation. *J Bone Joint Surg Am* 1948;30-A(2):263-273.
13. Pfahler M, Branner S, Refior HJ: The role of the bicipital groove in tendopathy of the long biceps tendon. *J Shoulder Elbow Surg* 1999;8(5):419-424.
14. Alpantaki K, McLaughlin D, Karagogeos D, Hadjipavlou A, Kontakis G: Sympathetic and sensory neural elements in the tendon of the long head of the biceps. *J Bone Joint Surg Am* 2005;87(7):1580-1583.
15. Sanders B, Lavery KP, Pennington S, Warner JJ: Clinical success of biceps tenodesis with and without release of the transverse humeral ligament. *J Shoulder Elbow Surg* 2012;21(1):66-71.
16. Lutton DM, Gruson KI, Harrison AK, Gladstone JN, Flatow EL: Where to tenodese the biceps: Proximal or distal? *Clin Orthop Relat Res* 2011;469(4):1050-1055.
17. Neviaser AS, Glashow JL, Parsons BO, Gladstone JN, Flatow EL: Paper #17: Landmarks for placement and tensioning during arthroscopic suprapectoral biceps tenodesis. *Closed Meeting Proceedings.* White Sulphur Springs, WV, American Shoulder and Elbow Surgeons, October 12-15, 2011, p 5.
18. Kumar VP, Satku K, Balasubramaniam P: The role of the long head of biceps brachii in the stabilization of the head of the humerus. *Clin Orthop Relat Res* 1989;(244):172-175.
19. Itoi E, Kuechle DK, Newman SR, Morrey BF, An KN: Stabilising function of the biceps in stable and unstable shoulders. *J Bone Joint Surg Br* 1993;75(4):546-550.
20. Youm T, ElAttrache NS, Tibone JE, McGarry MH, Lee TQ: The effect of the long head of the biceps on glenohumeral kinematics. *J Shoulder Elbow Surg* 2009;18(1):122-129.
21. Warner JJ, McMahon PJ: The role of the long head of the biceps brachii in superior stability of the glenohumeral joint. *J Bone Joint Surg Am* 1995;77(3):366-372.

22. Rodosky MW, Harner CD, Fu FH: The role of the long head of the biceps muscle and superior glenoid labrum in anterior stability of the shoulder. *Am J Sports Med* 1994;22(1):121-130.
23. Levy AS, Kelly BT, Lintner SA, Osbahr DC, Speer KP: Function of the long head of the biceps at the shoulder: Electromyographic analysis. *J Shoulder Elbow Surg* 2001;10(3):250-255.
24. Yamaguchi K, Riew KD, Galatz LM, Syme JA, Neviaser RJ: Biceps activity during shoulder motion: An electromyographic analysis. *Clin Orthop Relat Res* 1997;(336):122-129.
25. Sakurai G, Ozaki J, Tomita Y, Nishimoto K, Tamai S: Electromyographic analysis of shoulder joint function of the biceps brachii muscle during isometric contraction. *Clin Orthop Relat Res* 1998;(354):123-131.
26. Jobe FW, Moynes DR, Tibone JE, Perry J: An EMG analysis of the shoulder in pitching: A second report. *Am J Sports Med* 1984;12(3):218-220.
27. Soifer TB, Levy HJ, Soifer FM, Kleinbart F, Vigorita V, Bryk E: Neurohistology of the subacromial space. *Arthroscopy* 1996;12(2):182-186.
28. Maier D, Jaeger M, Suedkamp NP, Koestler W: Stabilization of the long head of the biceps tendon in the context of early repair of traumatic subscapularis tendon tears. *J Bone Joint Surg Am* 2007;89(8):1763-1769.
29. Favorito PJ, Harding WG III, Heidt RS Jr: Complete arthroscopic examination of the long head of the biceps tendon. *Arthroscopy* 2001;17(4):430-432.
30. Boileau P, Ahrens PM, Hatzidakis AM: Entrapment of the long head of the biceps tendon: the hourglass biceps—A cause of pain and locking of the shoulder. *J Shoulder Elbow Surg* 2004;13(3):249-257.
31. Depalma AF, Callery GE: Bicipital tenosynovitis. *Clin Orthop* 1954;(3):69-85.
32. Neer CS II, Horwitz BS: Fractures of the proximal humeral epiphysial plate. *Clin Orthop Relat Res* 1965;(41):24-31.
33. Warren RF: Lesions of the long head of the biceps tendon. *Instr Course Lect* 1985;34:204-209.
34. Mariani EM, Cofield RH, Askew LJ, Li GP, Chao EY: Rupture of the tendon of the long head of the biceps brachii: Surgical versus nonsurgical treatment. *Clin Orthop Relat Res* 1988;(228):233-239.
35. Gerber C, Sebesta A: Impingement of the deep surface of the subscapularis tendon and the reflection pulley on the anterosuperior glenoid rim: A preliminary report. *J Shoulder Elbow Surg* 2000;9(6):483-490.
36. Richards DP, Burkhart SS, Campbell SE: Relation between narrowed coracohumeral distance and subscapularis tears. *Arthroscopy* 2005;21(10):1223-1228.
37. Gerber C, Terrier F, Zehnder R, Ganz R: The subcoracoid space: An anatomic study. *Clin Orthop Relat Res* 1987;(215):132-138.
38. Sistermann R: The biceps tendon footprint. *Acta Orthop* 2005;76(2):237-240.

CHAPTER 3

Anatomy and Biomechanics: Biomechanics of the Biceps and Labrum

Cathryn D. Peltz, PhD
Steven Slotkin, MS
Vasilios Moutzouros, MD
Michael J. Bey, PhD

Introduction

The proximal biceps tendon, or long head of the biceps tendon, and the labrum form the biceps-labral complex, the mechanical function of which has been investigated using various in vivo, in vitro, and computed modeling studies. The in vivo function of these structures is somewhat controversial, at least partly because isolated ruptures (for example, of the proximal biceps tendon) occur rarely, and therefore, few opportunities exist to study the associated functional deficits. In addition, experimental techniques for studying these structures under dynamic, in vivo conditions are not well developed. In general, previous research has characterized the mechanical function of the biceps and labrum in terms of muscle activation patterns, soft-tissue mechanics, and glenohumeral joint mechanics. This chapter is a brief overview of existing research on the biomechanics of the proximal biceps tendon, labrum, and superior labrum anterior to posterior (SLAP) lesions.

Biomechanics of the Biceps

Muscle Activation Patterns

Electromyography (EMG) has been used extensively to evaluate biceps function during various activities. Previous research has demonstrated that biceps muscle activity ranges from 8% to 44% of maximum voluntary contraction (MVC) during the overhead baseball pitch, with peak muscle activity occurring during the arm deceleration phase that occurs after ball release.[1] Kelly et al[2] reported that biceps muscle activity ranges from 11% to 20% of MVC during overhead throwing in American football, with peak muscle activity also occurring during the deceleration and follow-through phases. Biceps muscle activity during the overhead tennis serve has been reported to range from 6% to 39% of MVC, with the peak muscle activity occurring during the cocking phase and significant activity (34% of MVC) occurring during the arm deceleration and follow-through phases.[3] Biceps activity during tennis forehand and back-

Dr. Bey or an immediate family member has received research or institutional support from DJ Orthopaedics and Nike. None of the following authors nor any immediate family member has received anything of value from or has stock or stock options held in a commercial company or institution related directly or indirectly to the subject of this chapter: Dr. Peltz, Mr. Slotkin, and Dr. Moutzouros.

hand strokes were found to be 86% and 45% of MVC, respectively, with appreciably lower levels of muscle activity occurring during the preparation and follow-through phases.[3] These data clearly indicate that the biceps muscle plays a substantial role in these complex athletic activities, but it is important to keep in mind that the biceps is a biarticulate muscle with both shoulder and elbow functions. Most EMG studies were not designed to discriminate between the role of the biceps at the shoulder and the elbow; therefore, ascertaining the specific role of the biceps at the shoulder using these results is difficult.

To more precisely evaluate biceps function during shoulder movement, EMG analysis of the biceps was performed using a brace to rigidly maintain the elbow and forearm in a fixed position.[4,5] Yamaguchi et al[5] investigated biceps muscle activity during 10 shoulder motions that represented various combinations of flexion/extension, internal/external rotation, and abduction. Biceps muscle activity was consistently less than 5% of MVC in control patients with uninjured shoulders and in patients with rotator cuff tears. Similarly, Levy et al[4] used indwelling EMG electrodes to demonstrate that biceps muscle activity was minimal or essentially absent (for example, less than approximately 5% MVC) during shoulder flexion, extension, abduction, external rotation, and internal rotation. These studies strongly suggest that biceps function at the shoulder is achieved through changes in passive tension that occur as a function of shoulder position, or through active contraction that is associated with elbow or forearm activity.

Soft-Tissue Mechanics

The role of the biceps has been characterized using cadaver or computational studies that investigated forces or strains placed on the biceps tendon. Braun et al[6] used a biplanar fluoroscopic system to track the three-dimensional position of small beads implanted in the biceps tendon of cadaver shoulder specimens. An 11-N load was applied to the distal biceps tendon and data were acquired from each specimen with the shoulder in nine positions that represented all combinations of glenohumeral elevation (neutral, 90° of forward flexion, and 90° of scapular plane abduction) and humeral rotation (neutral, 45° of internal rotation, and 45° of external rotation). By tracking the three-dimensional position of the implanted beads, the tendon excursion was calculated and expressed relative to a reference position with the shoulder in neutral elevation and rotation (**Figure 1**). Elevation and rotation both had a substantial effect on biceps tendon excursion. In particular, the position of forward flexion and internal rotation demonstrated the greatest tendon excursion (approximately 18 mm), followed by abduction and neutral rotation (approximately 16 mm). In contrast, the position of neutral elevation and external rotation demonstrated the least tendon excursion (approximately 5 mm of shortening), followed by forward flexion and external rotation (approximately 5 mm of tendon lengthening).

Similarly, Gramstad et al[7] assessed the effects of shoulder position on passive biceps tendon tension in six cadaver shoulder specimens. The investigators implanted an intratendinous force probe into the midsubstance of the biceps tendon, just distal to its origin on the labrum. Biceps tendon tension was quantified during elevation, adduction, forward flexion, coronal plane abduction, and extension, with the arm in neutral, maximum internal, and maximum external rotation in each position. These data were acquired under passive (no load) and active (55 N) biceps loading conditions. Tendon tension increased substantially in all arm positions except elevation, and was most pronounced in humeral extension and internal rotation with the elbow extended and the forearm pronated. This position is called the reach-back position because it corresponds to the arm position that occurs when reaching into the back seat of a car or reaching back to place the arm into a shirt sleeve. Differences in tendon tension due to changes in arm position were not detected when the 55-N biceps load was applied. This finding suggests that tensioning of the biceps tendon via active muscle contraction may mask any differences in biceps tendon tension that occur via changes in shoulder position alone.

Glenohumeral Joint Mechanics

Many cadaver experiments have attempted to define the mechanical role of the biceps, and these studies have generally concluded that the biceps plays a significant role in both translational (anterior/posterior, superior/inferior) and rotational glenohumeral joint stability. Several series of rigorous cadaver experiments were conducted, demonstrating that the biceps is an impor-

FIGURE 1

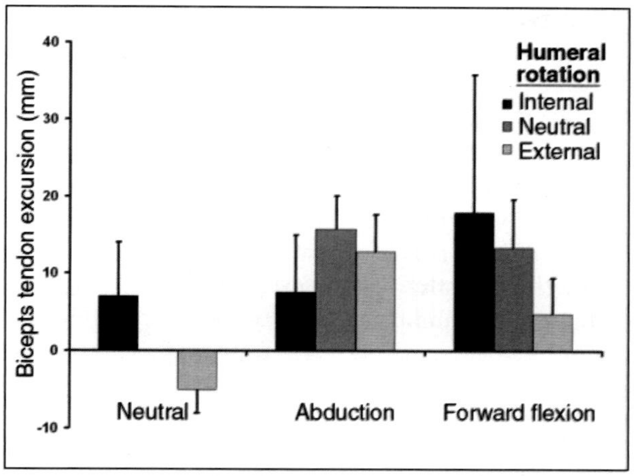

Graph measures the mean (±SD) tendon excursion. A biplanar fluoroscopic system was used to track the three-dimensional position of tantalum markers implanted in the biceps tendon of cadaver specimens. Biceps tendon excursion is influenced considerably by both shoulder position and humeral rotation. (Reproduced with permission from Braun S, Millett PJ, Yongpravat C, et al: Biomechanical evaluation of shear force vectors leading to injury of the biceps reflection pulley: A biplane fluoroscopy study on cadaveric shoulders. *Am J Sports Med* 2010;38[5]:1015-1024.)

tant stabilizer against anterior, posterior, and inferior glenohumeral joint translation.[8-10] Other cadaver experiments have reached similar conclusions: Pagnani et al[11] reported that biceps stabilization was most apparent at low-elevation to mid-elevation angles, Itoi et al[12,13] reported that the role of the biceps in anterior stability is substantially affected by shoulder position, and Kumar et al[14] suggested that the biceps may resist superior translation of the humerus.

In addition to translational stability, the long head of the biceps tendon has been shown to resist humeral rotation. Multiple studies have showed that the long head of the biceps tendon resists torsional forces placed on the shoulder, specifically with the arm in abduction and external rotation.[15,16] Similarly, Youm et al[17] investigated the effect of biceps loading on glenohumeral stability and concluded that increased loading of the biceps resulted in significantly decreased range of motion in internal and external rotation.

To further clarify the role of the long head of the biceps at the shoulder, Andrews et al[18] electrically stimulated the biceps muscle in five patients undergoing arthroscopic surgery while observing the biceps tendon, labrum, and glenohumeral joint. The contraction of the biceps muscle increased tension in the biceps tendon and compressed the humerus against the glenoid, but no substantial changes in glenohumeral joint motion were seen. More recently, Giphart et al[19] used a biplanar fluoroscopic system to investigate the role of the biceps in in vivo glenohumeral joint motion in five patients who had undergone unilateral biceps tenodesis. Glenohumeral joint motion was quantified bilaterally while simulating the late cocking phase of overhand throwing and lifting. Several significant differences in glenohumeral joint motion were reported between the uninjured shoulders and those that had undergone tenodesis, but these differences were small and not considered clinically relevant. The authors concluded that the long head of the biceps tendon appears to play a minimal role in glenohumeral joint kinematics during these simulated activities.

Although these and other cadaver experiments have contributed to the understanding of the mechanical role of the biceps, definitive conclusions regarding biceps tendon function are elusive for two reasons. First, considerable differences among previous studies are often reported in specific testing conditions. Factors including the shoulder positions tested, the number of muscles simulated, the magnitude of simulated muscle forces, the magnitude and mechanism of applied joint forces, and the conditions of the capsules and ligaments all influence the outcome of the study. Second, determining the extent to which cadaver experiments accurately re-create in vivo joint and muscle forces is difficult because those data are largely unknown. Furthermore, Levy et al[4] indicated that cadaver experiments are implicitly based on the theory that the biceps is actively contracting, even though EMG studies that eliminate elbow motion using a brace report little or no biceps muscle activity during shoulder motion.[4,5] Consequently, although the relative effect of the biceps on glenohumeral joint stability can certainly be appreciated from individual studies, caution should be used when generalizing the results of these studies with statements about in vivo biceps function.

Biomechanics of the Labrum and SLAP Lesions

Mechanisms of Injury

The etiology of SLAP injuries is not fully understood, but the two most commonly described mechanisms involve traction injuries due to either repetitive loading/trauma or a single traumatic load, or compression injuries such as falling on an outstretched arm. The repetitive loading/trauma theory is supported by data on the prevalence of labral injuries in baseball pitchers,[18,20,21] along with subsequent research indicating that the shoulder may be susceptible to injury at two critical moments of the throwing motion—the late cocking phase and the deceleration phase immediately after ball release—when the shoulder is subjected to high forces and torque.[22,23] Kuhn et al[24] conducted load-to-failure testing on cadaver biceps tendons with the shoulders placed in positions associated with the late cocking or deceleration phases of the throwing motion. Biceps-labral complex injuries occurred in 90% of specimens tested in the late cocking position but in only 20% of specimens tested in the deceleration position (**Figure 2**). Failure loads were also substantially lower in the late cocking position. Similarly, Shepard et al[25] reported biceps-labral complex failure at substantially lower loads in the late cocking position compared with the deceleration position. Bey et al[26] reported that a single rapidly applied force to the biceps can create a type II SLAP lesion, particularly when the humerus is displaced inferiorly relative to the glenoid. Although the cadaver studies described here were not designed to identify the specific injury mechanism that occurs under in vivo conditions, these studies—along with experimental[27] and computational[28] studies that have estimated strains in the biceps-labral complex—strongly suggest that repeated forces applied to the biceps tendon likely play a significant role in the development of SLAP injuries in overhead throwing athletes.

In contrast to traction injuries, Snyder et al[29] reported that compression injuries, such as those resulting from a fall on an outstretched arm, were the most common mechanism of injury. Under these circumstances, the humerus is thought to impact the glenoid and shear the biceps-labral complex from its attachment to the glenoid rim. Clavert et al[30] used five cadaver specimens to simulate falling on an outstretched arm and reported that type II SLAP lesions were more likely to occur when falling forward (all five specimens) than falling backward (two specimens).

Soft-Tissue Mechanics

Pradhan et al[27] performed a cadaver experiment to investigate the effects of simulated arm positions associated with the overhand throwing motion on superior labral strain. Cadaver specimens were mounted to a testing fixture, strain-sensing transducers were sutured to the anterior and posterior aspects of the superior labrum, and biceps muscle forces were applied in five arm positions based on previous EMG studies. Labral strain was recorded in five static arm positions associated with throwing motion: early cocking, late cocking, acceleration, deceleration, and follow-through. The authors reported that anterior and posterior labral strains were approximately twice as high in the late cocking phase as the other four phases, even though the applied biceps load in this position (26 N) was appreciably lower than the maximum biceps load (44 N) applied during deceleration. These data suggest that shoulder position may be more significant than biceps load in labral tissue mechanics.

Yeh et al[28] used a three-dimensional finite element model to investigate how shoulder position and biceps origin location influenced stress distribution in the superior labrum. In particular, the authors investigated four phases of the throwing motion (cocking, late cocking, acceleration, deceleration) and three locations of the biceps origin (anterior, posterior, central). A cadaver specimen was used to specify the orientation of the biceps tendon associated with each shoulder position. To evaluate the effects of arm position and biceps orientation on superior labral stresses, a standardized force was applied to the biceps tendon in each of the four shoulder positions. The deceleration phase demonstrated the highest stress for the central and anterior biceps origins, whereas the acceleration phase had the highest stress with the biceps in a posterior origin (**Figure 3**). Drury et al[31] also used finite element modeling to demonstrate that labral strains are significantly influenced by shoulder position. These computational studies indicate that shoulder position, biceps forces, and variations in the biceps origin all can potentially affect the stress distribution significantly in the superior labrum.

FIGURE 2

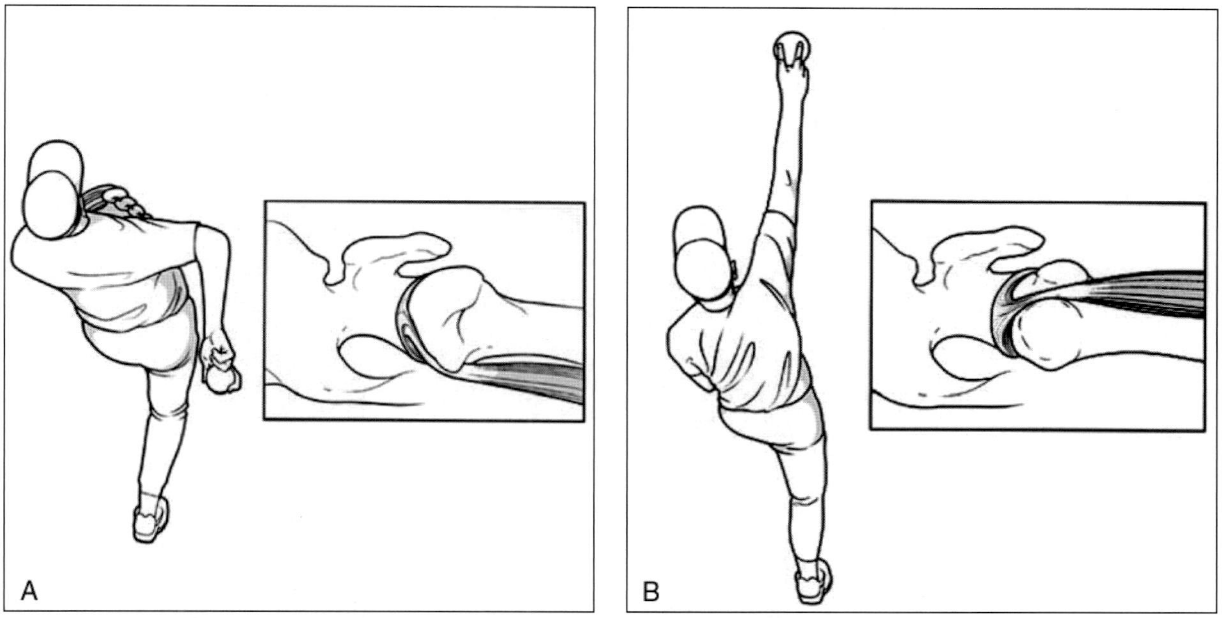

Illustration of the top view of the shoulder shows the orientation of the biceps tendon during the late cocking (**A**) and early deceleration (**B**) phases of the overhand throwing motion. (Reproduced with permission from Kuhn JE, Lindholm SR, Huston LJ, Soslowsky LJ, Blasier RB: Failure of the biceps superior labral complex: A cadaveric biomechanical investigation comparing the late cocking and early deceleration positions of throwing. *Arthroscopy* 2003;19[4]:373-379.)

Glenohumeral Joint Mechanics

Substantial research efforts have focused on characterizing the role of the labrum and the effect of labral injuries on glenohumeral joint mechanics.[32-37] For example, the labrum increases the depth of the glenoid socket by approximately 50%,[38] increases the load-bearing contact area,[39] and helps center the humeral head on the glenoid[40-42] by serving as an anchor point for the glenohumeral ligament and biceps tendon.[43,44] Studies focusing on the effect of labral injuries on joint mechanics have typically involved conducting a force-displacement test on the shoulder specimen in its native condition, simulating a labral injury, repeating the force-displacement protocol, and then, in some studies, repairing the simulated labral injury and repeating the protocol. These studies have used various shoulder positions and testing conditions to show that labral injury results in increased glenohumeral joint translation (primarily anteroinferiorly) and increased joint range of motion. The reported magnitude of the increased translation varies considerably. Panossian et al[35] reported that in response to a type II SLAP lesion, anterior translation increased 1 to 2 mm, whereas Burkhart et al[32] reported that anterior translation increased 7 to 8 mm. However, these differences may simply reflect the applied loading conditions specific to the particular study.

Muscle Activation Patterns

The extent to which clinical tests for diagnosing SLAP lesions provoke biceps muscle EMG activity has been documented by previous studies,[45-47] but relatively little is known about changes in muscle activation patterns following a biceps-labral complex injury. Horsley et al[48] investigated muscle activation patterns during rugby tackles and demonstrated that the biceps muscles of athletes with SLAP lesions activated later than muscles in the athlete's contralateral shoulder or of healthy control subjects. The implications of this finding are unclear, and further research is necessary to document the

FIGURE 3

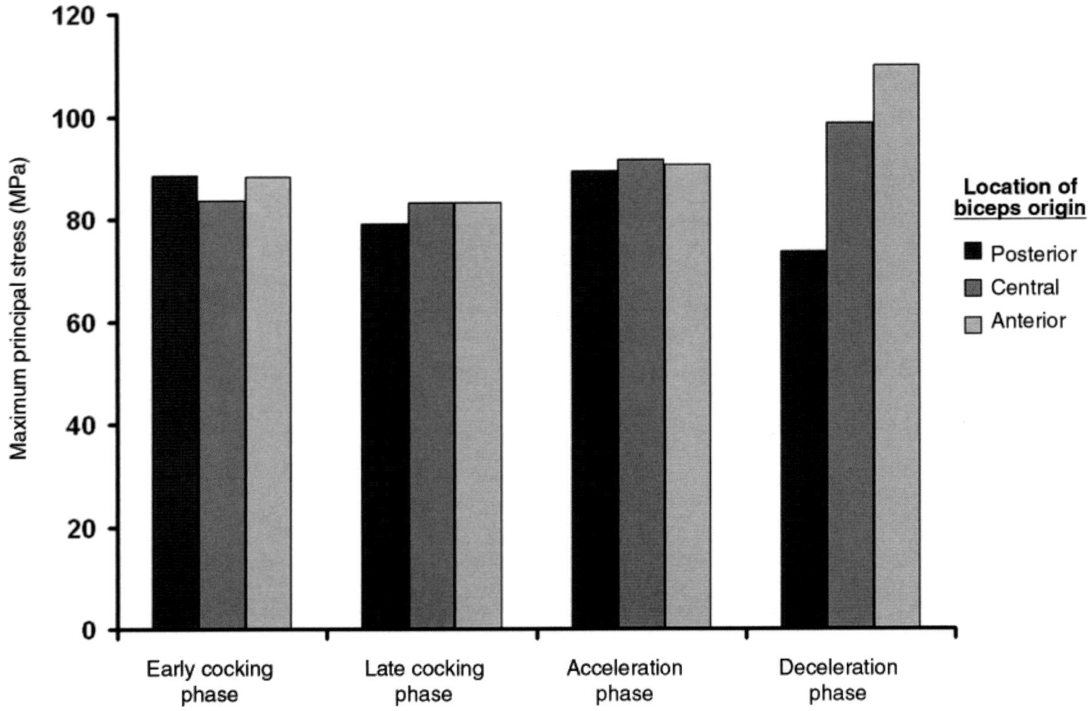

Finite element modeling shows that labral stresses are highest during the deceleration phase of the overhand throwing motion when the biceps has a central or anterior origin, and highest during the acceleration phase when the biceps has a posterior origin. (Reproduced with permission from Yeh ML, Lintner D, Luo ZP: Stress distribution in the superior labrum during throwing motion. *Am J Sports Med* 2005;33[3]:395-401.)

extent to which biceps muscle activity is influenced by biceps-labral complex injuries.

Conclusion

Considerable controversy exists regarding the mechanical function of the biceps-labral complex. For example, it is difficult to reconcile the findings of cadaver studies indicating that the biceps tendon plays a significant role in glenohumeral joint stability with in vivo studies showing that the biceps muscle has minimal activity at the shoulder when elbow motion is eliminated,[4,5] and that the effect of the biceps tendon on in vivo joint kinematics is minimal.[6] However, these controversies are excellent opportunities for future research, particularly for characterizing the specific mechanical role of the biceps tendon and labrum under in vivo conditions and relating these findings to conventional clinical measures of shoulder function. The advanced imaging techniques recently developed for quantifying dynamic joint motion[6,19,49-52] and soft-tissue mechanics[53-59] may provide the experimental capacity for studying the mechanical function of these tissues under in vivo conditions. Future research can potentially use these (and other) advanced experimental techniques to provide a more comprehensive understanding of the mechanisms of injury, the efficacy of injury prevention protocols, and the effects of surgical repair on dynamic shoulder function.

REFERENCES

1. Escamilla RF, Andrews JR: Shoulder muscle recruitment patterns and related biomechanics during upper extremity sports. *Sports Med* 2009;39(7):569-590.
2. Kelly BT, Backus SI, Warren RF, Williams RJ: Electromyographic analysis and phase definition of the overhead football throw. *Am J Sports Med* 2002;30(6): 837-844.
3. Ryu RK, McCormick J, Jobe FW, Moynes DR, Antonelli DJ: An electromyographic analysis of shoulder function in tennis players. *Am J Sports Med* 1988;16(5):481-485.
4. Levy AS, Kelly BT, Lintner SA, Osbahr DC, Speer KP: Function of the long head of the biceps at the shoulder: Electromyographic analysis. *J Shoulder Elbow Surg* 2001;10(3):250-255.
5. Yamaguchi K, Riew KD, Galatz LM, Syme JA, Neviaser RJ: Biceps activity during shoulder motion: An electromyographic analysis. *Clin Orthop Relat Res* 1997;(336):122-129.
6. Braun S, Millett PJ, Yongpravat C, et al: Biomechanical evaluation of shear force vectors leading to injury of the biceps reflection pulley: A biplane fluoroscopy study on cadaveric shoulders. *Am J Sports Med* 2010;38(5): 1015-1024.
7. Gramstad GG, Sears BW, Marra G: Variation of tension in the long head of the biceps tendon as a function of limb position with simulated biceps contraction. *Int J Shoulder Surg* 2010;4(1):8-14.
8. Blasier RB, Soslowsky LJ, Malicky DM, Palmer ML: Posterior glenohumeral subluxation: Active and passive stabilization in a biomechanical model. *J Bone Joint Surg Am* 1997;79(3):433-440.
9. Malicky DM, Soslowsky LJ, Blasier RB, Shyr Y: Anterior glenohumeral stabilization factors: Progressive effects in a biomechanical model. *J Orthop Res* 1996;14(2):282-288.
10. Soslowsky LJ, Malicky DM, Blasier RB: Active and passive factors in inferior glenohumeral stabilization: A biomechanical model. *J Shoulder Elbow Surg* 1997;6(4):371-379.
11. Pagnani MJ, Deng XH, Warren RF, Torzilli PA, O'Brien SJ: Role of the long head of the biceps brachii in glenohumeral stability: A biomechanical study in cadavera. *J Shoulder Elbow Surg* 1996;5(4):255-262.
12. Itoi E, Kuechle DK, Newman SR, Morrey BF, An KN: Stabilising function of the biceps in stable and unstable shoulders. *J Bone Joint Surg Br* 1993;75(4):546-550.
13. Itoi E, Newman SR, Kuechle DK, Morrey BF, An KN: Dynamic anterior stabilisers of the shoulder with the arm in abduction. *J Bone Joint Surg Br* 1994;76(5): 834-836.
14. Kumar VP, Satku K, Balasubramaniam P: The role of the long head of biceps brachii in the stabilization of the head of the humerus. *Clin Orthop Relat Res* 1989;(244):172-175.
15. Kuhn JE, Huston LJ, Soslowsky LJ, Shyr Y, Blasier RB: External rotation of the glenohumeral joint: Ligament restraints and muscle effects in the neutral and abducted positions. *J Shoulder Elbow Surg* 2005;14(Suppl 1): 39S-48S.
16. Rodosky MW, Harner CD, Fu FH: The role of the long head of the biceps muscle and superior glenoid labrum in anterior stability of the shoulder. *Am J Sports Med* 1994;22(1):121-130.
17. Youm T, ElAttrache NS, Tibone JE, McGarry MH, Lee TQ: The effect of the long head of the biceps on glenohumeral kinematics. *J Shoulder Elbow Surg* 2009;18(1):122-129.
18. Andrews JR, Carson WG Jr, McLeod WD: Glenoid labrum tears related to the long head of the biceps. *Am J Sports Med* 1985;13(5):337-341.
19. Giphart JE, Elser F, Dewing CB, Torry MR, Millett PJ: The long head of the biceps tendon has minimal effect on in vivo glenohumeral kinematics: A biplane fluoroscopy study. *Am J Sports Med* 2012;40(1):202-212.
20. Altchek DW, Dines DM: Shoulder injuries in the throwing athlete. *J Am Acad Orthop Surg* 1995;3(3):159-165.
21. Burkhart SS, Morgan CD, Kibler WB: Shoulder injuries in overhead athletes: The "dead arm" revisited. *Clin Sports Med* 2000;19(1):125-158.
22. Fleisig GS, Andrews JR, Dillman CJ, Escamilla RF: Kinetics of baseball pitching with implications about injury mechanisms. *Am J Sports Med* 1995;23(2): 233-239.
23. Fleisig GS, Barrentine SW, Escamilla RF, Andrews JR: Biomechanics of overhand throwing with implications for injuries. *Sports Med* 1996;21(6):421-437.
24. Kuhn JE, Lindholm SR, Huston LJ, Soslowsky LJ, Blasier RB: Failure of the biceps superior labral complex: A cadaveric biomechanical investigation comparing the late cocking and early deceleration positions of throwing. *Arthroscopy* 2003;19(4):373-379.

25. Shepard MF, Dugas JR, Zeng N, Andrews JR: Differences in the ultimate strength of the biceps anchor and the generation of type II superior labral anterior posterior lesions in a cadaveric model. *Am J Sports Med* 2004;32(5):1197-1201.
26. Bey MJ, Elders GJ, Huston LJ, Kuhn JE, Blasier RB, Soslowsky LJ: The mechanism of creation of superior labrum, anterior, and posterior lesions in a dynamic biomechanical model of the shoulder: The role of inferior subluxation. *J Shoulder Elbow Surg* 1998;7(4): 397-401.
27. Pradhan RL, Itoi E, Kido T, Hatakeyama Y, Urayama M, Sato K: Effects of biceps loading and arm rotation on the superior labrum in the cadaveric shoulder. *Tohoku J Exp Med* 2000;190(4):261-269.
28. Yeh ML, Lintner D, Luo ZP: Stress distribution in the superior labrum during throwing motion. *Am J Sports Med* 2005;33(3):395-401.
29. Snyder SJ, Karzel RP, Del Pizzo W, Ferkel RD, Friedman MJ: SLAP lesions of the shoulder. *Arthroscopy* 1990;6(4):274-279.
30. Clavert P, Bonnomet F, Kempf JF, Boutemy P, Braun M, Kahn JL: Contribution to the study of the pathogenesis of type II superior labrum anterior-posterior lesions: A cadaveric model of a fall on the outstretched hand. *J Shoulder Elbow Surg* 2004;13(1):45-50.
31. Drury NJ, Ellis BJ, Weiss JA, McMahon PJ, Debski RE: The impact of glenoid labrum thickness and modulus on labrum and glenohumeral capsule function. *J Biomech Eng* 2010;132(12):121003.
32. Burkart A, Debski RE, Musahl V, McMahon PJ: Glenohumeral translations are only partially restored after repair of a simulated type II superior labral lesion. *Am J Sports Med* 2003;31(1):56-63.
33. Mihata T, McGarry MH, Tibone JE, Fitzpatrick MJ, Kinoshita M, Lee TQ: Biomechanical assessment of Type II superior labral anterior-posterior (SLAP) lesions associated with anterior shoulder capsular laxity as seen in throwers: A cadaveric study. *Am J Sports Med* 2008;36(8):1604-1610.
34. Pagnani MJ, Deng XH, Warren RF, Torzilli PA, Altchek DW: Effect of lesions of the superior portion of the glenoid labrum on glenohumeral translation. *J Bone Joint Surg Am* 1995;77(7):1003-1010.
35. Panossian VR, Mihata T, Tibone JE, Fitzpatrick MJ, McGarry MH, Lee TQ: Biomechanical analysis of isolated type II SLAP lesions and repair. *J Shoulder Elbow Surg* 2005;14(5):529-534.
36. Patzer T, Habermeyer P, Hurschler C, et al: Increased glenohumeral translation and biceps load after SLAP lesions with potential influence on glenohumeral chondral lesions: A biomechanical study on human cadavers. *Knee Surg Sports Traumatol Arthrosc* 2011;19(10): 1780-1787.
37. Patzer T, Habermeyer P, Hurschler C, et al: The influence of superior labrum anterior to posterior (SLAP) repair on restoring baseline glenohumeral translation and increased biceps loading after simulated SLAP tear and the effectiveness of SLAP repair after long head of biceps tenotomy. *J Shoulder Elbow Surg* 2012;21(11): 1580-1587.
38. Howell SM, Galinat BJ: The glenoid-labral socket: A constrained articular surface. *Clin Orthop Relat Res* 1989;(243):122-125.
39. Soslowsky LJ, Flatow EL, Bigliani LU, Pawluk RJ, Ateshian GA, Mow VC: Quantitation of in situ contact areas at the glenohumeral joint: A biomechanical study. *J Orthop Res* 1992;10(4):524-534.
40. Fehringer EV, Schmidt GR, Boorman RS, et al: The anteroinferior labrum helps center the humeral head on the glenoid. *J Shoulder Elbow Surg* 2003;12(1):53-58.
41. Greis PE, Scuderi MG, Mohr A, Bachus KN, Burks RT: Glenohumeral articular contact areas and pressures following labral and osseous injury to the anteroinferior quadrant of the glenoid. *J Shoulder Elbow Surg* 2002;11(5):442-451.
42. Lazarus MD, Sidles JA, Harryman DT II, Matsen FA III: Effect of a chondral-labral defect on glenoid concavity and glenohumeral stability: A cadaveric model. *J Bone Joint Surg Am* 1996;78(1):94-102.
43. Cooper DE, O'Brien SJ, Warren RF: Supporting layers of the glenohumeral joint: An anatomic study. *Clin Orthop Relat Res* 1993;(289):144-155.
44. Jakanani GC, Botchu R, Rennie WJ: The MR arthrographic anatomy of the biceps labral insertion and its morphological significance with labral tears in patients with shoulder instability. *Eur J Radiol* 2012;81(11): 3390-3393.
45. Shanley KJ, Green RA, Taylor NF: An evaluation of the anatomical basis of the Biceps Load tests I and II for superior labral anterior and posterior (SLAP) lesions. *Clin Anat* 2008;21(7):647-651.

46. Swaringen JC, Mell AG, Langenderfer J, LaScalza S, Hughes RE, Kuhn JE: Electromyographic analysis of physical examination tests for type II superior labrum anterior-posterior lesions. *J Shoulder Elbow Surg* 2006;15(5):576-579.
47. Wood VJ, Sabick MB, Pfeiffer RP, Kuhlman SM, Christensen JH, Curtin MJ: Glenohumeral muscle activation during provocative tests designed to diagnose superior labrum anterior-posterior lesions. *Am J Sports Med* 2011;39(12):2670-2678.
48. Horsley IG, Herrington LC, Rolf C: Does a SLAP lesion affect shoulder muscle recruitment as measured by EMG activity during a rugby tackle? *J Orthop Surg Res* 2010;5:12.
49. Bey MJ, Kline SK, Zauel R, Lock TR, Kolowich PA: Measuring dynamic in-vivo glenohumeral joint kinematics: Technique and preliminary results. *J Biomech* 2008;41(3):711-714.
50. Bey MJ, Peltz CD, Ciarelli K, et al: In vivo shoulder function after surgical repair of a torn rotator cuff: Glenohumeral joint mechanics, shoulder strength, clinical outcomes, and their interaction. *Am J Sports Med* 2011;39(10):2117-2129.
51. Massimini DF, Li G, Warner JP: Glenohumeral contact kinematics in patients after total shoulder arthroplasty. *J Bone Joint Surg Am* 2010;92(4):916-926.
52. Massimini DF, Warner JJ, Li G: Non-invasive determination of coupled motion of the scapula and humerus—an in-vitro validation. *J Biomech* 2011;44(3):408-412.
53. De Zordo T, Chhem R, Smekal V, et al: Real-time sonoelastography: Findings in patients with symptomatic achilles tendons and comparison to healthy volunteers. *Ultraschall Med* 2010;31(4):394-400.
54. De Zordo T, Fink C, Feuchtner GM, Smekal V, Reindl M, Klauser AS: Real-time sonoelastography findings in healthy Achilles tendons. *AJR Am J Roentgenol* 2009;193(2):W134-8.
55. Drakonaki EE, Allen GM, Wilson DJ: Real-time ultrasound elastography of the normal Achilles tendon: Reproducibility and pattern description. *Clin Radiol* 2009;64(12):1196-1202.
56. Hawkins D, Lum C, Gaydos D, Dunning R: Dynamic creep and pre-conditioning of the Achilles tendon in-vivo. *J Biomech* 2009;42(16):2813-2817.
57. Korstanje JW, Selles RW, Stam HJ, Hovius SE, Bosch JG: Development and validation of ultrasound speckle tracking to quantify tendon displacement. *J Biomech* 2010;43(7):1373-1379.
58. O'Brien TD, Reeves ND, Baltzopoulos V, Jones DA, Maganaris CN: Mechanical properties of the patellar tendon in adults and children. *J Biomech* 2010;43(6):1190-1195.
59. Okotie G, Duenwald-Kuehl S, Kobayashi H, Wu MJ, Vanderby R: Tendon strain measurements with dynamic ultrasound images: Evaluation of digital image correlation. *J Biomech Eng* 2012;134(2):024504.

CHAPTER 4

Physical Examination of Superior Labrum Anterior to Posterior Lesions and the Biceps Tendon

Eric W. Tan, MD
Edward G. McFarland, MD

Introduction

The usefulness of the clinical examination of the shoulder is controversial despite increasing numbers of studies that have evaluated the various tests used by the clinician. Several important advances have been achieved in shoulder examination: Anterior shoulder instability is indicated by positive results for the anterior apprehension test (odds ratio, 20.22) and the relocation test (odds ratio, 10.35).[1] Full-thickness rotator cuff tears in patients older than 60 years are indicated by positive results for the painful arc and drop arm signs, as well as weakness in external rotation (odds ratio, 28.00).[2] In patients older than 65 years, a positive impingement sign, weakness in external rotation, and supraspinatus weakness indicated a 98% chance that the patient had a full-thickness rotator cuff tear.[3]

This degree of certainty does not exist in attempts to diagnose biceps tendon abnormalities, including partial tears of the biceps tendon, biceps tenosynovitis, biceps instability, and superior labrum anterior to posterior (SLAP) lesions.[4,5] Many previously described tests for diagnosing these entities are sensitive, but not very specific, for biceps abnormality.[4,5] No single mechanism of injury or clinical history is diagnostic for a biceps tear or a SLAP lesion, so clinicians rely more on physical examination and imaging to help diagnose biceps abnormalities. Considering the results of several examination techniques together may be beneficial in diagnosing particular types of SLAP lesions.[4,6-8]

This chapter reviews which physical examination techniques are beneficial and which are not in the diagnosis of biceps tendon abnormalities or SLAP lesions. Because the examination of biceps tendon abnormalities and SLAP lesions are topics of interest to clinicians who treat patients with shoulder problems, several systematic reviews and meta-analyses that provide more detail are referenced in this chapter. This topic is controversial, and not all investigations reached the same conclusions. This chapter clarifies some of these uncertainties and reports on the current status of the physical examination for biceps and SLAP abnormalities.

Dr. McFarland or an immediate family member serves as a paid consultant to or is an employee of Stryker, DePuy-Mitek, and DePuy, a Johnson & Johnson company; has received research or institutional support from DePuy-Mitek Corporation; and has received nonincome support (such as equipment or services), commercially derived honoraria, or other non–research-related funding (such as paid travel) from DePuy-Mitek. Neither Dr. Tan nor any immediate family member has received anything of value from or has stock or stock options held in a commercial company or institution related directly or indirectly to the subject of this chapter.

TABLE 1 Differential Diagnosis of Anterior Shoulder Pain

Acromioclavicular joint pathology
Impingement syndrome
Rotator cuff tendinitis
Rotator cuff tears
Long head of the biceps tendinopathy
Superior labrum anterior to posterior tears
Subacromial bursitis
Glenohumeral arthritis
Adhesive capsulitis
Glenohumeral instability
Cervical spine pathology
Humeral head osteonecrosis

Reproduced from Nho SJ, Strauss EJ, Lenart BA, et al: Long head of the biceps tendinopathy: Diagnosis and management. *J Am Acad Orthop Surg* 2010;18(11): 645-656.

PAIN DISTRIBUTION

Although pain isolated to the anterior shoulder that radiates down the arm is frequently called biceps pain, the reality is that practically no method exists to convincingly verify that pain in the anterior shoulder originates only in the biceps tendon. Biceps tendon abnormalities rarely occur in isolation, that is, without some other injury. Furthermore, rotator cuff and biceps tendon abnormalities increase in frequency with age, so it is difficult to ascribe the symptoms of anterior shoulder pain to the biceps tendon in many patients with coexisting rotator cuff disease. Nho et al[9] examined 12 abnormalities that can cause anterior shoulder pain (**Table 1**), but this list of possible causes may not be exhaustive. Several structures converge on the superior bicipital groove, including the superior subscapularis tendon, the anterior supraspinatus tendon, the superior glenohumeral ligament, the coracohumeral ligament, and the biceps tendon, so even when pain in the anterior shoulder seems localized to the bicipital groove, especially superiorly, the cause cannot be definitively assigned to one or more structures. Diagnostic injections of local anesthetic into the bicipital groove, even under imaging guidance, may alleviate anterior shoulder pain from these other structures, so the injections may not accurately reflect biceps abnormalities in the superior bicipital groove.[10]

Similarly, SLAP lesion types are so diverse that no single pain pattern is diagnostic for the entire spectrum of SLAP lesions. Powell et al[11] described 10 types of SLAP lesions, but type II is the most common pattern seen during arthroscopic evaluation of the shoulder. Burkhart et al[12] divided type II lesions into three variants, and suggested that the posterior variant (the biceps torn from the superior glenoid tubercle and posterior labrum, with the anterior and superior labrum intact) is more painful posteriorly and superiorly in the shoulder. This observation has not been verified by any study. The active compression test for diagnosing SLAP lesions[13] requires the patient to discriminate between pain deep in the shoulder and pain at the acromioclavicular joint. Patients often cannot reliably identify the origin of the pain, so although pain deep in the shoulder may be highly suspicious for a SLAP lesion, it is not diagnostic.

PALPATION

The bicipital groove lies approximately 1 cm anterior to the equator of the humeral head.[14] As a result, when the arm is at the side in internal rotation, the bicipital groove lies near the anterior shoulder joint. Palpation with the arm in this position does not discriminate the biceps tendon from the anterior joint line. As a result, Matsen et al[15] recommended placing the arm in neutral rotation when palpating the biceps tendon. However, the authors of this chapter recommend external rotation of approximately 30°, which moves the bicipital groove away from the anterior shoulder joint. With the arm in this position and by moving the elbow through flexion and extension, the biceps can sometimes be felt under one's finger, but the accuracy of this recommendation has not been established.

Gill et al[16] evaluated the clinical usefulness of palpation of the biceps tendon in the bicipital groove. Palpation was neither sensitive nor specific for the diagnosis of partial biceps tears. However, the study was limited because no isolated biceps tendon tears were reported, and all patients in the experimental group (which included patients with partial biceps tendon tears and various degrees of rotator cuff abnormality) were compared with a group of patients with rotator cuff disease only. Although the clinician might want to believe that he or she can palpate the biceps tendon accurately, this ability has not yet been established by any clinical study.

Clicking in the Shoulder

Two biceps abnormalities may cause clicking in the shoulder: a SLAP lesion and subluxation of the long head of the biceps tendon. Crepitus and clicking around the shoulder are notoriously ambiguous because they are difficult to isolate as originating from one particular structure. McFarland et al[17] found that 3% of patients with SLAP lesions had a click on examination, but this percentage was not statistically different from that of patients in the control group who had a click but no SLAP lesion (1%). The authors concluded that clicking on examination was not a feature unique to SLAP lesions.

Michener et al[7] found that for a patient who had a history of popping, clicking, or catching in the shoulder, the likelihood ratio for a positive result for the anterior glide test (**Figure 1**) increased the probability that a patient would have a type II, III, or IV SLAP lesion. Without that history, the authors found that the anterior glide test had no diagnostic utility for diagnosing a SLAP lesion, which is consistent with previous reports.[8,16] However, Michener et al[7] also found that a history of popping, clicking, or catching in the shoulder did not increase the diagnostic utility of the crank test or the active compression test when examining for a SLAP lesion.

Similarly, other authors suggested that clicking in the anterior shoulder with circumduction of the shoulder in internal and external rotation indicates biceps tendon instability.[18,19] Although this finding seems ingrained in the lore of the shoulder examination, the validity of this finding and its clinical utility has not been established. Because biceps instability is rarely diagnosed, no study exists in the literature that confirms the reliability or clinical usefulness of this test.

Boileau et al[20] suggested that localized swelling can develop in the biceps tendon that causes tendon catching and entrapment in the bicipital groove. In this setting, patients had reduced active and passive elevation of the arm, and any attempt to push beyond the obstruction caused pain to increase. This test was repeated with the patient under anesthesia, and arm elevation was restored once the intra-articular portion of the tendon was removed arthroscopically. No study evaluating this phenomenon or the clinical utility of this test has been published.

FIGURE 1

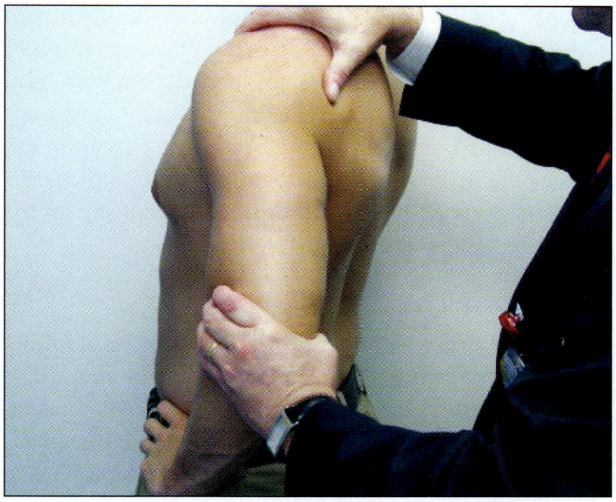

Photograph shows the anterior slide test, which is performed with the patient standing and the hand of the affected extremity on the hip with the hand pointing backward. The examiner applies an axial load on the shoulder anteriorly and superiorly, which the patient resists. A positive test result is indicated by pain or clicking in the shoulder. (Reproduced with permission from McFarland EG: Examination of the biceps tendon and superior labrum anterior and posterior [SLAP] lesions, in Kim TK, Park HB, El Rassi G, Gill H, Keyurapan E, eds: *Examination of the Shoulder: The Complete Guide.* New York, NY, Thieme, 2006, pp 213-243.)

Physical Examination Tests

Before evaluating the various clinical examination tests for the biceps tendon or superior labrum, it should be noted that the cause of the pain associated with these tests is still unknown. The heaviest concentrations of pain fibers in the shoulder are located in the subacromial bursa, followed by the biceps tendon.[21] The labrum has few pain nerve fibers, suggesting that pain with provocative tests is, in some manner, secondary to stretching or irritation of the biceps tendon. Another theory is that the pain with some of these maneuvers is the result of tension placed on the biceps tendon at its attachment onto the superior glenoid.[4] It is possible that some of these maneuvers produce biceps tendon pain with both mechanisms, but the exact mechanism in most maneuvers remains unknown. Therefore, these tests were examined for their usefulness for the diagnosis of biceps abnormalities, SLAP lesions, or both, depending on the literature for that specific test.

The Speed Test

The Speed test is performed with the patient standing and with the arm in 90° of forward flexion and 10° to 15° of horizontal extension, the elbow in full extension, and the forearm in full supination. Although it is probably the oldest and best-known test for biceps tendon abnormality, many studies have found this test to be neither sensitive nor specific.[22-24] Overall, the Speed test is not clinically helpful for the identification of biceps tendon abnormalities.

The Speed test has also been studied as a possible examination for SLAP lesions.[6,8] Oh et al[8] found a sensitivity of 32% and a specificity of 66% for correct diagnosis of a type II SLAP lesion, but if a positive Speed test result was combined with positive results for the compression rotation and active compression tests, the sensitivity remained low at 25% but the specificity increased to 90%. Kibler et al[6] found that the Speed test had a sensitivity of 29% and a specificity of 69% for SLAP lesions. Therefore, the Speed test alone is ineffective in the diagnosis of SLAP lesions, although it may have some utility when combined with other tests.

The Yergason Test

The Yergason test, first described in 1931 as a test for biceps abnormality, was formerly called the supination sign.[25] The test is performed with the patient standing with the arm at the side and the elbow in 90° of flexion. The examiner provides resistance to forearm supination, and pain over the bicipital groove indicates a positive result.

Surprisingly few studies have been conducted on the clinical utility of the Yergason test, partly because biceps tendon abnormality without coexisting abnormalities is uncommon. In a 2008 meta-analysis, Hegedus et al[5] reported that no study met the criteria for the analysis of the Yergason test. Kibler et al[6] reported a sensitivity of 41% and a specificity of 79% for biceps tendon injuries that included tendinopathy of the biceps midsubstance or at the biceps insertion. For SLAP lesions, the Yergason test had a sensitivity of 26% and a specificity of 70%. The odds ratios suggest that the Yergason test has a low sensitivity for SLAP lesions and biceps tendon abnormalities.

The Active Compression Test

The active compression test[13] has been described as a test for SLAP lesions and acromioclavicular joint abnormality, but not for lesions of the biceps tendon alone. The active compression test is performed with the patient standing with the arm in 90° of forward flexion and 20° of horizontal adduction, the elbow in full flexion, and the forearm in full pronation (**Figure 2**). In this position, the patient resists a downward force and is asked to identify any pain to the acromioclavicular joint or deep in the shoulder. This test was reported to have a sensitivity of 100% and a specificity of 98.5% for diagnosis of a SLAP lesion.[13]

Subsequent studies included a wider spectrum of patients and could not duplicate these results.[8,17,26,27] Systematic reviews and meta-analysis of the active compression test indicate that it is sensitive but not specific for SLAP lesions.[5,28,29] Overreliance on this test may result in an overdiagnosis of a SLAP tear because a positive result for this test can indicate various shoulder conditions.

The Compression Rotation Test

The compression rotation test was intended to be an examination for a SLAP lesion and was based on the concept that a labral tear would cause mechanical symptoms similar to those of a torn meniscus in the knee. The patient is placed in the supine position, and the arm is placed in 90° of abduction and neutral rotation. The shoulder is moved through internal and external rotation with compression applied to the joint. A positive test result is indicated by pain or clicking in the joint. This test has not been found to be clinically useful for diagnosing SLAP lesions.[17]

The Biceps Load II Test

The biceps load II test is a variation of the biceps load I test, which diagnoses labral lesions in patients with anterior shoulder instability. The biceps load I test

FIGURE 2

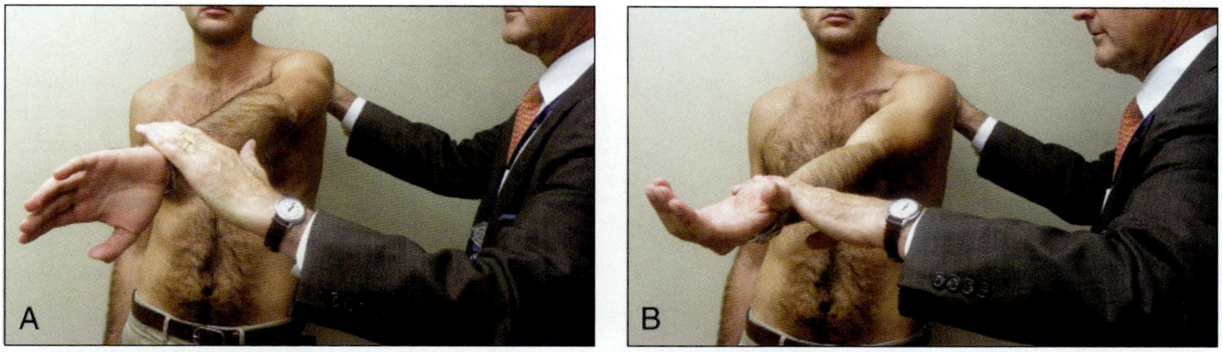

The O'Brien active compression test is performed with the patient standing and the arm in 90° of forward flexion, 15° to 20° of adduction, and in maximum internal rotation. **A,** The patient resists a downward force applied by the examiner. A positive result is indicated by pain deep in the shoulder or the examiner feeling a click in the shoulder. **B,** The test is repeated with the arm in external rotation and with the thumb facing up. A positive result is indicated by the patient reporting less pain or relief of pain with the test performed in the thumb-up position.

was used to diagnose labral tears in any location in the glenoid, not just SLAP lesions. The biceps load II test refines the diagnosis specifically to SLAP lesions in patients without instability.[30,31] The biceps load II test is performed with the patient in the supine position and with the arm in 120° of abduction, at the end range of external rotation, and at maximum supination (**Figure 3**). The examiner provides resistance to elbow flexion and supination simultaneously. A positive test result is indicated if the patient reports pain or increased pain with resisted elbow flexion and resisted supination. Kim et al[30,31] reported a sensitivity of 88% and a specificity of 96% for the biceps load II test to detect SLAP lesions.

Oh et al[8] reported a sensitivity of 30% and a specificity of 42% for the biceps load II test; however, combining it with other positive test results raised the specificity to more than 90% although the sensitivity was less than 32%. Cook et al[26] reported a sensitivity of 67%, but a specificity of 51%. Of the examination tests studied by the authors, the biceps load II test had the highest positive likelihood ratio of 1.7 and a low negative likelihood ratio of 0.39.

The Dynamic Labral Shear Test

The dynamic labral shear test can be performed with the patient sitting or in the supine position. The arm is elevated in the plane of the body from 70° to 120° while an anteriorly directed force, similar to that used in the anterior apprehension test, is applied[6] (**Figure 4**). A positive test result is indicated by pain and/or painful clicking in the posterior joint line between 70° and 120° of abduction.

The only two studies conducted of this test have contradictory results.[6,26] This discrepancy may relate to variations in how the test was performed. Both studies essentially exerted an anterior force on the arm through a range of motion between 90° and 120° of abduction. Kibler et al[6] found that this test had a sensitivity of 72% and specificity of 98% for SLAP tears. A positive test result for the dynamic shear test indicated a likelihood ratio of 31.0 that the patient had a SLAP tear (essentially diagnostic).

In contrast, Cook et al[26] also evaluated patients using the dynamic labral shear test and correlated their findings with subsequent arthroscopic surgery. The test had a sensitivity of 92% but a specificity of only 20% for SLAP tears; a positive test result indicated a likelihood ratio of only 1.1, and therefore is not considered diagnostic.

The dynamic labral shear test may be difficult to perform or interpret in individuals with traumatic anterior shoulder instability because the testing position may elicit substantial apprehension and pain. Further study is needed to determine the clinical utility of the dynamic labral shear test in the examination for SLAP lesions.

FIGURE 3

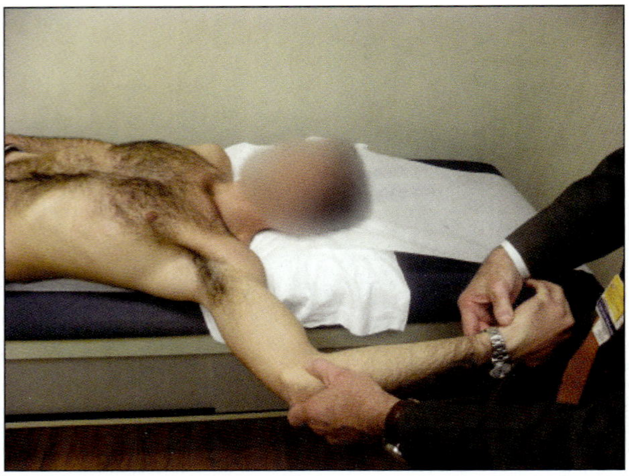

The biceps load II test is performed with the patient in the supine position and the arm in 120° of abduction. The arm is placed in maximum external rotation and supination and the patient resists forearm supination and elbow flexion. A positive test result is indicated by pain deep in the shoulder.

FIGURE 4

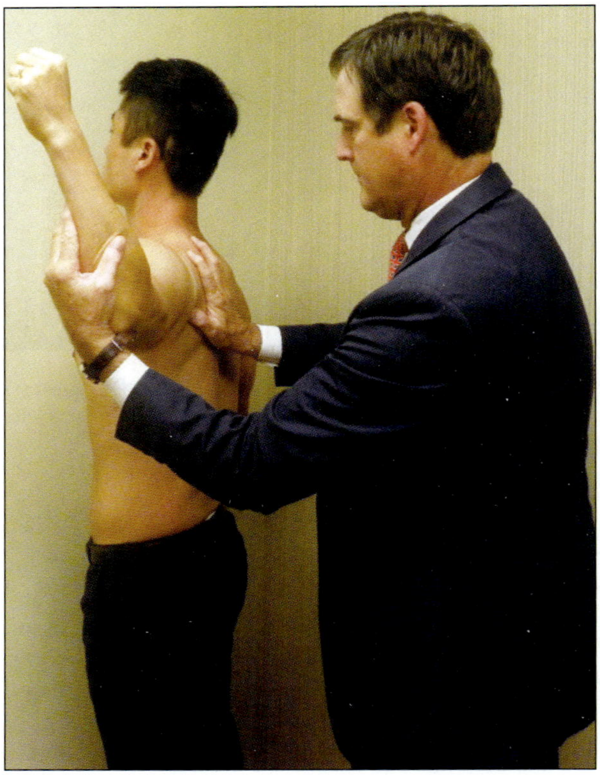

The dynamic shear test is performed with the patient standing or in the supine position. The arm is elevated in the sagittal plane from 60° to 120° as a force is directed anteriorly in the shoulder by the examiner. A positive test result is indicated by pain or clicking between 90° and 120°.

Combinations of Tests

Several studies have evaluated whether a combination of physical examination tests for biceps tears or SLAP lesions improves the clinical and diagnostic results of these tests.[6,16] Oh et al[8] found that no combination of 2 examination tests from the 10 that were studied increased the diagnostic accuracy for SLAP lesions. However, the authors found that three positive test results increased the sensitivity to 75% and the specificity to 90% for a SLAP tear. On a practical level, this schema would require an examiner to commit a long list of tests to memory or tabulate the results of these tests in the clinic or preoperatively. Cook et al[26] evaluated five SLAP examination tests and found that no combination increased the diagnostic accuracy of the tests for SLAP tears. Kibler et al[6] studied eight examination techniques and found that combining the dynamic labral shear test and the active compression test optimized the ability to diagnose a SLAP lesion.

Conclusion

The diagnosis of biceps tendon tears and SLAP lesions on physical examination is difficult for several reasons: the coexistence of other lesions with SLAP lesions, the variable history of SLAP lesions, the ambiguity of clicking or popping in the shoulder, the nonspecific pain pattern of these lesions, and the lack of specificity for many of the tests. The dynamic shear test has some promise in supporting a diagnosis of a SLAP tear, but the diametrically opposed results reported for this test warrant caution. Combining tests may improve the sensitivity to 75% and the specificity to as high as 90% for type II SLAP lesions,[8] but not all studies have confirmed this finding. Although the physical examination tests for SLAP lesions have limitations, careful examination of the patient for associated injuries is paramount. An optimal combination of history, physical examination findings, and radiographic findings may make the diagnosis of a SLAP lesion or biceps tendon injury more reliable. However, until that combination is determined, failed medical or nonsurgical treatment is the primary indication for surgical treatment.

References

1. Farber AJ, Castillo RC, Clough M, Bahk M, McFarland EG: Clinical assessment of three common tests for traumatic anterior shoulder instability. *J Bone Joint Surg Am* 2006;88(7):1467-1474.
2. Park HB, Yokota A, Gill HS, El Rassi G, McFarland EG: Diagnostic accuracy of clinical tests for the different degrees of subacromial impingement syndrome. *J Bone Joint Surg Am* 2005;87(7):1446-1455.
3. Murrell GA, Walton JR: Diagnosis of rotator cuff tears. *Lancet* 2001;357(9258):769-770.
4. McFarland EG: Examination of the biceps tendon and superior labrum anterior and posterior (SLAP) lesions, in Kim TK, Park HB, El Rassi G, Gill H, Keyurapan E, eds: *Examination of the Shoulder: The Complete Guide.* New York, NY, Thieme, 2006, pp 213-243.
5. Hegedus EJ, Goode A, Campbell S, et al: Physical examination tests of the shoulder: A systematic review with meta-analysis of individual tests. *Br J Sports Med* 2008;42(2):80-92.
6. Kibler WB, Sciascia AD, Hester P, Dome D, Jacobs C: Clinical utility of traditional and new tests in the diagnosis of biceps tendon injuries and superior labrum anterior and posterior lesions in the shoulder. *Am J Sports Med* 2009;37(9):1840-1847.
7. Michener LA, Doukas WC, Murphy KP, Walsworth MK: Diagnostic accuracy of history and physical examination of superior labrum anterior-posterior lesions. *J Athl Train* 2011;46(4):343-348.
8. Oh JH, Kim JY, Kim WS, Gong HS, Lee JH: The evaluation of various physical examinations for the diagnosis of type II superior labrum anterior and posterior lesion. *Am J Sports Med* 2008;36(2):353-359.
9. Nho SJ, Strauss EJ, Lenart BA, et al: Long head of the biceps tendinopathy: Diagnosis and management. *J Am Acad Orthop Surg* 2010;18(11):645-656.
10. Hashiuchi T, Sakurai G, Morimoto M, Komei T, Takakura Y, Tanaka Y: Accuracy of the biceps tendon sheath injection: Ultrasound-guided or unguided injection? A randomized controlled trial. *J Shoulder Elbow Surg* 2011;20(7):1069-1073.
11. Powell SE, Nord KD, Ryu RK: The diagnosis, classification, and treatment of SLAP lesions. *Oper Tech Sports Med* 2012;20(1):46-56.
12. Burkhart SS, Morgan CD, Kibler WB: The disabled throwing shoulder: Spectrum of pathology: Part I. Pathoanatomy and biomechanics. *Arthroscopy* 2003;19(4):404-420.
13. O'Brien SJ, Pagnani MJ, Fealy S, McGlynn SR, Wilson JB: The active compression test: A new and effective test for diagnosing labral tears and acromioclavicular joint abnormality. *Am J Sports Med* 1998;26(5):610-613.
14. Hertel R, Knothe U, Ballmer FT: Geometry of the proximal humerus and implications for prosthetic design. *J Shoulder Elbow Surg* 2002;11(4):331-338.
15. Matsen FA III, Kirby RM: Office evaluation and management of shoulder pain. *Orthop Clin North Am* 1982;13(3):453-475.
16. Gill HS, El Rassi G, Bahk MS, Castillo RC, McFarland EG: Physical examination for partial tears of the biceps tendon. *Am J Sports Med* 2007;35(8):1334-1340.
17. McFarland EG, Kim TK, Savino RM: Clinical assessment of three common tests for superior labral anterior-posterior lesions. *Am J Sports Med* 2002;30(6):810-815.
18. Abbot CL, Saunders JB: Acute traumatic dislocation of the tendon of long head of biceps brachii: A report of six cases with operative findings. *Surgery* 1939;6:817-840.
19. O'Donoghue DH: Injuries of the shoulder girdle, in O'Donoghue DH, ed: *Treatment of Injuries to Athletes.* Philadelphia, PA, WB Saunders, 1976, pp 142-243.
20. Boileau P, Ahrens PM, Hatzidakis AM: Entrapment of the long head of the biceps tendon: The hourglass biceps—a cause of pain and locking of the shoulder. *J Shoulder Elbow Surg* 2004;13(3):249-257.
21. Soifer TB, Levy HJ, Soifer FM, Kleinbart F, Vigorita V, Bryk E: Neurohistology of the subacromial space. *Arthroscopy* 1996;12(2):182-186.
22. Bennett WF: Specificity of the Speed's test: Arthroscopic technique for evaluating the biceps tendon at the level of the bicipital groove. *Arthroscopy* 1998;14(8):789-796.
23. Holtby R, Razmjou H: Accuracy of the Speed's and Yergason's tests in detecting biceps pathology and SLAP lesions: Comparison with arthroscopic findings. *Arthroscopy* 2004;20(3):231-236.
24. Karlsson J: Physical examination tests are not valid for diagnosing SLAP tears: A review. *Clin J Sport Med* 2010;20(2):134-135.

25. Yergason RM: Supination sign. *J Bone Joint Surg Am* 1931;13(1):160.
26. Cook C, Beaty S, Kissenberth MJ, Siffri P, Pill SG, Hawkins RJ: Diagnostic accuracy of five orthopedic clinical tests for diagnosis of superior labrum anterior posterior (SLAP) lesions. *J Shoulder Elbow Surg* 2012;21(1):13-22.
27. Kim TK, Queale WS, Cosgarea AJ, McFarland EG: Clinical features of the different types of SLAP lesions: An analysis of one hundred and thirty-nine cases. *J Bone Joint Surg Am* 2003;85-A(1):66-71.
28. Abrams GD, Safran MR: Diagnosis and management of superior labrum anterior posterior lesions in overhead athletes. *Br J Sports Med* 2010;44(5):311-318.
29. Calvert E, Chambers GK, Regan W, Hawkins RH, Leith JM: Special physical examination tests for superior labrum anterior posterior shoulder tears are clinically limited and invalid: A diagnostic systematic review. *J Clin Epidemiol* 2009;62(5):558-563.
30. Kim SH, Ha KI, Ahn JH, Kim SH, Choi HJ: Biceps load test II: A clinical test for SLAP lesions of the shoulder. *Arthroscopy* 2001;17(2):160-164.
31. Kim SH, Ha KI, Han KY: Biceps load test: A clinical test for superior labrum anterior and posterior lesions in shoulders with recurrent anterior dislocations. *Am J Sports Med* 1999;27(3):300-303.

CHAPTER 5

Imaging of the Superior Labrum and the Proximal Biceps Tendon

Alissa J. Burge, MD
Hollis G. Potter, MD

Introduction

Imaging evaluation of the shoulder provides a noninvasive means of diagnosing labral and proximal biceps pathology. The choice of modality and imaging protocol depends on the suspected pathology and, to a lesser extent, on patient factors such as contraindications to certain types of imaging. Each modality has strengths and weaknesses in the evaluation of certain types of tissues and pathologic processes, and complementary modalities may be combined for a comprehensive evaluation of suspected pathology. Imaging techniques typically used to evaluate the shoulder include MRI, magnetic resonance and CT arthrography, CT, ultrasonography, and radiography.

Imaging Modalities and Techniques

Magnetic Resonance Imaging

MRI provides the most comprehensive evaluation of the shoulder, combining superior soft-tissue depiction with the ability to simultaneously evaluate osseous pathology. MRI of the shoulder is best performed at 1.5 or 3.0 T using a dedicated surface coil, with images routinely obtained in the axial, oblique coronal, and oblique sagittal planes relative to the anatomic axis of the shoulder. Imaging protocols vary by institution but should include a combination of pulse sequences optimized to allow both sensitive detection of mobile water and high-resolution depiction of morphology. The authors of this chapter achieved this using a protocol consisting of a single oblique coronal fat-suppressed image (inversion recovery [IR] or T2 with fat saturation), followed by oblique coronal, axial, and oblique sagittal moderate echo time fast spin-echo (FSE) images in three planes (**Table 1**).

Each imaging plane provides valuable information regarding the imaged structures, although certain structures are best evaluated in specific planes. The teres minor, infraspinatus, and supraspinatus tendons, as well as the superior labrum, including the biceps-labral complex, inferior labrum, glenohumeral ligaments, and glenohumeral articular cartilage, are easily evaluated in the oblique coronal plane. The subscapularis, long head of the biceps (LHB) tendon, anterior and posterior labrum, rotator interval, acromioclavicular joint, and glenohumeral cartilage are easily evaluated in the axial plane. In the oblique sagittal plane, the rotator cuff tendons and their muscle bellies may be viewed in cross

Dr. Potter or an immediate family member serves as a paid consultant to or is an employee of Smith & Nephew and Biomet; and has received research or institutional support from General Electric Healthcare. Neither Dr. Burge nor any immediate family member has received anything of value from or has stock or stock options held in a commercial company or institution related directly or indirectly to the subject of this chapter.

TABLE 1 Parameters and Common Abbreviations for Routine 1.5-T Imaging of the Shoulder

Imaging Parameter	Coronal Fast IR	Oblique Coronal FSE	Oblique Sagittal FSE	Axial FSE
Repetition time (TR, msec)	5,000	4,000	4,000	4,000
Echo time (TE, msec)	17	34	34	34
Time to inversion (TI, msec)	150	NA	NA	NA
Receiver bandwidth (BW, kHz)	31.25	31.25	31.25	31.25
Echo train length (ETL)	7	10	10	9
No. of excitations (NEX)	2	2	2	2
Field of view (FOV, cm)	16	16	16	15
Matrix	256 × 192	512 × 384	512 × 224	512 × 384
Slice/gap (mm)	3/0	3/0	4.0/0.5	3.5/0
No phase wrap (NPW)	Yes	Yes	Yes	Yes
Frequency	R/L	R/L	A/P	R/L

A/P = anterior to posterior, FSE = fast spin-echo, IR = inversion recovery, NA = not applicable, R/L = right to left.

section, facilitating evaluation for selective denervation. The sagittal plane also allows evaluation of the rotator interval, including the superior glenohumeral ligament (SGHL), coracohumeral ligament (CHL), and coracoclavicular ligament. Given the curvilinear architecture of both the labrum and the proximal biceps tendon, complete evaluation of these structures requires scrutiny in multiple imaging planes, particularly the oblique coronal and axial planes. Knowledge of the expected normal morphology and the signal intensity characteristics of a given structure imaged in multiple planes and using various pulse sequences is key to accurate image interpretation, facilitating the differentiation between normal anatomy and pathology.

Various advanced MRI techniques may be used for certain applications. The periodically rotated overlapping parallel lines with enhanced reconstruction pulse sequence, which involves radial sampling of parallel data lines rotating about the center of k-space (the raw data matrix of each MRI slice), is used to reduce the severity of motion artifact in patients who are unable to remain motionless, increasing image quality and diagnostic yield.[1]

Early chondral degeneration may be evaluated using quantitative MRI techniques that can detect changes in chondral matrix elements, including proteoglycan and collagen, before the development of gross morphologic degeneration is visible on conventional imaging sequences. These techniques include T2 mapping, which is sensitive to changes in collagen orientation and free water content, as well as spin lattice relaxation in the rotating frame (T1ρ), which is sensitive to proteoglycan depletion.[2,3] Delayed gadolinium-enhanced MRI of cartilage is a similar technique that uses intravenous gadolinium-based contrast material to assess proteoglycan depletion in cartilage.[3] In the postoperative patient with metal hardware, various techniques may be used to reduce metal susceptibility artifact, some of which involve modification of the acquisition parameters to optimize conventional sequences, and some of which use specialized advanced methods.

Magnetic Resonance Arthrography

Magnetic resonance arthrography has been advocated as a more sensitive method for the detection of chondral and labral pathology than noncontrast MRI. Although some authors have described an advantage in the detection of chondral and labral defects following the intra-articular administration of gadolinium-based contrast material, others have achieved statistically equivalent or superior sensitivity and specificity using high-resolution noncontrast techniques.[4] The advantage of any technique's accuracy depends largely on the experience and preference of the interpreting radiologist. Therefore, the optimal technique in a given situation is determined by the convention of the institution. The authors of this chapter advocate high-resolution noncontrast imaging to provide sensitive detection of chondral and labral lesions while simultaneously allowing direct visualization of the synovium and sensitive evaluation of chondral signal changes in the absence of focal chondral defects.

CT Arthrography

CT arthrography may be used when MRI is contraindicated, such as in patients with pacemakers, those with severe claustrophobia, and obese patients who exceed imager capacity. This technique may provide information regarding the integrity of the rotator cuff, articular cartilage, and capsulolabral-ligamentous complex, but it does not provide the soft-tissue contrast necessary for the comprehensive evaluation of these structures. Additionally, this technique involves subjecting the patient to both ionizing radiation and intra-articular contrast injection and is therefore best used when MRI is contraindicated.[5,6]

Ultrasonography

Although MRI provides the most complete evaluation of the soft tissues of the shoulder, ultrasonography is a useful modality for the assessment of the more superficial soft-tissue structures, including the rotator cuff and the LHB tendon. The advantages of ultrasonography include the ability to perform dynamic diagnostic imaging, as well as image-guided interventions such as steroid injections. Accurate ultrasonographic evaluation of the shoulder is highly operator dependent, requiring knowledge of anatomy and familiarity with certain pitfalls specific to ultrasonography such as anisotropy. Comprehensive clinical ultrasonographic evaluation of the shoulder requires a standardized scanning protocol that incorporates a checklist of key structures.[7]

Radiography

Although radiography does not depict the superior labrum or the LHB tendon directly, it is often the first imaging modality performed and may exclude other types of pathology such as calcific tendinosis and mineralized intra-articular bodies. Multiple views are typically obtained when evaluating the shoulder; the specific views are generally determined by the suspected pathology. Certain views provide optimal visualization of commonly injured or pathologic anatomic structures; multiple views from different angles help localize pathology.

Normal Imaging Anatomy

The Superior Labrum and Biceps-Labral Complex

The glenoid labrum is a rim of fibrous and fibrocartilaginous tissue that adds depth to the glenoid fossa, thereby augmenting joint stability, and provides an attachment point for the glenohumeral ligaments and the LHBT. Because it is composed of fibrous tissue and fibrocartilage, normal labral tissue has a uniform low signal intensity on routine clinical MRI sequences. The labrum has a roughly ovoid contour and a typically triangular cross section. In the sagittal plane, the labrum may be visualized as a clock face, with the 12 o'clock position as superior and the 3 o'clock position as anterior. Alternatively, the various portions of the labrum may be referred to by anatomic position: direct superior, anterosuperior, anteroinferior, direct inferior, posteroinferior, and posterosuperior.[8] Anatomic variation is common within the labrum; most variants involve the anterosuperior portion. Commonly described anterosuperior labral variants include the sublabral foramen, sublabral sulcus, and small focal defects confined to the anterosuperior labrum, as well as the Buford complex, a hypoplastic anterosuperior labrum with compensatory thickening of the middle glenohumeral ligament. Familiarity with common anatomic variants prevents misinterpreting them as pathology.[9,10]

The intra-articular portion of the LHB tendon originates at the superior aspect of the glenoid and labrum and varies in the degree to which it originates from osseous versus labral tissue. The biceps-labral complex, or biceps anchor, is the labral origin of the LHB tendon (**Figure 1**). A degree of normal variation occurs in both the anteroposterior location of the tendon's origin on

FIGURE 1

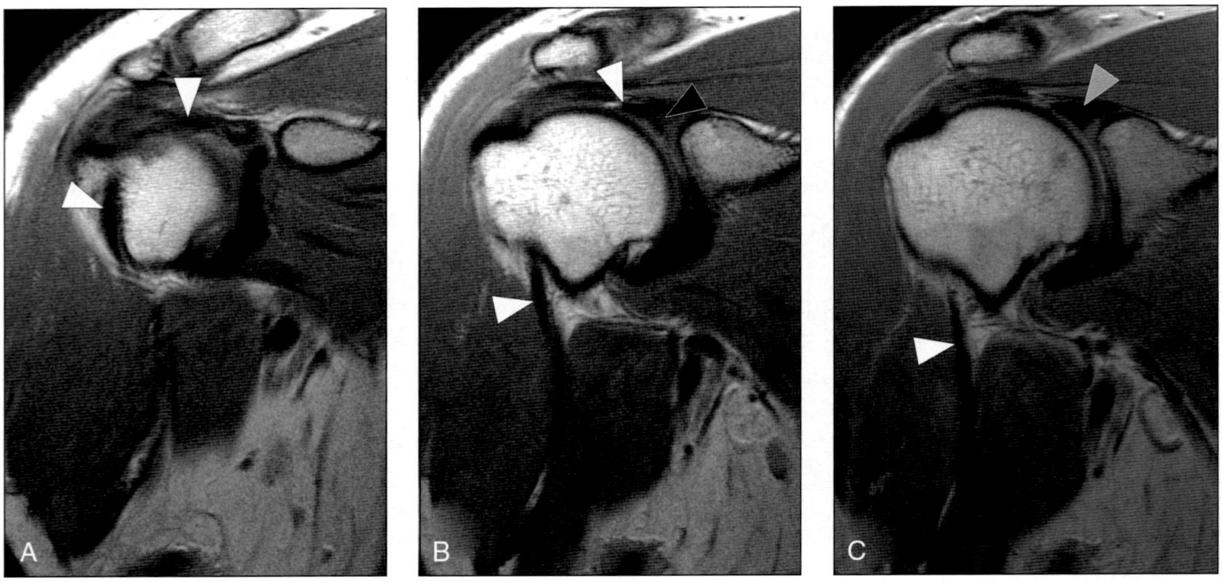

Oblique coronal fast spin-echo MRIs obtained in a 24-year-old man demonstrate the superior labral anatomy (black arrowhead), proximal biceps tendon (white arrowheads), and biceps-labral complex (gray arrowhead). **A**, Anteriorly, in the rotator cuff interval, the biceps tendon curves around the humeral head and enters the proximal bicipital groove. **B**, More posteriorly, the biceps tendon extends from its origin at the superior labrum proximally and can be visualized within the distal bicipital groove. **C**, Slightly more posteriorly, the biceps-labral complex is visible proximally, and the more distal extent of the proximal biceps tendon is visible at the level of the proximal humeral shaft.

the superior labrum and in the morphology of the attachment of the biceps-labral complex to the underlying glenoid rim.[9,10] Additionally, accessory tendon origins may exist, most commonly originating at the rotator cuff at the anterior margin of the supraspinatus.[11,12] Accessory muscle heads, which tend to originate most often from the humeral diaphysis, have also been described, but are extremely rare.[13]

The Rotator Cuff Interval and Biceps Pulley

The term rotator cuff interval refers to the gap between the supraspinatus and infraspinatus tendons at the anterior aspect of the shoulder. This space is traversed by multiple structures, including the LHB tendon, CHL, and SGHL. The biceps pulley is a U-shaped confluence of predominantly ligamentous structures, formed largely from the CHL and SGHL, with lesser contributions from the supraspinatus and subscapularis tendons. Located in the lateral aspect of the rotator interval, the biceps pulley forms a supportive sling for the distal aspect of the intra-articular LHBT as it exits the joint.[12,14,15]

The Extra-Articular Biceps Tendon and Bicipital Groove

As the LHB tendon exits the glenohumeral joint, it enters the biceps tendon sheath within the osseous bicipital groove (**Figure 1**). The roof of the groove is formed by a convergence of tendon fibers extending from the supraspinatus and infraspinatus tendons, with a possible fascial contribution from the pectoralis major tendon; this structure has been referred to as the transverse humeral ligament, although it is a confluence of fibers from multiple structures, and not a separate ligament.[12] Within the biceps tendon sheath, the vincula, a small synovial/vascular band, may be present, traversing the interval from between the anterior LHB tendon to the tendon sheath. Synovial fluid may decompress into the tendon sheath, given its contact with the glenohumeral joint space.

FIGURE 2

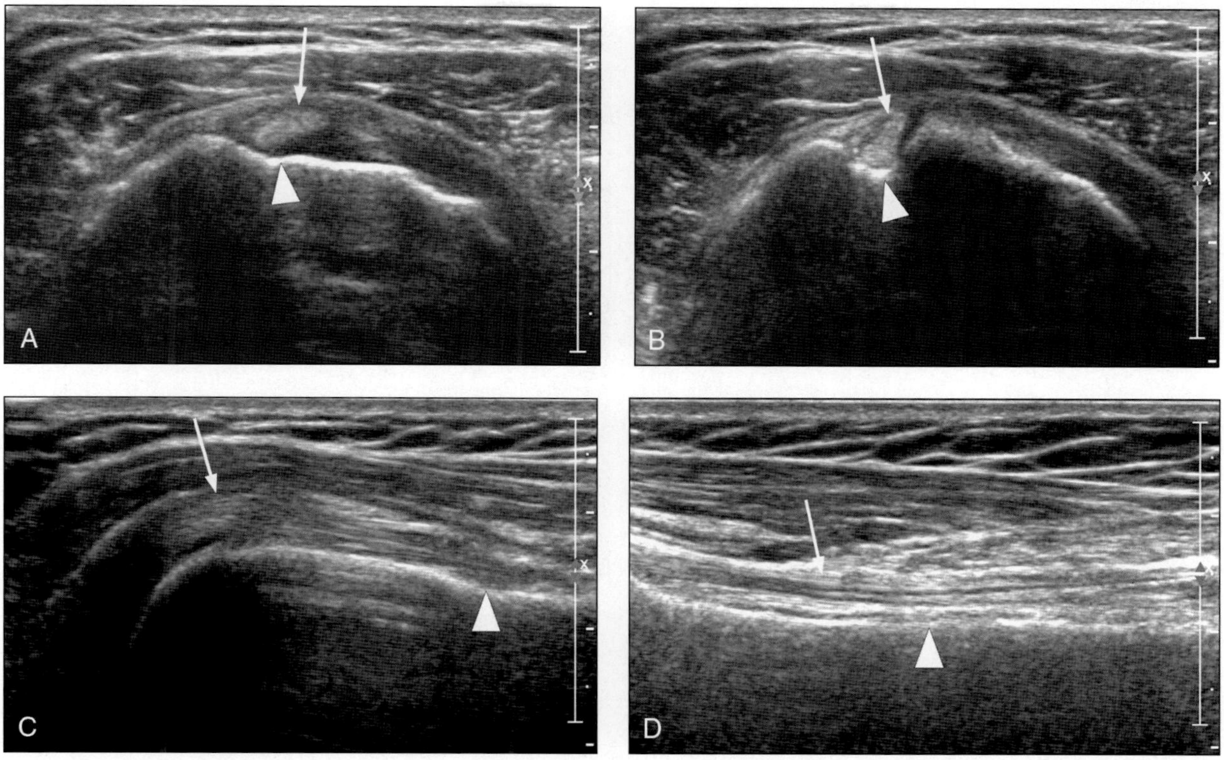

Ultrasonographic images demonstrate normal biceps anatomy in a 46-year-old man. The proximal biceps tendon (arrows) entering (**A**, short axis; **C**, long axis) and within (**B**, short axis; **D**, long axis) the bicipital groove (arrowheads).

Ultrasonography

On ultrasonography, normal tendons and ligaments should appear hyperechoic and fibrillar. The LHB tendon may be visualized within the bicipital groove, but evaluation of the proximal extent of the LHB tendon is limited. During ultrasonographic examination of the proximal biceps, the transducer is placed transversely across the bicipital groove, which is readily identified given its characteristic osseous contour. In the short axis, the LHB tendon appears as a rounded structure within the groove; the fibrillar anatomy of the tendon manifests as a speckled pattern. On completion of the short-axis evaluation, the transducer is rotated 90° to visualize the tendon in the long axis, where the fibrillar architecture is reflected as a pattern of hyperechoic parallel lines (**Figure 2**). Tendon pathology is reflected in changes in echogenicity and morphology; however, proper sonographic technique must be used to avoid false-positive diagnoses related to anisotropy, which may cause the tendon to appear artifactually hypoechoic, mimicking pathology. To avoid artifact related to anisotropy, the ultrasound transducer must be oriented perpendicular to the tendon by rocking or angling the transducer to achieve the proper orientation.[7]

Superior Labrum and Proximal Biceps Tendon Pathology

The Superior Labrum and Biceps-Labral Complex

A superior labrum anterior to posterior (SLAP) lesion is a superior labral tear, with a variable degree of anteroposterior extension and possible propagation into surrounding structures (see chapter 7). Since the original

FIGURE 3

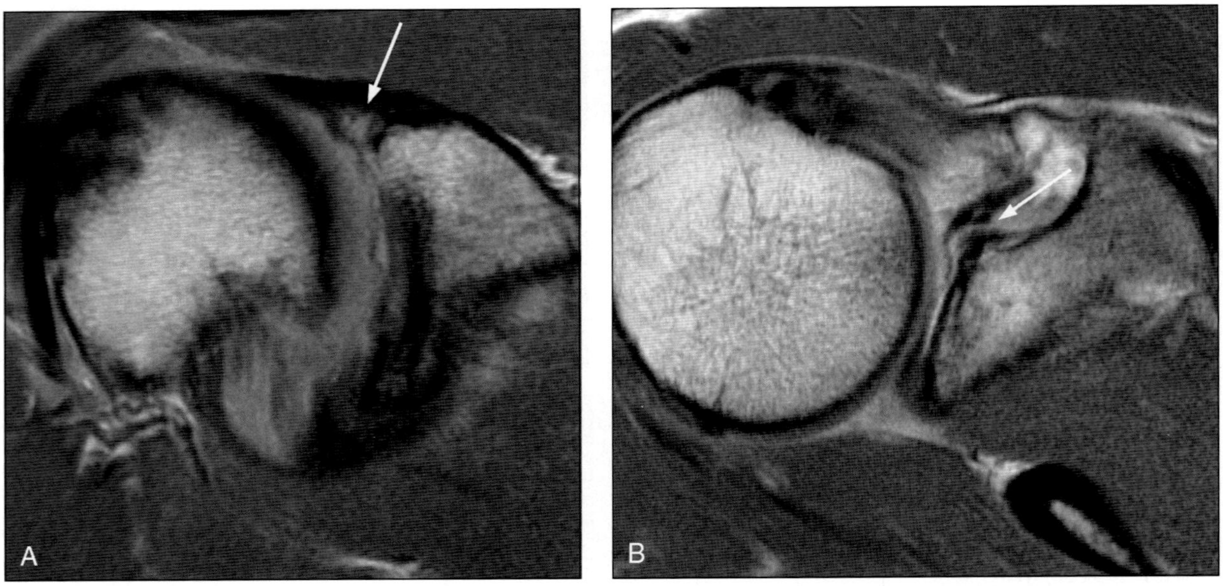

Oblique coronal (**A**) and axial (**B**) fast spin-echo MRIs of the shoulder in a 55-year-old man demonstrate a tear across the base of the superior labrum (arrow, **A**) extending to the anterosuperior labrum (arrow, **B**).

description of these tears in throwing athletes by Andrews et al[16] and the coining of the term SLAP by Snyder et al,[17] who described and classified the first 4 types of SLAP tears, the original classification system has been expanded to include at least 10 types of tears.[18] The common factor among these injuries is the involvement of the superior labrum and the biceps-labral complex.

MRI findings vary based on the type of SLAP tear. A type I tear, described as superior labral fraying without involvement of the LHB tendon, appears as intrasubstance signal hyperintensity without a frank labral tear, typically best visualized in the oblique coronal plane. The remaining SLAP injury subtypes represent frank superior labral tears, manifesting as focal linear signal hyperintensity and/or labral detachment, with varied degrees and directions of extension, the full characterization of which requires high-resolution multiplanar evaluation. Type II SLAP tears are the most common, consisting of a superior labral tear with involvement of the LHB tendon[18] (**Figures 3** and **4**).

Although the classification of SLAP tears provides insight into the type of injury, mechanism, and probable therapeutic options, precise classification of these lesions may not always be possible on imaging, and not all referring clinicians are familiar with the classification system. Therefore, when reporting these types of injuries, rather than providing a numeric classification, it is generally more important to provide an accurate description of the injury, including location and anteroposterior extent, involvement of the proximal LHB tendon and surrounding structures, the morphology of the tear including any displacement, and any associated injuries.[8]

Associated injuries depend on the injury mechanism. Tears associated with repetitive overhead motion such as throwing, including types I and II, may be seen in the setting of accompanying imaging features of posterior impingement such as rotator cuff tears and Bennett lesions. Type V and VII tears, which occur in the setting of anterior glenohumeral dislocation, generally occur in the setting of other injuries associated with anterior translation, including Hill-Sachs lesions and anterior capsular injury. Similarly, type VIII tears, which may occur in the setting of acute posterior glenohumeral dis-

FIGURE 4

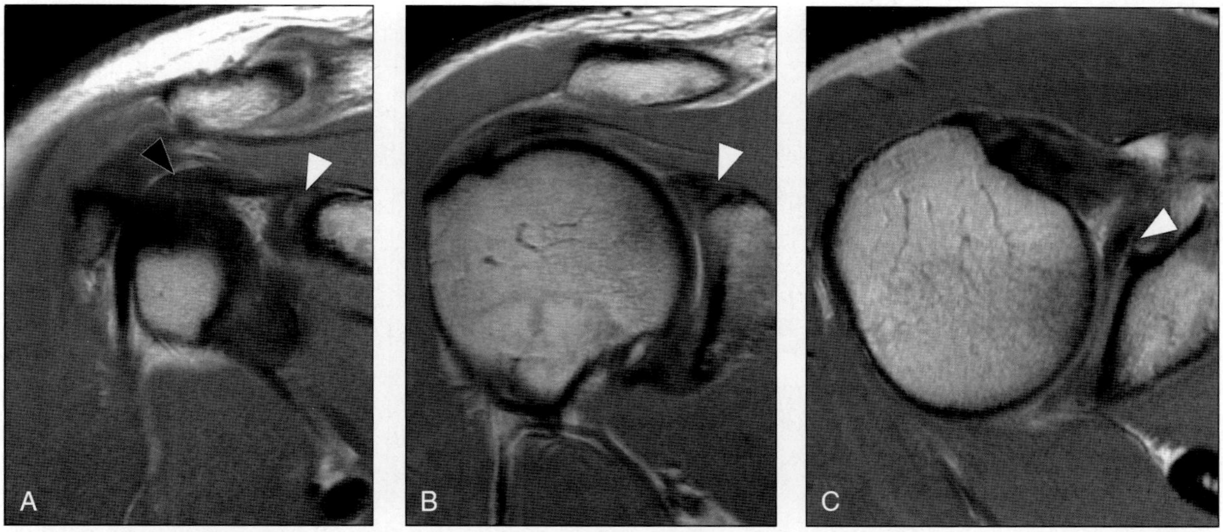

Oblique coronal (**A, B**) and axial (**C**) fast spin-echo MRIs of the shoulder in a 26-year-old pitcher demonstrate a tear across the base of the superior labrum (white arrowhead, **A**), undercutting the biceps-labral complex (white arrowhead, **B**), and extending to the anterosuperior labrum (white arrowhead, **C**). Note the proximal biceps tendon within the rotator interval (black arrowhead, **A**), just anterior to its origin at the biceps-labral complex.

location, may therefore be accompanied by associated injuries such as reverse Hill-Sachs lesions and posterior capsular injury. A fall on an outstretched hand may result in a type III, IV, or VI SLAP tear, whereas types IX and X most commonly result from severe trauma; associated imaging findings therefore depend on the type and severity of the traumatic injury.[18]

The Rotator Cuff Interval and Biceps Pulley

The biceps pulley and the fibers of the subscapularis and supraspinatus tendons stabilize the intra-articular LHB tendon within the rotator cuff interval; disruption of these structures may therefore result in instability of the LHB tendon. The biceps pulley complex can be divided into two functional units: a medial complex located along the inferomedial aspect of the LHB tendon and composed of superficial CHL and deep SGHL fibers, and a lateral complex located at the superolateral aspect of the LHB tendon that includes fibers of the lateral CHL.[12] Injury to the pulley structures may be subtle, both on imaging studies and at surgery, and localized imaging of lesions specific to the pulley components may be impossible.[14,19] Secondary signs of pulley injury may prove more easily identifiable and include injury of the superior subscapularis and anterior supraspinatus tendons, focal chondral wear adjacent to the bicipital groove, and medial subluxation of the LHB tendon (**Figure 5**). Various classifications of biceps instability have been developed based on supporting structures that have been disrupted and the direction of LHB tendon displacement.[12]

The LHB Tendon

The proximal biceps tendon is subjected to a variety of mechanical stresses during normal range of motion, particularly at the level of the biceps pulley and within the bicipital groove. These forces may lead to tendinosis, partial tears, and complete tendon rupture. Given its complex course, the LHB tendon is best evaluated in multiple planes. However, axial images provide cross-sectional evaluation of a large portion of the tendon. Biceps tendinosis may be primary in nature, resulting from attritional changes, or secondary to impingement or instability.[12] Tendinosis manifests as tendon hyperintensity and thickening on MRI; ancillary findings of impingement or tendon instability also may be present. Fluid dis-

FIGURE 5

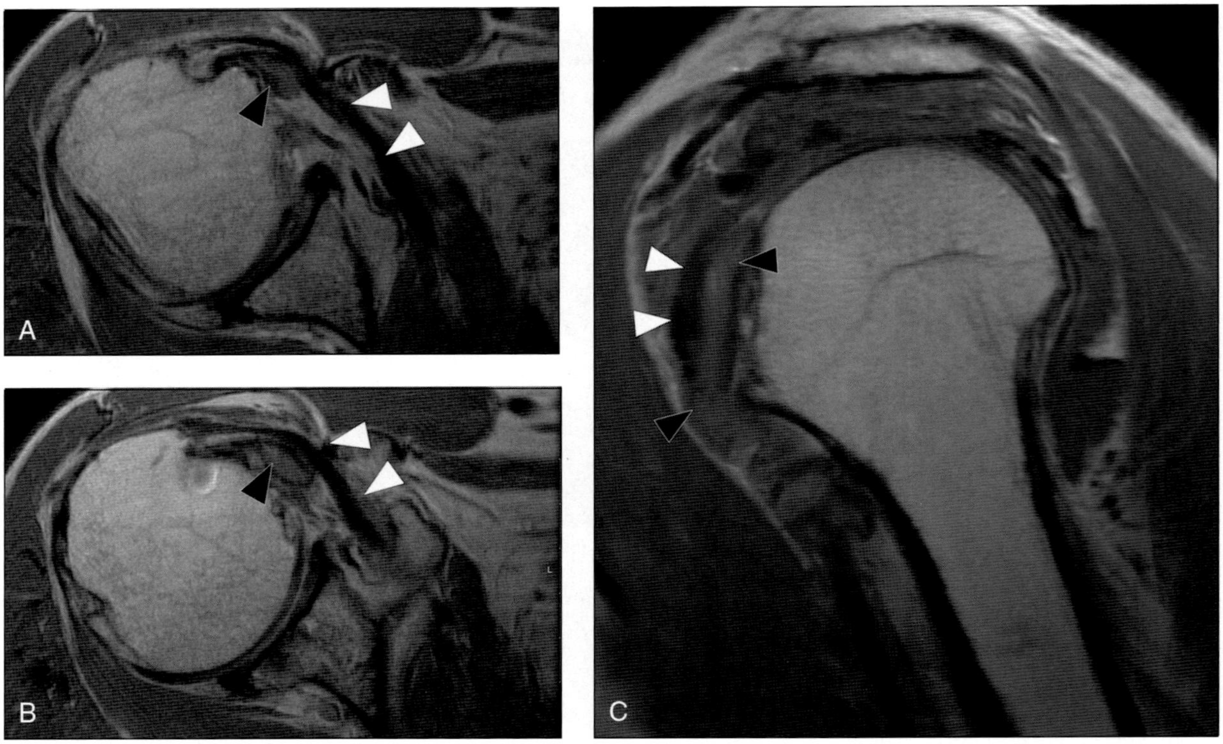

Axial (**A, B**) and oblique sagittal (**C**) fast spin-echo MRIs of the shoulder in a 75-year-old man demonstrate an intrasubstance tear of the subscapularis (white arrowheads), allowing medial subluxation of the degenerated and chronically torn biceps tendon (black arrowheads).

tention and adhesions of the biceps tendon sheath may be present in the setting of associated tenosynovitis. Although it more commonly involves the rotator cuff, calcific tendinosis, or hydroxyapatite depositional disease, may also occur in the LHB tendon, and is also amenable to ultrasonographically guided lavage (**Figure 6**). Tendinosis resulting in focal thickening of the proximal biceps in an hourglass configuration may occur in the region of the entrance to the bicipital groove, a condition termed "hourglass biceps," which is thought to represent a compensatory mechanism related to underlying degenerative pathology. This focal thickening may result in pain and locking during range of motion.[12] Biceps tendinosis may predispose the patient to a partial tear or complete tendon rupture (**Figure 7**). Although a partial tendon tear commonly manifests as a longitudinal split of the degenerated tendon, it may also be evident as tendon attenuation or a focal contour abnormality. Spontaneous complete proximal biceps rupture typically occurs in older patients in the setting of tendon degeneration, and is evident on imaging as complete discontinuity of the tendon, often with distal retraction of the torn tendon, yielding an empty tendon sheath proximally.

Combination Injuries

Combinations of the aforementioned injuries may be evident on imaging, reflecting the close anatomic and biomechanical relationships between these structures. Bennett[20] documented an association between SLAP tears and medial biceps pulley injury in a retrospective arthroscopic study, noting that the two coexisted in 43% of patients. Braun et al[21] reported a significant association between proximal biceps injury and biceps pulley and SLAP tears, as well as with hourglass defor-

FIGURE 6

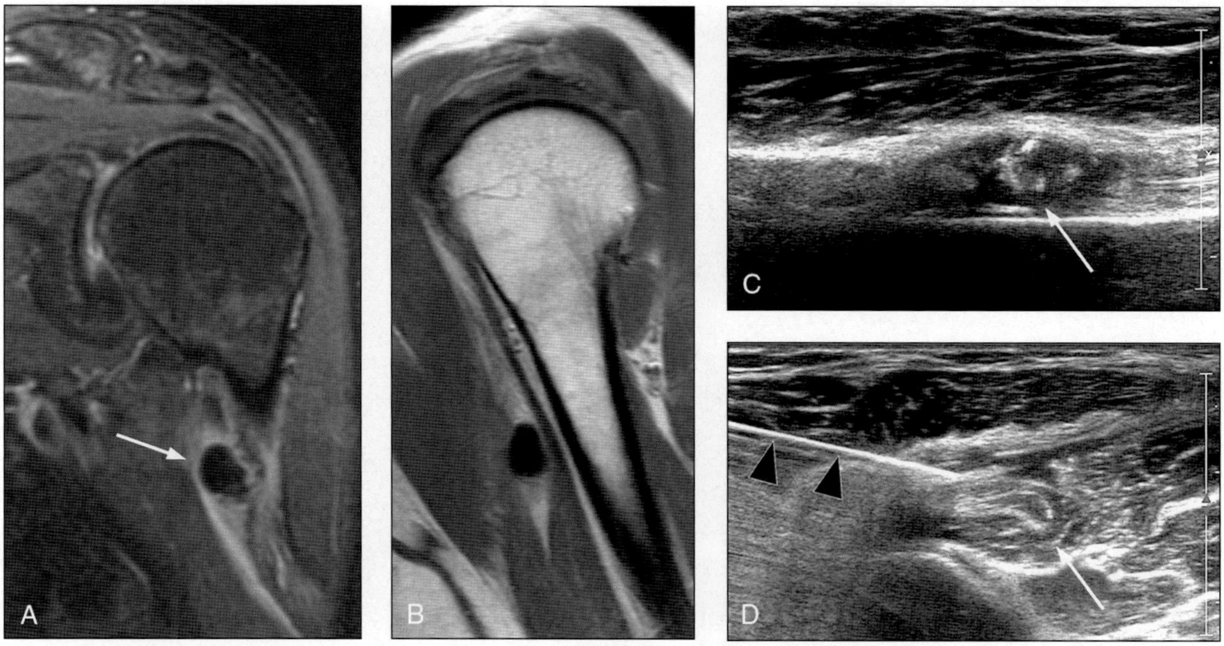

Coronal inversion recovery (IR) (**A**) and sagittal fast spin-echo (**B**) MRIs of the shoulder in a 61-year-old woman demonstrate a large focus of mineralization (arrow) within the biceps tendon sheath, consistent with hydroxyapatite deposition. Long-axis ultrasonographic images (**C, D**) also show the mineralized focus (arrows), with subsequent ultrasonographically guided lavage performed (arrowheads indicate the needle).

mity. Additionally, the authors reported a 79% prevalence of pulley tears in patients with torn rotator cuffs, particularly those with injury to the supraspinatus and subscapularis tendons.

Postoperative Imaging

MRI of the postoperative shoulder requires knowledge of the surgical intervention performed to allow implementation of proper pulse parameter modifications, if necessary, such as in the presence of metallic hardware, as well as to allow the interpreting radiologist to remain cognizant of the expected range of normal and pathologic findings specific to the surgical procedure. Techniques for reducing metal susceptibility artifact when using conventional pulse sequences include widening the receiver bandwidth, aligning the frequency encoding axis along the long axis of the implant, and oversampling in the frequency direction. Additional improvement in image quality may be obtained by decreasing the voxel size and increasing the number of excitations. When metal is present, 3T imaging should be avoided because the degree of susceptibility artifact generated by a particular piece of hardware is directly proportional to the strength of the main magnetic field. Additionally, fat suppression using frequency-selective methods such as fat saturation generally fail in the presence of metal because of local field inhomogeneities; nonfrequency-selective short tau inversion recovery sequences yield more uniform fat suppression in this setting.[22,23]

When the amount of metallic hardware present exceeds the ability of parameter modifications to create a diagnostic image, specialized pulse sequences designed to largely eliminate metal artifact can be used. These include multiacquisition variable-resonance image combination (MAVRIC) and slice-encoding for metal artifact correction (SEMAC). MAVRIC uses multiple acquisitions at varying off-resonance spectral frequency bins, which are subsequently postprocessed to create

FIGURE 7

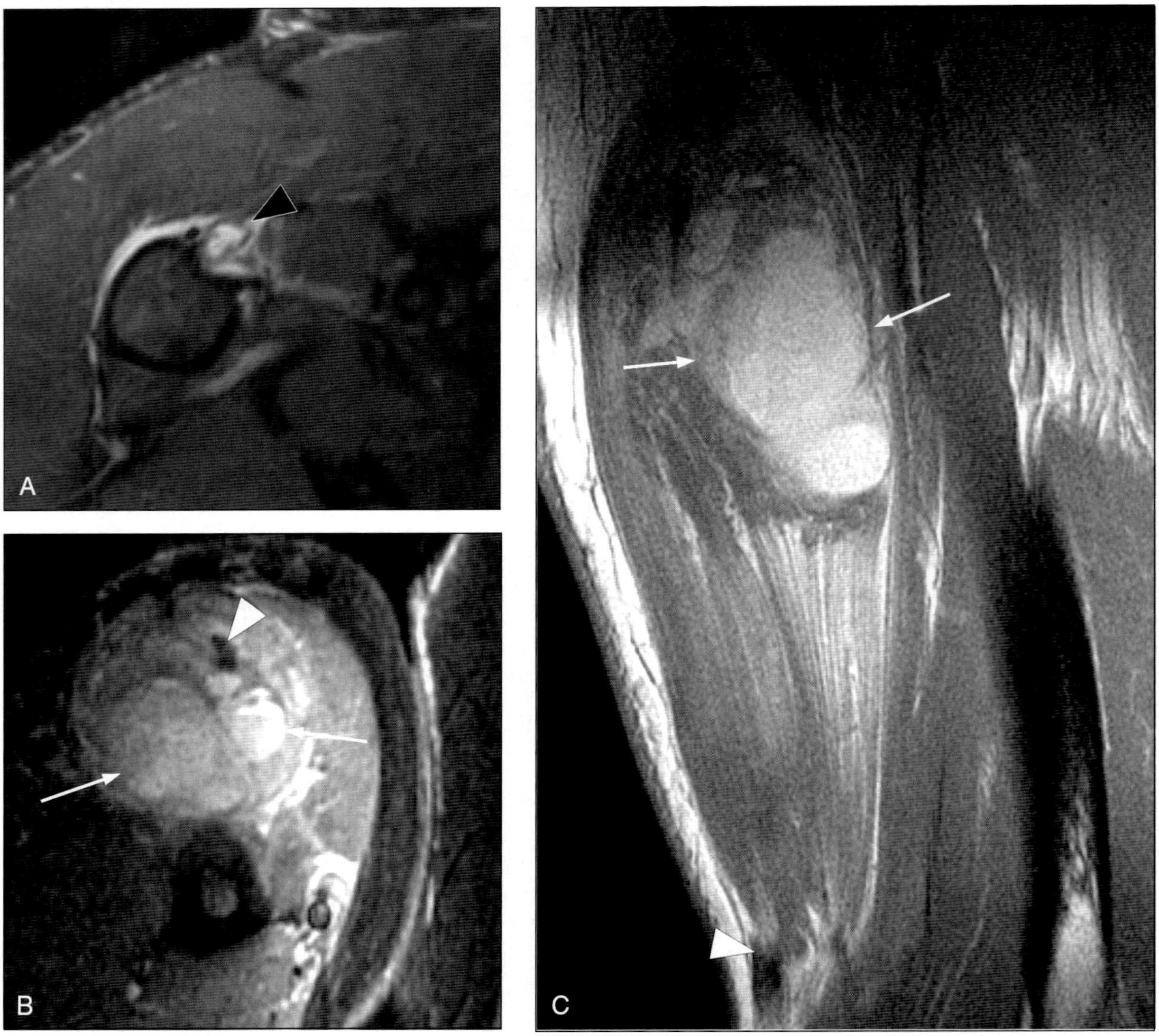

Axial IR (**A, B**) and sagittal fast spin-echo (**C**) MRIs of the shoulder and upper arm in a 53-year-old man demonstrate complete proximal biceps rupture manifested by an empty biceps tendon sheath proximally (black arrowhead), with prominent intramuscular hemorrhage (arrows), and retraction of the distal tendon stump (white arrowhead).

images largely free of susceptibility artifact. SEMAC uses view angle tilting plus a phase-encoding step in the Z-axis (the axis of the main magnetic field), diminishing the degree of susceptibility artifact via robust spatial encoding.[23,24]

SLAP Repair

The management of SLAP tears depends on the type and severity of the tear and any associated injuries, as well as on patient factors. Options range from nonsurgical treatment to surgical repair and stabilization of the

FIGURE 8

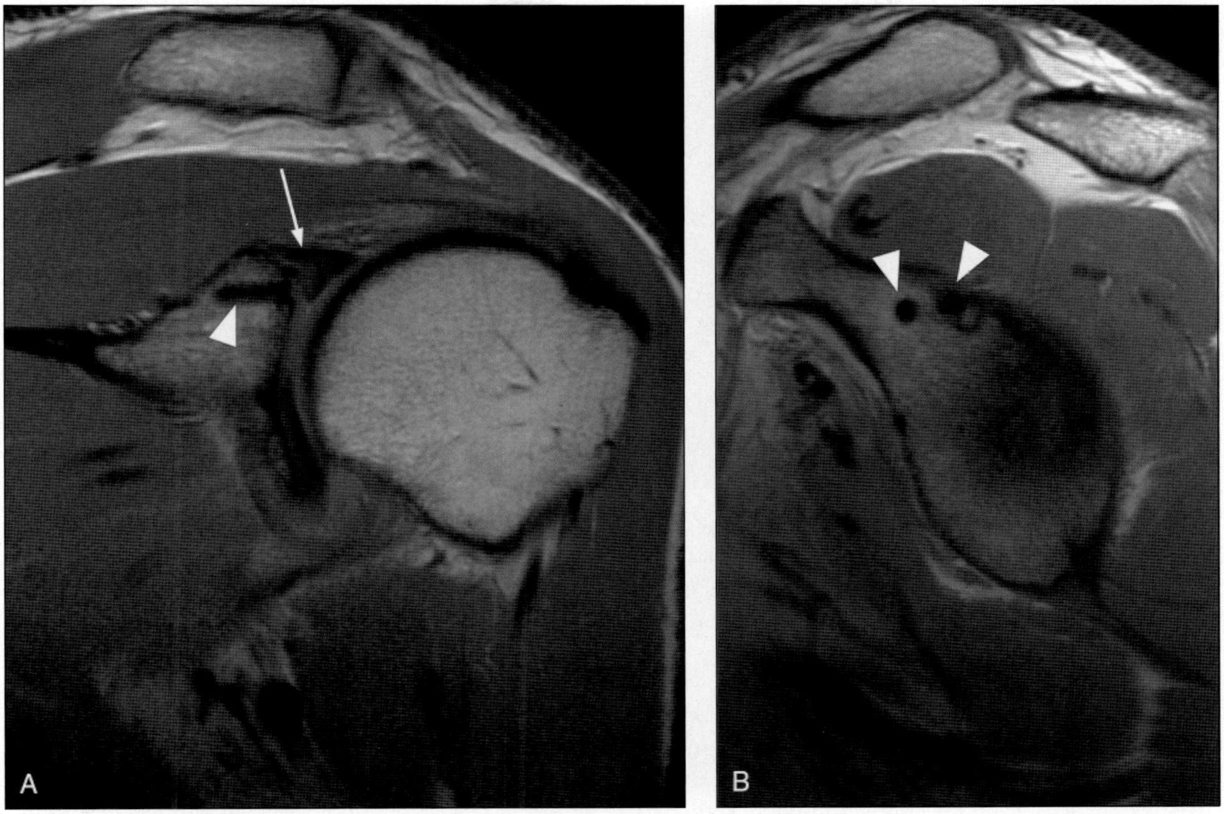

Oblique coronal (**A**) and sagittal (**B**) MRIs of the shoulder in a 42-year-old man following superior labral repair with anchors along the superior glenoid (arrowheads). The repaired portion of the labrum (arrow) is somewhat hyperintense; however, no fragmentation or fluid imbibition is present to suggest retear.

shoulder. A type I tear may be managed nonsurgically or with débridement, depending on the severity of the tear. A type II lesion, which involves the LHB tendon, generally warrants surgical repair of the torn superior labrum and the LHB tendon.[18,25,26] Various fixation techniques may be used to reattach the torn labrum, including transosseous sutures, arthroscopic suture anchors, staples, and screws; the MRI appearance of a particular fixation device depends on its degree of ferromagnetism: less ferrous anchors such as titanium generate less susceptibility artifact, and nonmetallic anchors such as plastic generate no susceptibility. At postoperative MRI, a normal, repaired labrum may appear truncated if concurrently débrided, enlarged, or abnormal in contour or signal (**Figure 8**). A recurrent or residual tear manifests as fluid imbibition into the substance of the repaired labrum, labral detachment, or labral fragmentation. Capsular thickening is an expected finding and may be related to postoperative scar or capsular tightening.[27,28] If a significant LHB tendon injury was present at the time of surgery, biceps tenotomy or tenodesis also may have been performed. If a SLAP tear was sustained during glenohumeral dislocation, concomitant surgical procedures may include augmentation of osseous Bankart lesions using bone graft or coracoid transfer, as well as graft augmentation of large Hill-Sachs lesions.

FIGURE 9

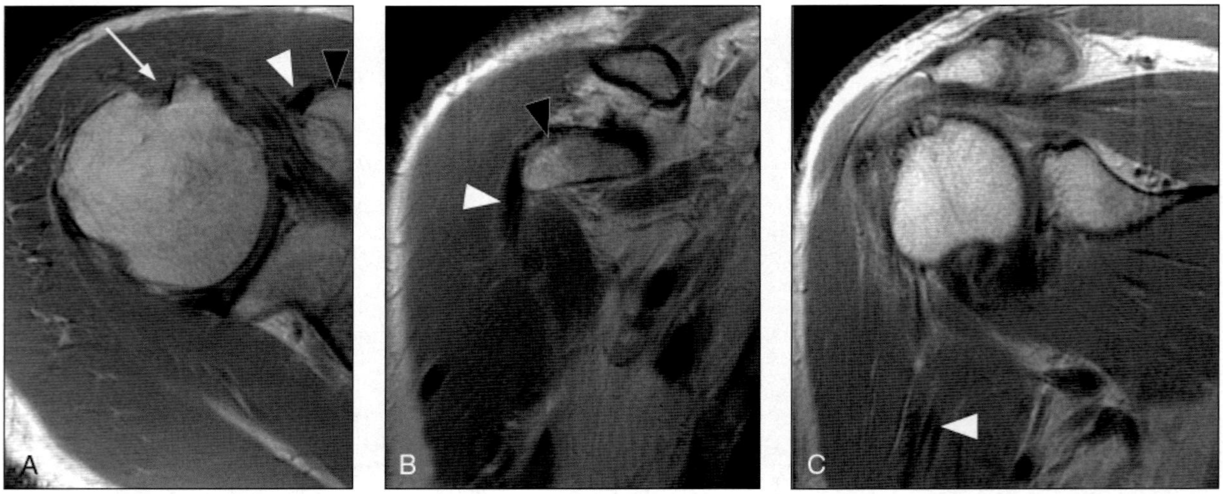

Axial (**A**) and oblique coronal (**B, C**) periodically rotated overlapping parallel lines with enhanced reconstruction images in a 64-year-old man following biceps tendon transfer demonstrate an empty bicipital groove (arrow) with transfer of the proximal biceps tendon (white arrowheads) to the coracoid (black arrowheads). Distally, the biceps tendon–muscle junction is medially displaced relative to the expected anatomic position (white arrowhead, **C**).

Biceps Tenotomy and Tenodesis

Painful biceps tendinosis and partial tears may initially be managed nonsurgically with rest, NSAIDs, intra-articular corticosteroid injections, and physical therapy. If nonsurgical management fails, surgical intervention may be considered. Additionally, patients with biceps instability may be considered for surgical intervention initially because nonsurgical treatment options for these patients are limited. The two most common surgical procedures used in the treatment of proximal biceps pain are tenotomy and tenodesis. During tenotomy, the LHB tendon is severed, typically just distal to its origin at the superior labrum and supraglenoid tubercle. This procedure is typically chosen over tenodesis in older, low-demand individuals; however, if cosmesis is of significant concern, tenodesis may be a better option, given the high rate of Popeye deformity (distal retraction of the biceps with associated focal bulge) associated with tenotomy.[29] Postoperative imaging following tenotomy reveals discontinuity of the proximal LHB tendon at its origin, with retraction of the cut tendon distally. Tenodesis involves performing an initial tenotomy and subsequently fixing the cut LHB tendon either to soft tissue or to bone. Although more extensive postoperative rehabilitation is necessary following tenodesis, the advantages include improved cosmesis and some preservation of biceps function.[29] Various surgical techniques may be used to perform tenodesis, either arthroscopic or open, with intertubercular or subpectoral fixation. The postoperative imaging appearance depends on the surgical technique used and the type of fixation device used.[30,31] On imaging, as with tenotomy, the proximal biceps appears discontinuous at its origin; however, the cut end of the tendon is fixed either proximally within the bicipital groove, as with intertubercular tenodesis, or more distally on the humeral shaft, as with subpectoral tenodesis.[27,28] For biceps instability, in addition to performing tenotomy or tenodesis, the subscapularis is also repaired. Subscapularis repair performed in this setting without treating the LHB tendon predisposes the subscapularis repair to rupture.[32]

Biceps Transfer

Although encountered less commonly than biceps tenotomy or tenodesis, transfer of the LHB tendon to the conjoint tendon at the coracoid process may be

FIGURE 10

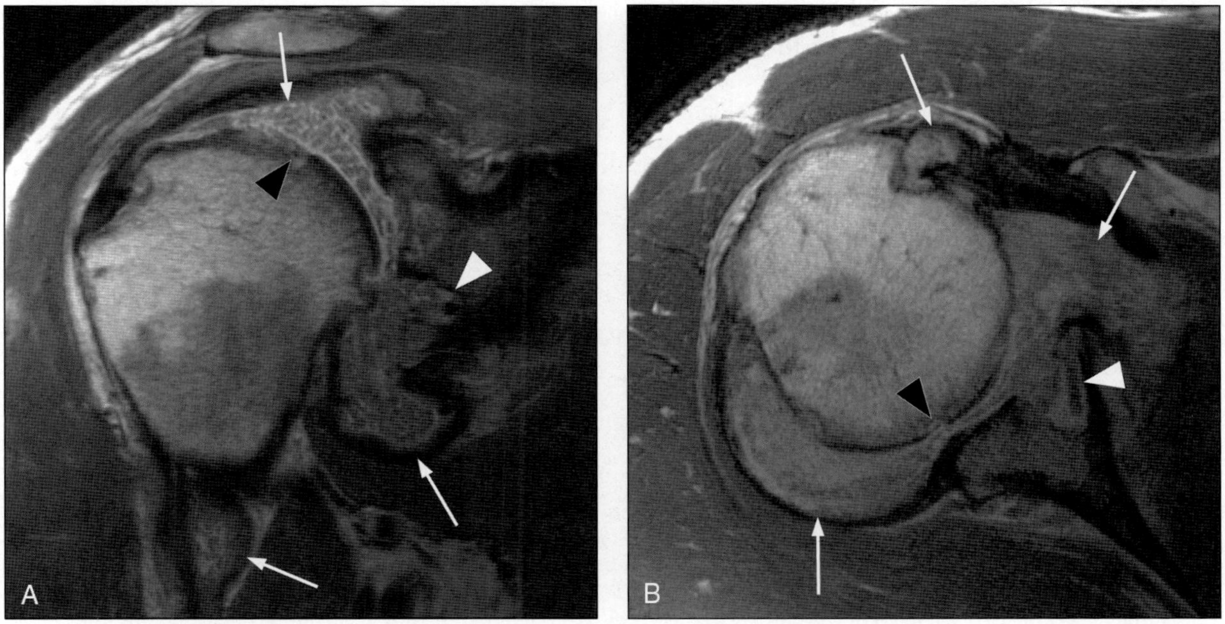

Oblique coronal (**A**) and axial (**B**) fast spin-echo MRIs of the shoulder in a 34-year-old man following labral repair demonstrate severe inflammatory synovitis (arrows) distending the capsule and decompressing into the biceps tendon sheath, with aggressive erosion yielding extensively denuded cartilage (black arrowheads) and osseous resorption about the glenoid anchors (white arrowheads); subsequent joint aspiration revealed joint infection with *Propionibacterium acnes.*

performed for similar indications (for example, painful tendinosis and/or instability after failed nonsurgical management). The procedure entails biceps tenotomy at its origin, followed by acromioplasty to expose the conjoint tendon, to which the LHB tendon is then sutured. Similar to tenotomy and tenodesis, postoperative imaging following biceps transfer will demonstrate the absence of a normal biceps origin, but in this case, the cut LHB tendon will be fixed on the coracoid[33] (**Figure 9**).

Complications

Complications that may be seen on postoperative imaging include general surgical complications such as infection and hemorrhage, or may be specific to the procedure performed, including failure of the repair or graft, retear of the repaired structure, or hardware malposition or failure. Joint infection appears on MRI as a pronounced inflammatory synovitis, commonly with hyperintense, lamellated synovial thickening; associated soft-tissue edema and lymphadenopathy are common ancillary findings[34] (**Figure 10**). Soft-tissue edema and small amounts of hemorrhage are expected findings postoperatively; however, large, loculated fluid collections such as seromas and hematomas should be considered abnormal, and the surrounding soft-tissue and neurovascular structures should be scrutinized for possible impingement by these fluid collections.

Conclusion

Although various imaging modalities may be used to evaluate the shoulder, MRI provides a particularly efficacious combination of soft-tissue and osseous evaluation, with proper imaging technique achieving superior soft-tissue contrast, high-resolution depiction of morphology, and sensitive detection of mobile water. Optimized conventional sequencing provides accurate, reliable imaging in a routine clinical setting, and the application of advanced imaging techniques may provide additional valuable information in specific clinical situations. Noncontrast MRI is an excellent modality for the evaluation of the superior labrum, rotator cuff interval, and LHB tendon, achieving sensitive and specific detection of superior labral lesions, as well as evaluation of the full spectrum of pathology occurring in the proximal LHB tendon, from SLAP lesions to biceps pulley injury to LHB tendon pathology. Knowledge of the expected normal signal characteristics and morphology of these structures on MRI is paramount in imaging evaluation, facilitating recognition of pathologic processes.

References

1. Dietrich TJ, Ulbrich EJ, Zanetti M, Fucentese SF, Pfirrmann CW: PROPELLER technique to improve image quality of MRI of the shoulder. *AJR Am J Roentgenol* 2011;197(6):W1093-W1100.
2. Koff MF, Potter HG: Noncontrast MR techniques and imaging of cartilage. *Radiol Clin North Am* 2009;47(3):495-504.
3. Jazrawi LM, Alaia MJ, Chang G, Fitzgerald EF, Recht MP: Advances in magnetic resonance imaging of articular cartilage. *J Am Acad Orthop Surg* 2011;19(7):420-429.
4. Connell DA, Potter HG, Wickiewicz TL, Altchek DW, Warren RF: Noncontrast magnetic resonance imaging of superior labral lesions: 102 cases confirmed at arthroscopic surgery. *Am J Sports Med* 1999;27(2): 208-213.
5. Fritz J, Fishman EK, Small KM, et al: MDCT arthrography of the shoulder with datasets of isotropic resolution: Indications, technique, and applications. *AJR Am J Roentgenol* 2012;198(3):635-646.
6. Kim YJ, Choi JA, Oh JH, Hwang SI, Hong SH, Kang HS: Superior labral anteroposterior tears: accuracy and interobserver reliability of multidetector CT arthrography for diagnosis. *Radiology* 2011;260(1):207-215.
7. Jacobson JA: Shoulder US: Anatomy, technique, and scanning pitfalls. *Radiology* 2011;260(1):6-16.
8. Chang D, Mohana-Borges A, Borso M, Chung CB: SLAP lesions: Anatomy, clinical presentation, MR imaging diagnosis and characterization. *Eur J Radiol* 2008;68(1):72-87.
9. Dunham KS, Bencardino JT, Rokito AS: Anatomic variants and pitfalls of the labrum, glenoid cartilage, and glenohumeral ligaments. *Magn Reson Imaging Clin N Am* 2012;20(2):213-228, x.
10. Fitzpatrick D, Walz DM: Shoulder MR imaging normal variants and imaging artifacts. *Magn Reson Imaging Clin N Am* 2010;18(4):615-632.
11. Dierickx C, Ceccarelli E, Conti M, Vanlommel J, Castagna A: Variations of the intra-articular portion of the long head of the biceps tendon: A classification of embryologically explained variations. *J Shoulder Elbow Surg* 2009;18(4):556-565.
12. Morag Y, Bedi A, Jamadar DA: The rotator interval and long head biceps tendon: Anatomy, function, pathology, and magnetic resonance imaging. *Magn Reson Imaging Clin N Am* 2012;20(2):229-259, x.
13. Sookur PA, Naraghi AM, Bleakney RR, Jalan R, Chan O, White LM: Accessory muscles: Anatomy, symptoms, and radiologic evaluation. *Radiographics* 2008;28(2):481-499.
14. Hunt SA, Kwon YW, Zuckerman JD: The rotator interval: anatomy, pathology, and strategies for treatment. *J Am Acad Orthop Surg* 2007;15(4):218-227.
15. Nakata W, Katou S, Fujita A, Nakata M, Lefor AT, Sugimoto H: Biceps pulley: Normal anatomy and associated lesions at MR arthrography. *Radiographics* 2011;31(3):791-810.
16. Andrews JR, Carson WG Jr, McLeod WD: Glenoid labrum tears related to the long head of the biceps. *Am J Sports Med* 1985;13(5):337-341.
17. Snyder SJ, Karzel RP, Del Pizzo W, Ferkel RD, Friedman MJ: SLAP lesions of the shoulder. *Arthroscopy* 1990;6(4):274-279.
18. Modarresi S, Motamedi D, Jude CM: Superior labral anteroposterior lesions of the shoulder: Part 2, mechanisms and classification. *AJR Am J Roentgenol* 2011;197(3):604-611.
19. Krupp RJ, Kevern MA, Gaines MD, Kotara S, Singleton SB: Long head of the biceps tendon pain: Differential diagnosis and treatment. *J Orthop Sports Phys Ther* 2009;39(2):55-70.
20. Bennett WF: Correlation of the SLAP lesion with lesions of the medial sheath of the biceps tendon and intra-articular subscapularis tendon. *Indian J Orthop* 2009;43(4):342-346.
21. Braun S, Horan MP, Elser F, Millett PJ: Lesions of the biceps pulley. *Am J Sports Med* 2011;39(4):790-795.
22. Potter HG, Foo LF: Magnetic resonance imaging of joint arthroplasty. *Orthop Clin North Am* 2006;37(3):361-373, vi-vii.

23. Hayter CL, Koff MF, Shah P, Koch KM, Miller TT, Potter HG: MRI after arthroplasty: comparison of MAVRIC and conventional fast spin-echo techniques. *AJR Am J Roentgenol* 2011;197(3):W405-W411.
24. Koch KM, Hargreaves BA, Pauly KB, Chen W, Gold GE, King KF: Magnetic resonance imaging near metal implants. *J Magn Reson Imaging* 2010;32(4):773-787.
25. Brockmeier SF, Voos JE, Williams RJ III, et al: Outcomes after arthroscopic repair of type-II SLAP lesions. *J Bone Joint Surg Am* 2009;91(7):1595-1603.
26. Knesek M, Skendzel JG, Dines JS, Altchek DW, Allen AA, Bedi A: Diagnosis and management of superior labral anterior posterior tears in throwing athletes. *Am J Sports Med* 2013;41(2):444-460.
27. Bancroft LW, Wasyliw C, Pettis C, Farley T: Postoperative shoulder magnetic resonance imaging. *Magn Reson Imaging Clin N Am* 2012;20(2):313-325, xi.
28. Jacobson JA, Miller B, Bedi A, Morag Y: Imaging of the postoperative shoulder. *Semin Musculoskelet Radiol* 2011;15(4):320-339.
29. Barber FA, Field LD, Ryu RK: Biceps tendon and superior labrum injuries: Decision making. *Instr Course Lect* 2008;57:527-538.
30. Moros C, Levine WN, Ahmad CS: Suture anchor and percutaneous intra-articular transtendon biceps tenodesis. *Sports Med Arthrosc* 2008;16(3):177-179.
31. Provencher MT, LeClere LE, Romeo AA: Subpectoral biceps tenodesis. *Sports Med Arthrosc* 2008;16(3):170-176.
32. Friedman DJ, Dunn JC, Higgins LD, Warner JJ: Proximal biceps tendon: Injuries and management. *Sports Med Arthrosc* 2008;16(3):162-169.
33. Drakos MC, Verma NN, Gulotta LV, et al: Arthroscopic transfer of the long head of the biceps tendon: Functional outcome and clinical results. *Arthroscopy* 2008;24(2):217-223.
34. Plodkowski AJ, Hayter CL, Miller TT, Nguyen JT, Potter HG: Lamellated hyperintense synovitis: Potential MR imaging sign of an infected knee arthroplasty. *Radiology* 2013;266(1):256-260.

CHAPTER 6

Nonsurgical Treatment of Superior Labrum Anterior to Posterior and Biceps Injuries

W. Ben Kibler, MD

Introduction

Determining the most effective treatment of superior labrum anterior to posterior (SLAP) tears has proved to be a difficult task. The current surgical treatment algorithms have demonstrated mixed outcomes,[1,2] which have been the impetus for a more extensive study of the role of rehabilitation in these injuries preoperatively, postoperatively, or as definitive treatment. Nevertheless, few reports demonstrate a benefit of rehabilitation for the treatment of SLAP tears.[3] To be effective, rehabilitation protocols must be developed to treat the full spectrum of labral injuries. Rehabilitation will not "heal" altered labral anatomy, but will enhance the patient's physiology and mechanics so that the shoulder recovers the functional stability necessary for specific tasks.

Although most SLAP injuries occur as a result of sports activities, they can also occur in the industrial athlete during the course of normal work activities (see chapter 16). SLAP injuries are best understood in the context of the disabled throwing [working] shoulder,[4] which suggests that SLAP injuries are part of a physiologic and pathomechanical process that is responsible for the clinical presentation. This directs attention to the many areas of the body in which alterations have been found that can be treated through rehabilitation. Resolution of these alterations appears to be associated with favorable clinical outcomes. The most common alterations occur in the proximal kinetic chain, the scapula, and glenohumeral rotation. This chapter reviews the pathophysiologic alterations associated with labral injuries and describes rehabilitation protocols for treatment.

The Role of the Kinetic Chain

Studies have clearly established that the forces and loads that have been demonstrated in the overhead throwing motion or in working activities are developed and regulated through a sequential, coordinated, task-specific kinetic chain of force development, and a kinematic chain of sequential body positions and motions.[5,6] This creates a unifying concept to understand the mechanics of the overhead throwing or working motion. The term kinetic chain collectively describes the results of both chains. The kinetic chain has several functions: (1) using integrated programs of muscle activation to temporarily link multiple body segments into one functional segment (for example, the back leg in the cocking stance and push-off, the arm in the long axis of rotation before ball release or ball impact, and both legs as a proximal base for precision arm and hand movement) to decrease the degrees of freedom in the entire motion;[5-7] (2) pro-

Dr. Kibler or an immediate family member serves as an unpaid consultant to Alignmed; has stock or stock options held in Alignmed; and serves as a board member, owner, officer, or committee member of the International Society of Arthroplasty, Knee Surgery, and Orthopaedic Sports Medicine and the American Orthopaedic Society for Sports Medicine.

viding a stable proximal base for distal arm mobility; (3) maximizing force development in the large muscles of the core and transferring it to the hand;[7,8] (4) producing interactive moments at distal joints that develop more force and energy than the joint itself could develop and decreasing the magnitude of the applied loads at the distal joint;[5,9,10] and (5) producing torque that decreases deceleration forces.[5,10,11]

Maximizing kinetic chain involvement decreases the distal loads[5] and increases the efficiency of the resulting motions.[12] Kinetic chain deficits are discovered on physical examination in most patients with SLAP injuries. Deficits in hip abductor or extensor strength, hip rotation flexibility, or core strength weakness have been identified in 50% of SLAP injuries.[13,14] These deficits can be identified by using the single-leg stability series as a screening method. The single-leg stability series assesses the patient's ability to control the trunk and body over the planted leg and has two components: the single-leg standing balance test, which evaluates dynamic control of position, and the single-leg squat test, which evaluates dynamic control of motion.

For the standing balance test, the patient places his or her hands over the chest and stands on one leg with no other verbal cue. Deviations such as a Trendelenburg posture or internal or external rotation of the weight-bearing limb indicate an inability to control posture and correlated with proximal core weakness, especially in the gluteus medius. The single-leg squat is the next progressive evaluation. Assuming the same starting point as the standing balance test, the patient performs repetitive partial or half-squats, returning to the standing position after each half-squat with no other verbal cues. Deviations in the quality of the movement are assessed in a manner similar to that of the standing balance test. A Trendelenburg posture, which may not be noted with standing balance, may be elicited by a single-leg squat. During the single-leg squat test, the patient may also use the arms for balance or may go into an exaggerated flexed or rotated posture, termed corkscrewing, to put greater tension on the gluteal or short rotator muscles to compensate for muscle weakness.[15]

The Role of the Scapula

Labral injury[4] occurs in association with scapular dyskinesis in a significant percentage of patients and workers with disabled throwing/working shoulder.[4,16] Treating the dyskinesis has been shown to decrease impingement symptoms,[17] improve rotator cuff strength,[18] and decrease symptoms in labral injury. Scapular alterations, another manifestation of scapular dyskinesis, can be evaluated by using a clinical observation method.[19,20]

The testing protocol starts with an evaluation of inflexibility (pectoralis minor tightness[21] and humeral rotation deficit). Scapular resting position and dynamic motion can be evaluated by observing the scapula as the arms move into forward flexion and descent.[19] Medial border prominence is characterized as "yes" (observed, scapular dyskinesis is present) or "no" (not observed, dyskinesis is not present). The effect of dyskinesis on symptoms can be estimated by corrective maneuvers. The scapular assistance test creates posterior tilt and can decrease external impingement symptoms[22] (**Figure 1**). The scapular retraction test[22] and/or the scapular reposition test[23] creates external rotation and posterior tilt and can increase demonstrated rotator cuff strength and decrease internal impingement symptoms in labral injury[24] (**Figure 2**).

Forward scapular posture has been implicated as a negative factor for successful nonsurgical treatment of a SLAP injury. This posture results from weaker posterior scapular muscles and tight pectoralis minor muscles.[21] Clinical assessment by observation and palpation of the tight anterior structures and measurement using the double square method can be performed and has been shown to be clinically reliable.[25] With the patient standing against a wall, the distance between the wall and the anterior acromion is measured.

The Role of Altered Glenohumeral Rotation

Glenohumeral internal rotation deficit (GIRD) and total range of motion deficit (TROMD) are seen in virtually all patients with SLAP injury and have been found to be predictive of future injury in asymptomatic patients.[26] Precise, reproducible measurement is possible with specific protocols that stabilize the scapula and measure glenohumeral motion with either a goniometer or inclinometer.[27,28]

GIRD has multiple definitions. Early studies defined GIRD as less than 25° of internal rotation or a side-to-side asymmetry greater than 20°.[4] More recent studies

FIGURE 1

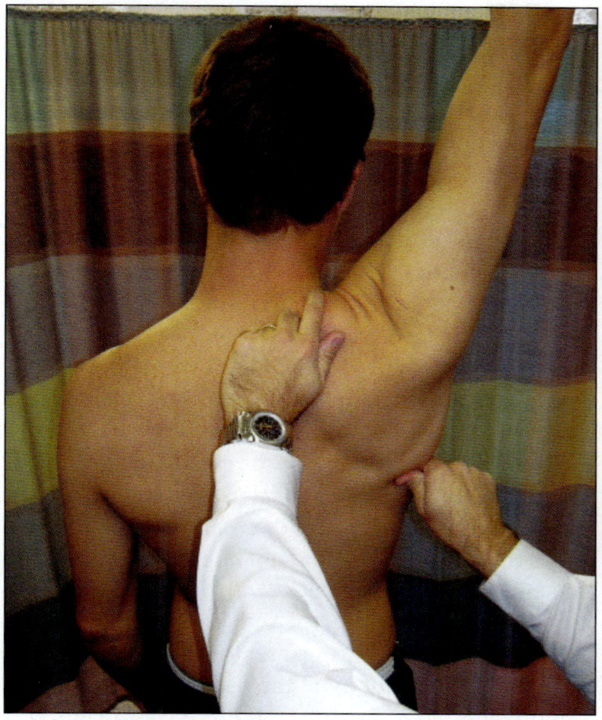

Photograph shows increased arm elevation during the scapular assistance test to demonstrate the dysfunctional scapula.

FIGURE 2

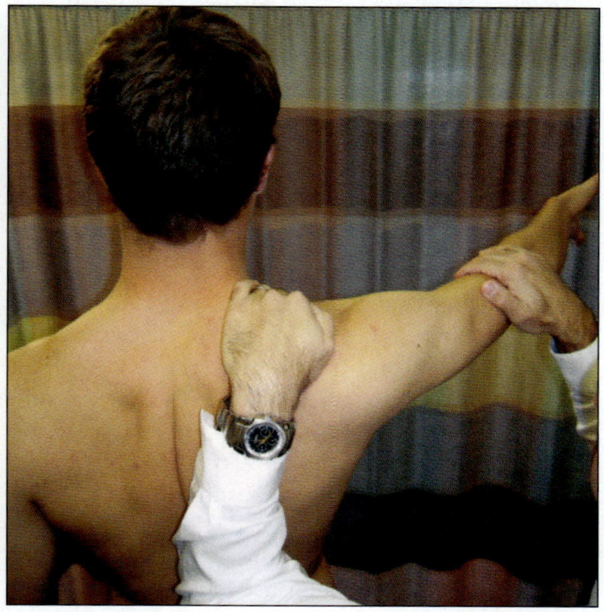

Photograph shows manual stabilization of the scapula during the scapular retraction test, or "empty can" muscle test.

have established more precise definitions.[26] GIRD has been defined as side-to-side asymmetry greater than 18°, and TROMD has been defined as side-to-side asymmetry greater than 5°. Although GIRD and TROMD may be considered predictive for shoulder injury, they are not considered solely causative. GIRD and TROMD alter the normal glenohumeral kinematics and place increased load on adjacent joint structures, and may be considered components of the shoulder at increased risk of injury.[29]

Several factors have been implicated as causes of the alterations linked to GIRD and TROMD. Capsuloligamentous changes that may result from scar tissue related to chronic tensile overload altering glenohumeral kinematics have been well documented.[4,30] A thickened posterior capsule may be demonstrated on the MRIs of patients with superior labral injuries, and may be identified by using physical examination and therapeutic techniques for the detection and correction of capsular components of joint mobility.[31] However, these changes do not occur uniformly and do not explain the high percentage of patients without thickened capsules on imaging, the acute changes in glenohumeral internal rotation observed after a throwing exposure,[32] or the frequently rapid alteration in glenohumeral internal rotation measurements with stretching programs.[33] These dynamic changes indicated a strong muscular component in the causation of GIRD.

The muscular component of GIRD is related to acute and chronic responses to strain that affect joint range of motion. An acute response to repetitive tensile strain in eccentric muscle contractions, which is actually "sarcomere popping," characterized by separation of the sarcomere ends, has been demonstrated.[34] This muscle damage releases intramuscular calcium, which mediates fibril contraction, resulting in muscle shortening. This process peaks between 4 and 18 hours after throwing and is modifiable with gentle stretching at 12 hours.

In contrast, a chronic muscle response to muscular strain is thixotropy, or increased muscle stiffness mediated by the exposure history of the muscle.[34] Repetitive exposure to strain can result in increased stiffness within the muscles that can affect joint motion, and is not related to neurologic changes. The thixotropic response is modifiable by stretching within certain ranges and velocities.

Another muscle response relates to the architectural design of the rotator cuff muscles. The pennation angle of these muscles optimizes their efficiency at producing force through a short midrange of motion in abduction and internal rotation but diminishes their capacity to withstand large changes in length.[35] Experimental data suggest that increases in strain rate or strain length of these muscles beyond their normal physiologic limits induces muscular responses that increase internal stiffness and decrease range of motion.[35] An exercise program directed at increasing the eccentric endurance of posterior rotator cuff and increasing the resistance to length change has been associated with preserving glenohumeral internal rotation during one baseball season (W. Ben Kibler, MD, unpublished data, 2013).

The Labrum And Injuries In Throwers

The actual role of the labrum as part of the normal mechanisms for functional shoulder stability has been the source of some confusion. Enhancing knowledge of these roles helps implement rehabilitation strategies.

The role of the labrum in shoulder function has been traditionally explained as an attachment site for the biceps, a bumper to deepen the glenohumeral socket and to improve stability by minimizing glenohumeral translation, and to help increase capsular tension.[36] However, the role of the labrum may actually be more complex. The role of the superior labrum as a mechanical bumper is controversial. In one study, the mechanical glenohumeral translation increased only 10% after superior labral resection,[37] meaning that the superior labrum likely has other functions in addition to a role in mechanical stability. Biomechanical studies have highlighted three additional important functions for the labrum:[36,37] (1) as a deformable structure with high compliance to more evenly distribute contact pressures between two surfaces, increase boundary lubrication, and maximize concavity/compression characteristics (as with a washer between two surfaces); (2) as a pressure sensor maximizing proprioceptive feedback; and (3) as an attachment site to optimize the tension for muscles and ligaments. Experimental labral release resulted in significant changes in capsular tension.[36] Another cadaver study using sequential cuts demonstrated that increased glenohumeral translation was restored to normal with posterior superior labral repair.

The intact labrum results in optimal glenohumeral kinematics during shoulder motion, creating a "best fit" glenohumeral articulation that enables stable ball-and-socket kinematics, and allows maximum force transfer from the core and legs through a stable linkage at the shoulder to the delivery mechanism (the hand). Optimizing the alignment of the humerus within the glenoid by smooth scapulohumeral rhythm and maximizing muscular strength and co-activation to create concavity compression may decrease the shoulder dysfunction created by labral injury and altered anatomy.

A comprehensive physical examination should reveal local and distant physiologic and biomechanical deficits that are commonly associated with SLAP injury. These deficits need to be corrected with treatment, and have been shown to decrease the disabled throwing shoulder dysfunction.[3,38] In addition, the results of several labral examination tests can suggest the presence of a labral injury.

Of the labral examination tests, the modified dynamic labral shear (DLS) test[39] has been shown to be of high clinical utility in the evaluation of labral injuries. The arm is moved into abduction and 90° of flexion, and then to more than 120° of abduction in the scapular plane and to the end range of external rotation. A shear load is applied to the joint by maintaining external rotation and horizontal abduction and lowering the arm from 120° to 60° of abduction. A positive test result is indicated by the reproduction of pain and/or a painful clicking or catching along the posterior joint line between 120° and 90° of abduction. The test has a sensitivity of 72%, a specificity of 98%, a positive predictive value of 97%, and a positive likelihood ratio of 31.6.[39] Other labral examination tests that have been advocated include the O'Brien active compression test, the relocation test (with pain as the indicator), and an anterior levering maneuver to place a posterior load and shear (Richard Hawkins, MD, unpublished data, 2013).

In addition, intra-articular examination tests can help determine the loss of labral roles. A positive result for the Hawkins test (a painful arc of motion, with no relief achieved from scapular posterior tilt in the scapular assistance test) indicates increased translation. A positive result for the O'Brien test indicates loss of the washer effect, increased biceps tension, and increased translation. The modified DLS test has been shown to have high clinical utility because it specifically replicates a peel-back phenomenon. A positive DLS test result indicates loss of biceps stability, loss of washer, and increased translation.

The physical examination can provide findings that help construct a comprehensive picture of the anatomic and physiologic deficits that exist and may cause or exacerbate the SLAP injury, and that should be the focus of a comprehensive rehabilitation program.

Nonsurgical Treatment of Labral Tears

Rehabilitation is often recommended and performed for the treatment of labral tears, but the outcomes have not been widely studied. Only one case series describes the results of nonsurgical treatment of SLAP lesions. Edwards et al[3] collected data using a survey with validated outcome measures of 305 patients with labral tears (response rate, 16.4% [50 patients]). Of these, 39 patients had symptomatic SLAP lesions diagnosed by a positive result for the O'Brien test, pain at the bicipital groove, and MRI follow-up greater than 1 year. All patients were treated nonsurgically with NSAIDs and a physical therapy protocol that focused on scapular stabilization and posterior capsule stretching. This protocol was considered successful in 19 patients (49%). In this group, 18 were active in sports before treatment and 15 participated in overhead sports. Of these 15, 10 (67%) returned to overhead athletics after nonsurgical treatment.

Similar findings were reported in a cohort of 76 Major League Baseball players.[38] These players all had SLAP lesions and all underwent physical therapy to treat the posterior capsule contracture (GIRD) and scapular rehabilitation. In this group, follow-up was greater than 1 year following treatment. Thirty-one patients (41%) were effectively managed nonsurgically; 28 (90%) returned to prior level of play.

In addition, in a population of active, nonprofessional athletes, 51% of SLAP injuries confirmed by examination and imaging became functionally asymptomatic after a 6- to 8-week guided rehabilitation program.[38] The programs have been specifically designed to treat kinetic chain and scapular deficits as well as muscle flexibility, strength, and strength balance deficits discovered on physical examination and described in the following paragraphs.[13,40]

Although the data are limited, nonsurgical treatment has been shown to be successful for several elite and recreational athletes with SLAP lesions. Rehabilitation should be focused on treating GIRD, TROMD, scapular dyskinesis, and kinetic chain deficits.

Rehabilitation

Rehabilitation can play a key role in modifying the dysfunction of the disabled throwing shoulder and reducing the need for surgery. The rehabilitation program has three primary focus points: the kinetic chain, shoulder mobility, and shoulder strengthening (**Table 1**).

Strengthening and stabilizing the core and the lower extremity musculature is critical because of their contributions to the throwing motion. No single exercise targets all abdominal muscles; therefore, a program for the anterior, lateral, and posterior torso should be undertaken. Mat exercises emphasizing endurance are a good start, and positions that limit stress to the shoulder should be considered. The athlete should be engaged in lower extremity and core exercises such as rotational chopping and lifting activities that simulate the demands of throwing.[41] Using unstable surfaces such as stability balls or foam mats has demonstrated increased core activation[42] and improvement in core strength, but has not necessarily carried over into functional tasks.

When the patient can safely perform arm motion and shoulder loads, the scapular stability series is an extremely effective set of exercises for the initiation of scapular retraction and depression. These exercises include the low row (**Figure 3**), inferior glide (**Figure 4**), lawnmower (**Figure 5**), and robbery (**Figure 6**) maneuvers, which include trunk extension, scapular retraction, and shoulder extension with the arm close to the side. These exercises may be started in an isometric fashion and progressed to isotonic, concentric, and eccentric work with rubber tubing. To appropriately challenge and enhance scapular muscle function, exercises should continue to focus on scapular retraction, depression,

TABLE 1 **Rehabilitation Program for SLAP and Biceps Injury**

Rehabilitation Program for SLAP and Biceps Injury
Kinetic chain
Leg drive and lower extremity strength
Hip mobility
Proximal core stability
Dynamic core strength/power
Scapular stabilization
Shoulder mobility
Restoring internal and external rotation deficits to achieve safe total range of motion
Treating joint restrictions in the spine and shoulder complex
Treating muscular flexibility imbalances in the spine and scapula
Arm strength and endurance
Restoring scapular motor control for functional and pain-free motion
Facilitating inhibited or weak scapular musculature
Integrating scapular exercises with functional tasks
Facilitating endurance and eccentric control by advanced shoulder and scapular exercises
Strengthening forearm, wrist, and hand

and external rotation while simultaneously integrating movements of the pelvis and trunk. Trunk position has been shown to positively affect arm motion and muscle activation; the single-leg squat performed during scapular retraction/depression exercises increases scapular muscle activation.[43,44]

The prevention and treatment of shoulder motion deficits is a critical component of any intervention program for throwing athletes. The glenohumeral internal rotation of the throwing shoulder should be within a mean of 18° (range, 13° to 20°) of the nondominant shoulder,[26] and the total range of motion in the throwing shoulder should be within 5° of the nondominant shoulder and not exceed 186° to avoid an increased risk of injury.[26] The goal of the intervention program

FIGURE 3

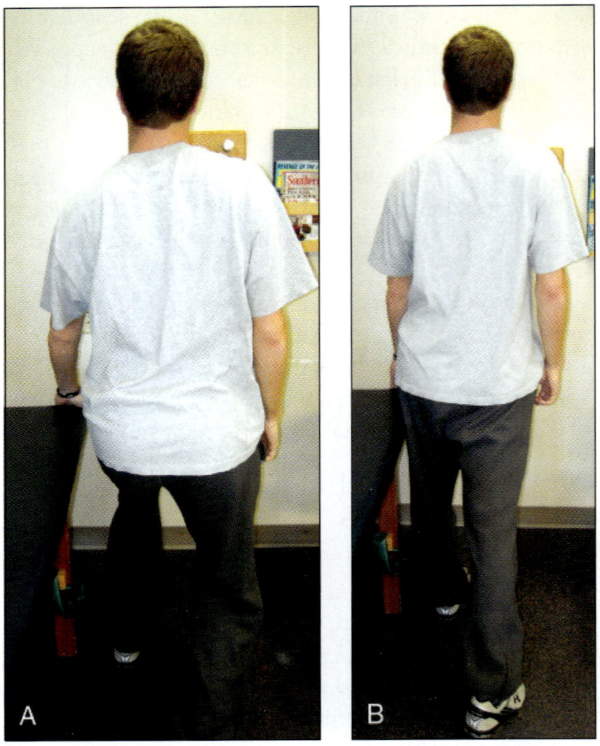

Photographs show the low row exercise. **A,** Starting position. **B,** The patient extends the hips and trunk to facilitate scapular retraction.

FIGURE 4

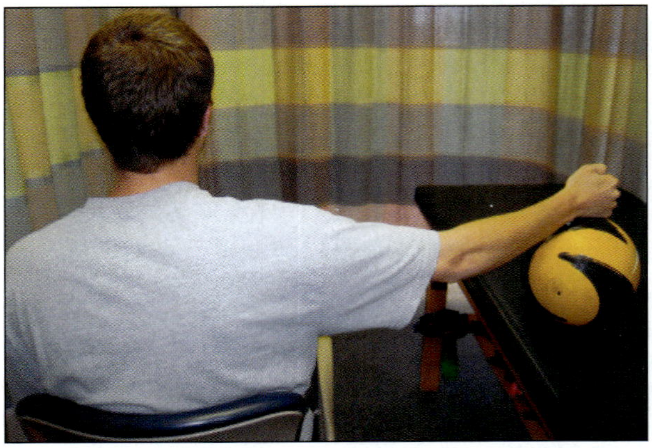

Photograph shows the active inferior glide exercise, which uses co-contraction of the shoulder and scapular muscles to help depress the humerus and scapula.

FIGURE 5

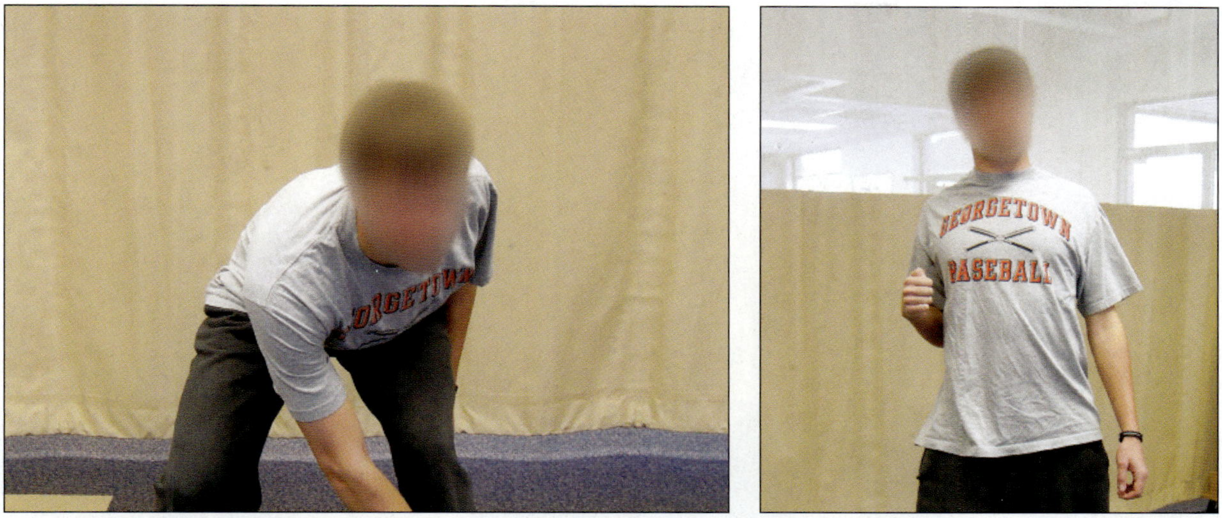

Photographs show the lawnmower exercise. **A,** Starting position. **B,** The patient extends the hips and trunk, followed by trunk rotation to facilitate scapular retraction.

is the restoration of range of motion to acceptable values. Deficits in glenohumeral internal rotation and total range of motion should be treated to restore safe range of motion; however, it is important to remember that range of motion is affected by throwing activities for at least 24 hours.[45] The cross-body stretch and sleeper stretch target the posterior shoulder musculature and capsule to effectively improve glenohumeral internal rotation and glenohumeral horizontal abduction.[33,46] Additional treatments include joint mobilizations,[47] muscle energy techniques, and soft-tissue mobilization. The assessment and treatment of glenohumeral horizontal abduction is becoming more important. Tyler et al[31] conducted a multimodal treatment approach that included posterior shoulder stretching and joint mobilization and demonstrated that change in glenohumeral horizontal abduction is as important as change in glenohumeral internal rotation for the reduction of symptoms.

Muscular adaptations that can alter scapular kinematics during elevation can occur because of tight anterior structures such as the pectoralis minor. Dominant-side pectoralis minor tightness has been identified in tennis players and is associated with increased scapular anterior tilt and scapular internal rotation.[21] Pectoralis minor tightness can be effectively treated with corner stretching exercises.[48]

Deficits in shoulder strength are predictive of future injury, particularly in external rotation and supraspinatus activation.[49] Athletes presenting with shoulder symptoms typically have strength deficits of the rotator cuff[50] and scapular musculature, which may present with various movement patterns.[51] Several treatment protocols have been developed for these deficits.[52] Initial management should focus on control of the scapular musculature, which facilitates stability and prepares the shoulder musculature for more dynamic and stressful exercises. Scapular setting exercises have been shown to primarily activate the trapezius musculature and can facilitate muscular balance between the scapular force couple of the serratus anterior and the upper and lower trapezius.[53,54] The scapular exercise program should focus on the rhomboids, lower trapezius, and middle trapezius musculature. Facilitation of serratus anterior and lower trapezius musculature can be targeted with isometric adduction and extension exercises, with continued focus on proper scapular orientation of posterior tilting and retraction.[55]

Upper extremity power and endurance are increased with high-repetition, long-lever exercises performed

FIGURE 6

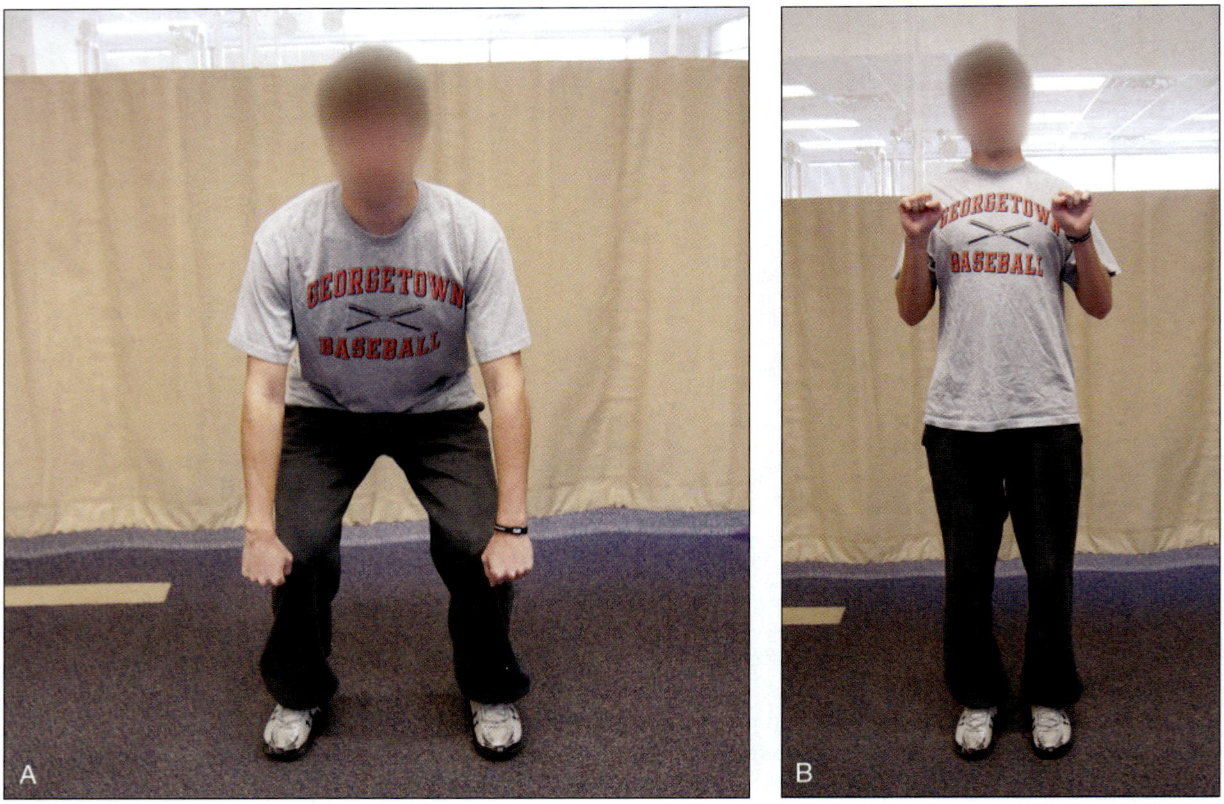

Photographs show the robbery maneuver. **A,** Starting position. **B,** The patient extends the hips and trunk to "place the elbows in the back pockets."

while standing and in the prone position. Maneuvers such as scaption and external rotation and horizontal abduction in the prone position are ideal for activating the muscles of the rotator cuff,[56] and should be used following the restoration and optimization of scapular function.

The exercise program is progressive, sequential, and divided into three phases based on the level of disability and tissue irritability that exists. Movement through the phases varies and is based on achieving functional capabilities rather than adhering to specific time frames. Phase 1, the acute phase, minimizes loads on the injured tissues by focusing on scapular and glenohumeral muscular activation, particularly in correcting the timing of muscular activation to ensure synchronous activation. Phase 2, the recovery phase, focuses on strengthening and restoring core, kinetic chain, and progressive isotonic strengthening. Phase 3, the functional phase, focuses on sport-specific actions, and includes endurance and ballistic exercises. Strengthening exercises are oriented toward endurance, with an emphasis on higher repetitions and lower resistance. The patient should demonstrate the ability to perform 3 to 4 sets of 15 to 20 repetitions for a given exercise, using proper form, before resistance is increased.

Conclusion

SLAP and biceps injuries are best evaluated and treated as components of the disabled throwing or working shoulder. Multiple physiologic and biomechanical alterations have been demonstrated in association with this clinical entity: strength and flexibility deficits in the proximal kinetic chain, including the hips, legs, and core; scapular dyskinesis; and alterations in glenohumeral rotation, in addition to the anatomic labral and/or biceps injury. Nonsurgical treatment has been shown to be beneficial in a significant number of cases and should be considered in the initial treatment protocols.

REFERENCES

1. Yung PS, Fong DT, Kong MF, et al: Arthroscopic repair of isolated type II superior labrum anterior-posterior lesion. *Knee Surg Sports Traumatol Arthrosc* 2008;16(12):1151-1157.
2. Kim SH, Ha KI, Kim SH, Choi HJ: Results of arthroscopic treatment of superior labral lesions. *J Bone Joint Surg Am* 2002;84-A(6):981-985.
3. Edwards SL, Lee JA, Bell JE, et al: Nonoperative treatment of superior labrum anterior posterior tears: Improvements in pain, function, and quality of life. *Am J Sports Med* 2010;38(7):1456-1461.
4. Burkhart SS, Morgan CD, Kibler WB: The disabled throwing shoulder: Spectrum of pathology Part I. Pathoanatomy and biomechanics. *Arthroscopy* 2003;19(4):404-420.
5. Putnam CA: Sequential motions of body segments in striking and throwing skills: Descriptions and explanations. *J Biomech* 1993;26(Suppl 1):125-135.
6. Davids K, Glazier P, Araújo D, Bartlett R: Movement systems as dynamical systems: The functional role of variability and its implications for sports medicine. *Sports Med* 2003;33(4):245-260.
7. Lintner D, Noonan TJ, Kibler WB: Injury patterns and biomechanics of the athlete's shoulder. *Clin Sports Med* 2008;27(4):527-551.
8. Elliott BC, Marshall R, Noffal G: Contributions of upper limb segment rotations during the power serve in tennis. *J Appl Biomech* 1995;11:433-442.
9. Hirashima M, Yamane K, Nakamura Y, Ohtsuki T: Kinetic chain of overarm throwing in terms of joint rotations revealed by induced acceleration analysis. *J Biomech* 2008;41(13):2874-2883.
10. Fleisig GS, Barrentine SW, Escamilla RF, Andrews JR: Biomechanics of overhand throwing with implications for injuries. *Sports Med* 1996;21(6):421-437.
11. Young JL, Herring SA, Press JM, Casazza BA: The influence of the spine on the shoulder in the throwing athlete. *J Back Musculoskeletal Rehabil* 1996;7:5-17.
12. Davis JT, Limpisvasti O, Fluhme D, et al: The effect of pitching biomechanics on the upper extremity in youth and adolescent baseball pitchers. *Am J Sports Med* 2009;37(8):1484-1491.
13. Burkhart SS, Morgan CD, Kibler WB: The disabled throwing shoulder: Spectrum of pathology Part III. The SICK scapula, scapular dyskinesis, the kinetic chain, and rehabilitation. *Arthroscopy* 2003;19(6):641-661.
14. Kibler WB, Press J, Sciascia AD: The role of core stability in athletic function. *Sports Med* 2006;36(3):189-198.
15. Crossley KM, Zhang WJ, Schache AG, Bryant A, Cowan SM: Performance on the single-leg squat task indicates hip abductor muscle function. *Am J Sports Med* 2011;39(4):866-873.
16. Warner JJ, Micheli LJ, Arslanian LE, Kennedy J, Kennedy R: Scapulothoracic motion in normal shoulders and shoulders with glenohumeral instability and impingement syndrome: A study using Moiré topographic analysis. *Clin Orthop Relat Res* 1992;(285):191-199.
17. Michener LA, Walsworth MK, Burnet EN: Effectiveness of rehabilitation for patients with subacromial impingement syndrome: A systematic review. *J Hand Ther* 2004;17(2):152-164.
18. Kibler WB: Rehabilitation of rotator cuff tendinopathy. *Clin Sports Med* 2003;22(4):837-847.
19. Kibler WB, Ludewig PM, McClure P, Uhl TL, Sciascia A: Scapular Summit 2009: Introduction. July 16, 2009, Lexington, Kentucky. *J Orthop Sports Phys Ther* 2009;39(11):A1-A13.
20. Uhl TL, Kibler WB, Gecewich B, Tripp BL: Evaluation of clinical assessment methods for scapular dyskinesis. *Arthroscopy* 2009;25(11):1240-1248.
21. Borstad JD, Ludewig PM: The effect of long versus short pectoralis minor resting length on scapular kinematics in healthy individuals. *J Orthop Sports Phys Ther* 2005;35(4):227-238.
22. Kibler WB: The role of the scapula in athletic shoulder function. *Am J Sports Med* 1998;26(2):325-337.
23. Tate AR, McClure PW, Kareha S, Irwin D: Effect of the Scapula Reposition Test on shoulder impingement symptoms and elevation strength in overhead athletes. *J Orthop Sports Phys Ther* 2008;38(1):4-11.
24. Kibler WB, Sciascia AD, Dome DC: Evaluation of apparent and absolute supraspinatus strength in patients with shoulder injury using the scapular retraction test. *Am J Sports Med* 2006;34(10):1643-1647.

25. Kibler WB, Sciascia AD: Current concepts: Scapular dyskinesis. *Br J Sports Med* 2010;44(5):300-305.
26. Wilk KE, Macrina LC, Fleisig GS, et al: Correlation of glenohumeral internal rotation deficit and total rotational motion to shoulder injuries in professional baseball pitchers. *Am J Sports Med* 2011;39(2):329-335.
27. Wilk KE, Reinold MM, Macrina LC, et al: Glenohumeral internal rotation measurements differ depending on stabilization techniques. *Sports Health* 2009;1(2): 131-136.
28. Kibler WB, Sciascia AD, Thomas SJ: Glenohumeral internal rotation deficit: Pathogenesis and response to acute throwing. *Sports Med Arthrosc* 2012;20(1):34-38.
29. Grossman MG, Tibone JE, McGarry MH, Schneider DJ, Veneziani S, Lee TQ: A cadaveric model of the throwing shoulder: A possible etiology of superior labrum anterior-to-posterior lesions. *J Bone Joint Surg Am* 2005;87(4):824-831.
30. Thomas SJ, Swanik CB, Higginson JS, et al: A bilateral comparison of posterior capsule thickness and its correlation with glenohumeral range of motion and scapular upward rotation in collegiate baseball players. *J Shoulder Elbow Surg* 2011;20(5):708-716.
31. Tyler TF, Nicholas SJ, Lee SJ, Mullaney M, McHugh MP: Correction of posterior shoulder tightness is associated with symptom resolution in patients with internal impingement. *Am J Sports Med* 2010;38(1):114-119.
32. Kibler WB, Sciascia AD, Moore SD: An acute throwing episode decreases shoulder internal rotation. *Clin Orthop Relat Res* 2012;470(6):1545-1551.
33. Laudner KG, Sipes RC, Wilson JT: The acute effects of sleeper stretches on shoulder range of motion. *J Athl Train* 2008;43(4):359-363.
34. Proske U, Morgan DL: Muscle damage from eccentric exercise: Mechanism, mechanical signs, adaptation and clinical applications. *J Physiol* 2001;537(Pt 2):333-345.
35. Butterfield TA: Eccentric exercise in vivo: Strain-induced muscle damage and adaptation in a stable system. *Exerc Sport Sci Rev* 2010;38(2):51-60.
36. Pagnani MJ, Warren RF: Instability of the shoulder, in Nicholas JA, Hershman EB, eds: *The Upper Extremity in Sports Medicine*. St Louis, MO, Mosby, 1995, pp 173-208.
37. Veeger HE, van der Helm FC: Shoulder function: The perfect compromise between mobility and stability. *J Biomech* 2007;40(10):2119-2129.
38. Kibler WB, Kuhn JE, Wilk K, et al: The disabled throwing shoulder: Spectrum of pathology-10-year update. *Arthroscopy* 2013;29(1):141, e26.
39. Ben Kibler W, Sciascia AD, Hester P, Dome D, Jacobs C: Clinical utility of traditional and new tests in the diagnosis of biceps tendon injuries and superior labrum anterior and posterior lesions in the shoulder. *Am J Sports Med* 2009;37(9):1840-1847.
40. Kibler WB, McMullen J, Uhl TL: Shoulder rehabilitation strategies, guidelines, and practice. *Oper Tech Sports Med* 2000;8(4):258-267.
41. Voight ML, Hoogenboom BJ, Cook G: The chop and lift reconsidered: Integrating neuromuscular principles into orthopedic and sports rehabilitation. *N Am J Sports Phys Ther* 2008;3(3):151-159.
42. Escamilla RF, Lewis C, Bell D, et al: Core muscle activation during Swiss ball and traditional abdominal exercises. *J Orthop Sports Phys Ther* 2010;40(5):265-276.
43. Maenhout A, Van Praet K, Pizzi L, Van Herzeele M, Cools A: Electromyographic analysis of knee push up plus variations: What is the influence of the kinetic chain on scapular muscle activity. *Br J Sports Med* 2010;44(14):1010-1015.
44. De May K, Danneels L, Cagnie B, Cools A: Are kinetic chain rowing exercises relevant in shoulder and trunk injury prevention training? *Br J Sports Med* 2011;45(4):320-321.
45. Reinold MM, Wilk KE, Macrina LC, et al: Changes in shoulder and elbow passive range of motion after pitching in professional baseball players. *Am J Sports Med* 2008;36(3):523-527.
46. McClure P, Balaicuis J, Heiland D, Broersma ME, Thorndike CK, Wood A: A randomized controlled comparison of stretching procedures for posterior shoulder tightness. *J Orthop Sports Phys Ther* 2007;37(3):108-114.
47. Manske RC, Meschke M, Porter A, Smith B, Reiman M: A randomized controlled single-blinded comparison of stretching versus stretching and joint mobilization for posterior shoulder tightness measured by internal rotation motion loss. *Sports Health* 2010;2(2):94-100.
48. Borstad JD, Ludewig PM: Comparison of three stretches for the pectoralis minor muscle. *J Shoulder Elbow Surg* 2006;15(3):324-330.
49. Byram IR, Bushnell BD, Dugger K, Charron K, Harrell FE Jr, Noonan TJ: Preseason shoulder strength measurements in professional baseball pitchers: Identifying play-

ers at risk for injury. *Am J Sports Med* 2010;38(7): 1375-1382.

50. Merolla G, De Santis E, Campi F, Paladini P, Porcellini G: Supraspinatus and infraspinatus weakness in overhead athletes with scapular dyskinesis: Strength assessment before and after restoration of scapular musculature balance. *Musculoskelet Surg* 2010;94(3):119-125.

51. Roy JS, Moffet H, McFadyen BJ: Upper limb motor strategies in persons with and without shoulder impingement syndrome across different speeds of movement. *Clin Biomech (Bristol, Avon)* 2008;23(10): 1227-1236.

52. Ellenbecker TS, Cools A: Rehabilitation of shoulder impingement syndrome and rotator cuff injuries: An evidence-based review. *Br J Sports Med* 2010;44(5): 319-327.

53. Ludewig PM, Cook TM: Alterations in shoulder kinematics and associated muscle activity in people with symptoms of shoulder impingement. *Phys Ther* 2000;80(3):276-291.

54. Ludewig PM, Reynolds JF: The association of scapular kinematics and glenohumeral joint pathologies. *J Orthop Sports Phys Ther* 2009;39(2):90-104.

55. Kibler WB, Sciascia AD, Uhl TL, Tambay N, Cunningham T: Electromyographic analysis of specific exercises for scapular control in early phases of shoulder rehabilitation. *Am J Sports Med* 2008;36(9):1789-1798.

56. Reinold MM, Wilk KE, Fleisig GS, et al: Electromyographic analysis of the rotator cuff and deltoid musculature during common shoulder external rotation exercises. *J Orthop Sports Phys Ther* 2004;34(7):385-394.

CHAPTER 7

Arthroscopic Findings: What Is a Clinically Significant Superior Labrum Anterior to Posterior Tear?

Brandon R. Vier, MD, LT, USN
Lucas S. McDonald, MD, MPH, LCDR, USN
James R. Bailey, MD, LCDR, USN
John W. McNeil II, BA
Matthew T. Provencher, MD, CDR, USN

Introduction

Superior labrum anterior to posterior (SLAP) tears of the shoulder are a continual challenge to diagnose and treat successfully. This chapter analyzes the causes, anatomy, diagnostic challenges, anatomic variants, and arthroscopic findings related to SLAP tears.

History and Classification

In 1985, shortly after the advent of arthroscopy, Andrews et al[1] described tears of the labrum. In 1990, the term SLAP was coined by Snyder et al.[2] The authors stratified SLAP lesions into four types, and these classic descriptions are currently being used (**Figure 1**). Type I involves a frayed superior labrum, likely a result of a degenerative mechanism. Type II involves a frayed superior labrum with an associated separation of the superior labrum and biceps tendon from the glenoid. Type III is a bucket-handle lesion of the superior labrum. Type IV is a bucket-handle lesion with extension into the biceps tendon.

In 1995, Maffet et al[3] reported that only 62% of SLAP lesions matched the four original categories, so three additional categories, types V through VII, were created (**Figure 2**). Type V is an injury to the anteroinferior labrum (Bankart lesion), with superior extension that involves the biceps tendon. Type VI is an unstable labral flap with separation of the biceps tendon. Type VII is an anterior extension of the SLAP lesion coursing under the middle glenohumeral ligament (MGHL). Several other SLAP tear types were described by Barber et al.[4] Type VIII is a type II lesion with posterior extension, type IX is a type II lesion with circumferential involve-

Dr. Provencher or an immediate family member serves as a board member, owner, officer, or committee member of the American Academy of Orthopaedic Surgeons, the American Orthopaedic Society for Sports Medicine, the American Shoulder and Elbow Surgeons, the Arthroscopy Association of North America, the International Society of Arthroscopy, Knee Surgery, and Orthopaedic Sports Medicine, the San Diego Shoulder Institute, and the Society of Military Orthopaedic Surgeons. None of the following authors nor any immediate family member has received anything of value from or has stock or stock options held in a commercial company or institution related directly or indirectly to the subject of this chapter: Dr. Vier, Dr. McDonald, Dr. Bailey, and Mr. McNeil.

FIGURE 1

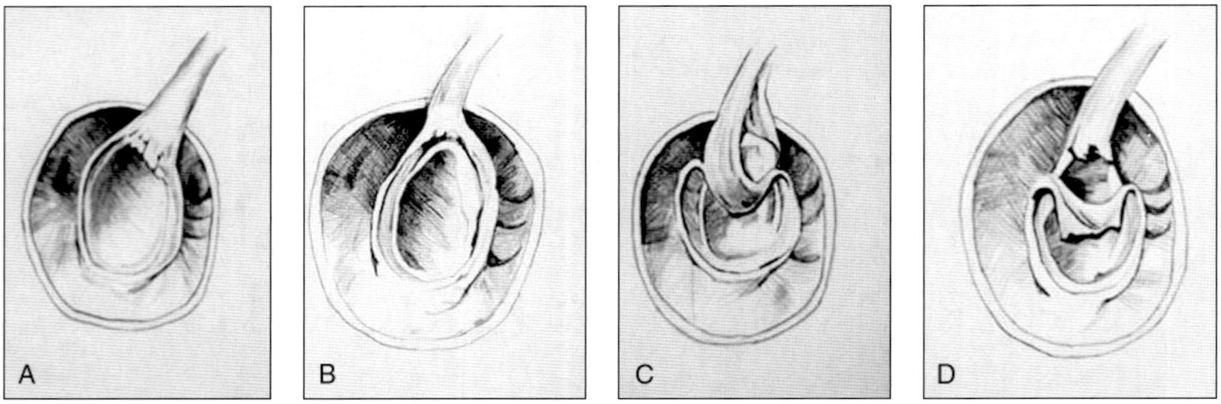

Snyder classification for types of SLAP lesions. **A,** type I. **B,** type II. **C,** type III. **D,** type IV. (Adapted with permission from Snyder SJ, Karzel RP, Del Pizzo W, Ferkel RD, Friedman MJ: SLAP lesions of the shoulder. *Arthroscopy* 1990;6[4]:274-279.)

FIGURE 2

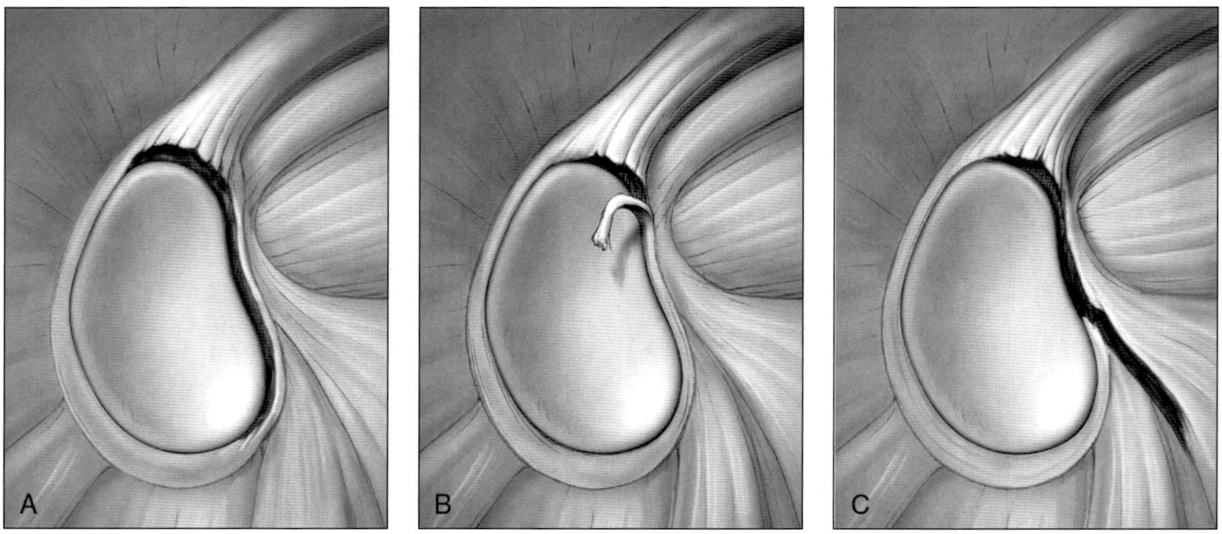

Modification of SLAP lesion classification. **A,** Type V. **B,** Type VI. **C,** Type VII. (Reproduced with permission from Maffet MW, Gartsman GM, Moseley B: Superior labrum-biceps tendon complex lesions of the shoulder. *Am J Sports Med* 1995;23[1]:93-98.)

ment of the labrum, and type X is a type II lesion with posterior and inferior separation of the labrum.

SLAP tear subtypes have also been described. In 1998, Morgan et al[5] further stratified type II SLAP tears based on anatomic location of the lesion. The authors found that type II lesions were almost evenly divided among anterior, posterior, and combined anterior-posterior locations (**Figure 3**). Additionally, Choi and Kim[6] described a unique lesion, similar to a type II tear, also involving injury to the articular cartilage. The classification of SLAP tears is summarized in **Table 1**.

SLAP tears can be associated with other shoulder pathology. Mileski and Snyder[7] found that 72% of patients with SLAP tears had concomitant pathologies: 29% had

FIGURE 3

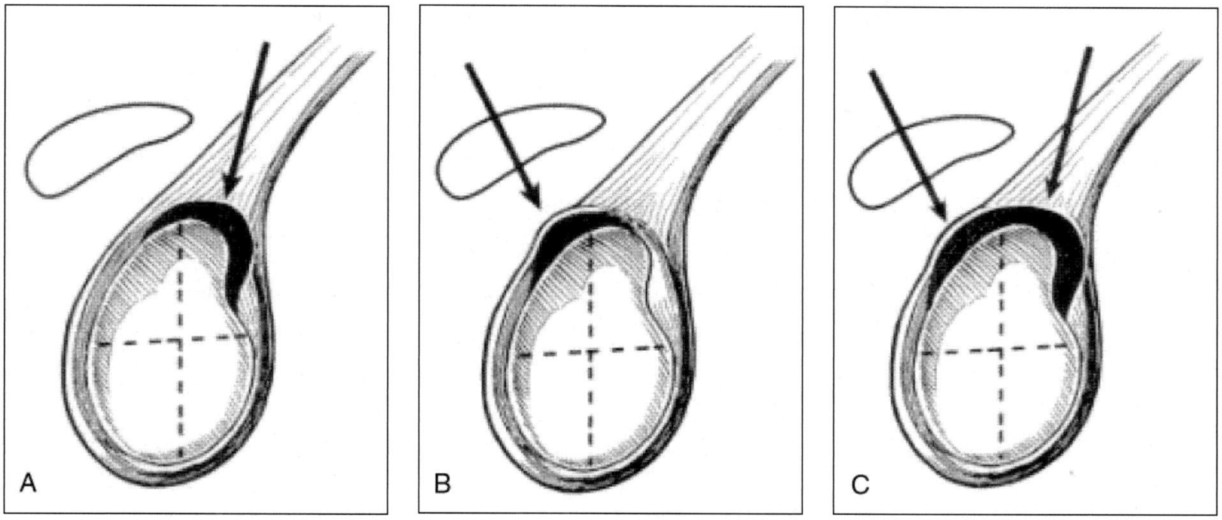

Illustration shows position of SLAP tear (arrows) in relation to long head of the biceps tendon origin. **A,** Posterior SLAP tear. **B,** Anterior SLAP tear. **C,** Anterior-posterior SLAP tear. (Reproduced with permission from Morgan CD, Burkhart SS, Palmeri M, Gillespie M: Type II SLAP lesions: Three subtypes and their relationships to superior instability and rotator cuff tears. *Arthroscopy* 1998;14[6]:553-565.)

partial rotator cuff tears, 11% had complete rotator cuff tears, 22% had Bankart lesions, 10% had humeral head pathology, and 16% had acromioclavicular joint degeneration.

Causal Factors

Multiple mechanisms have been proposed to cause SLAP tears. In a cadaver model, Bey et al[8] reproduced type II SLAP tears with biceps tendon traction by means of inferior subluxation. A cadaver study conducted by Clavert et al[9] demonstrated a possible shearing mechanism from a fall onto an outstretched hand. Multiple studies have shown repetitive overhead throwing, specifically the late cocking phase, to be associated with SLAP tear development.[10-13] Burkhart and Morgan[14] suggested a peel-back mechanism in which rotational forces about the bicep tendon, caused by abduction and external rotation, create a torsional force transmitted through the tendon that ultimately peels the posterior labrum from the glenoid[15] (**Figure 4**).

Diagnostic Challenges

SLAP tears can be very difficult to diagnose clinically. The symptoms of a SLAP tear are often nonspecific but can include anterior shoulder pain, clicking, or instability. Therefore, a patient's history may not always be a very useful diagnostic tool. Furthermore, no reliable, reproducible physical examination maneuvers exist. Multiple tests have been described in the literature, including the active compression, Speed, anterior slide, crank, and Yergason tests.[16-20] However, a recent meta-analysis by Hegedus et al[21] showed no single test had sufficient sensitivity and specificity for the detection of SLAP tears. The active compression test had the highest sensitivity (67%); however, the specificity was only 37%. The Yergason test had the highest specificity (95%); however, the sensitivity was only 12%. Although arthroscopy is generally considered the gold standard for the diagnosis of SLAP tears, no clear consensus exists regarding the interobserver and intraobserver reliability of arthroscopic diagnosis.[22-24] MRI, magnetic resonance arthrography, and CT arthrography have all been explored as radiologic adjuncts in the diagnosis of SLAP tears. Magnetic resonance arthrography is the current modality of choice, with sensitivity as high as 96% and specificity as high as 85%, although these percentages may be artificially high given the normal anatomic variants that may be interpreted as false-positive results.[25-27]

TABLE 1 Classification of SLAP Tears

SLAP Tear Type	Description
I	Frayed labrum with intact biceps anchor
II	Separation of superior labrum and biceps anchor (anterior, posterior, or combined anterior-posterior)
III	Bucket-handle tear not involving the biceps anchor
IV	Bucket-handle tear extending into the biceps tendon
V	Anteroinferior labral (Bankart) lesion with superior extension into the biceps tendon
VI	Labral flap with separation of the biceps tendon
VII	Anterior extension under the MGHL
VIII	Type II lesion with posterior extension
IX	Type II lesion with circumferential extension
X	Type II lesion with posterior inferior extension

MGHL = middle glenohumeral ligament, SLAP = superior labrum anterior to posterior.

FIGURE 4

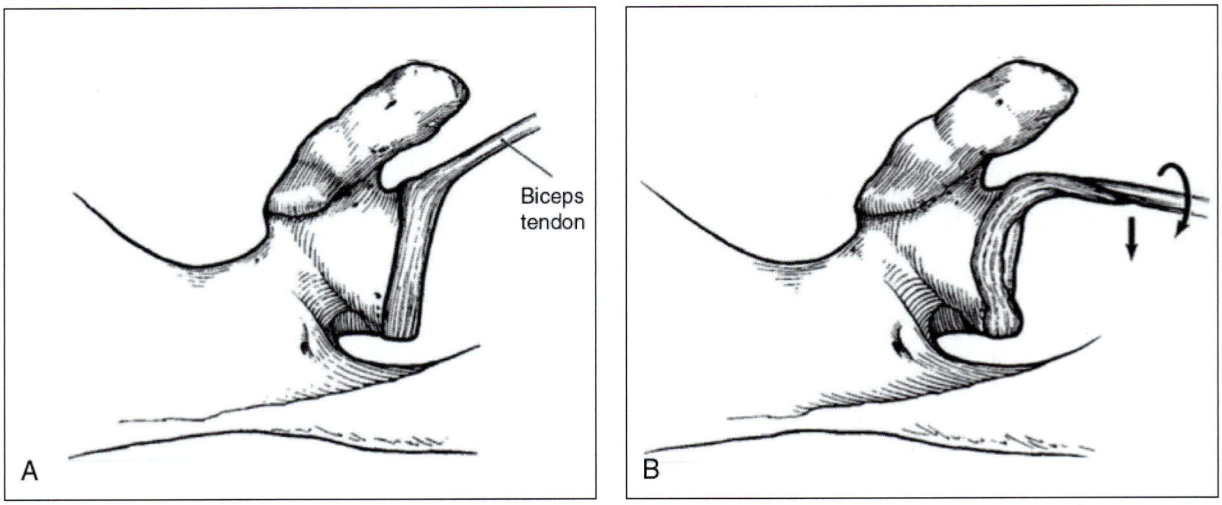

Illustration shows the peel-back mechanism of a SLAP injury from a coronal view. **A,** Anatomic position with the biceps tendon at rest. **B,** The arm in abduction (arrow) and external rotation (curved arrow) increases stress and peel-back forces on the SLAP region at the long head of the biceps tendon origin. (Reproduced with permission from Burkhart SS, Morgan CD, Kibler WB: The disabled throwing shoulder: Spectrum of pathology. Part II: Evaluation and treatment of SLAP lesions in throwers. *Arthroscopy* 2003;19[5]:531-539.)

Normal Anatomy

The labrum is composed of fibrous tissue, with a fibrocartilaginous transition zone that connects it to the glenoid.[28] The labrum is an essential component for the maintenance of glenohumeral stability, effectively increasing the surface area of glenoid articulation with the humeral head. Additionally, the labrum is the attachment site for the glenohumeral ligaments and the origin of the long head of the biceps (LHB) tendon. Typically, the biceps anchor is continuous with the labrum and is lined by synovium from its origin at the supraglenoid tubercle. The superior, middle, and inferior glenohumeral ligaments are also continuous with the anterior labrum and contribute to shoulder stability.[29] The MGHL has the most anatomic variations of the glenohumeral ligaments, but typically originates from the supraglenoid tubercle and courses at a 45° angle to the subscapularis tendon.[30] It is classically thought of as sheet-like, although it can have several variants.

Anatomic Variants

Several anatomic variants of the superior labrum can be identified arthroscopically.[31-33] Identification of these variants as nonpathologic is essential because inadvertent repair may result in overconstraining a functionally normal shoulder.[34] The most common variants are the sublabral recess, the sublabral foramen, the Buford complex, and variations of the MGHL. In patients with an anatomic variant in one shoulder, 50% were found to have an anatomic variant in the contralateral shoulder, although 75% of these were a different type of variant.[33]

The superior labrum can also have a meniscoid appearance in up to 15% of shoulders, where it is loosely attached to the glenoid, not unlike the meniscus in the knee[4,30] (**Figure 5, A**). With meniscoid variants, careful arthroscopic probing shows the LHB tendon firmly attached to normal glenoid cartilage even though the labrum itself may be mobile. Traction of the LHB tendon does not result in arching of the labrum.

The sublabral recess is a sulcus between the superior labrum and the glenoid cartilage found between the 11 o'clock and 1 o'clock positions (**Figure 5, B**). The sublabral recess has been identified in up to 73% of cadavers, with a sulcus measuring at least 2 mm in 39%.[35,36] A fetal cadaver study by Fealy et al[37] revealed that some separation between the glenoid and superior labrum was evident in gestation as early as 22 weeks.[38]

The sublabral foramen, or sublabral hole, is located more anteriorly, from the 12 o'clock to the 3 o'clock position, and is a complete separation of the labrum and glenoid[34] (**Figure 5, C**). The sublabral foramen has an incidence as high as 18.5% in arthroscopic studies and 16.0% in cadaver studies.[39,40] Both the sublabral recess and sublabral foramen can be difficult to distinguish from a true SLAP tear; however, these anatomic variants are usually asymptomatic.

The Buford complex is an absence of the anterosuperior labrum associated with a cord-like MGHL (**Figure 5, D**). The Buford complex has been identified in 1.5% to 6.0% of arthroscopic cases.[39,41] Additionally, the MGHL can be very narrow and may be accompanied by a hypertrophic inferior glenohumeral ligament.[30]

Although these anatomic variants do not contribute to glenohumeral instability, they may predispose patients to SLAP lesions by means of altered biomechanics. Ilahi et al[33] found the incidence of SLAP lesions to be twice as high in patients with some variant of the anterosuperior labrum.

Arthroscopic Findings

Type I SLAP Tear

A type I SLAP tear is a frayed superior labrum with a normal attachment of the labrum to the glenoid and a normal-appearing biceps tendon (**Figure 6**). The superior labrum and biceps anchor remain immobile with arthroscopic probing. The literature varies widely on the percentage of type I SLAP lesions, ranging from 11% to 74%.[2,42] Type I lesions likely represent normal degenerative changes and are largely asymptomatic.

Type II SLAP Tear

Most SLAP tears that require surgical treatment are type II. These lesions have a degenerative appearance and a frayed labrum, along with associated separation of the labrum and the LHBT root from the glenoid (**Figure 7**). Type II tears can be further defined by the anatomic position of the separation: anterior, posterior, or combined anterior-posterior. An excessively frayed type I lesion should not be confused with a type II lesion. Débridement of the frayed portion may help properly visualize the superior labrum and biceps anchor. Arthroscopic

FIGURE 5

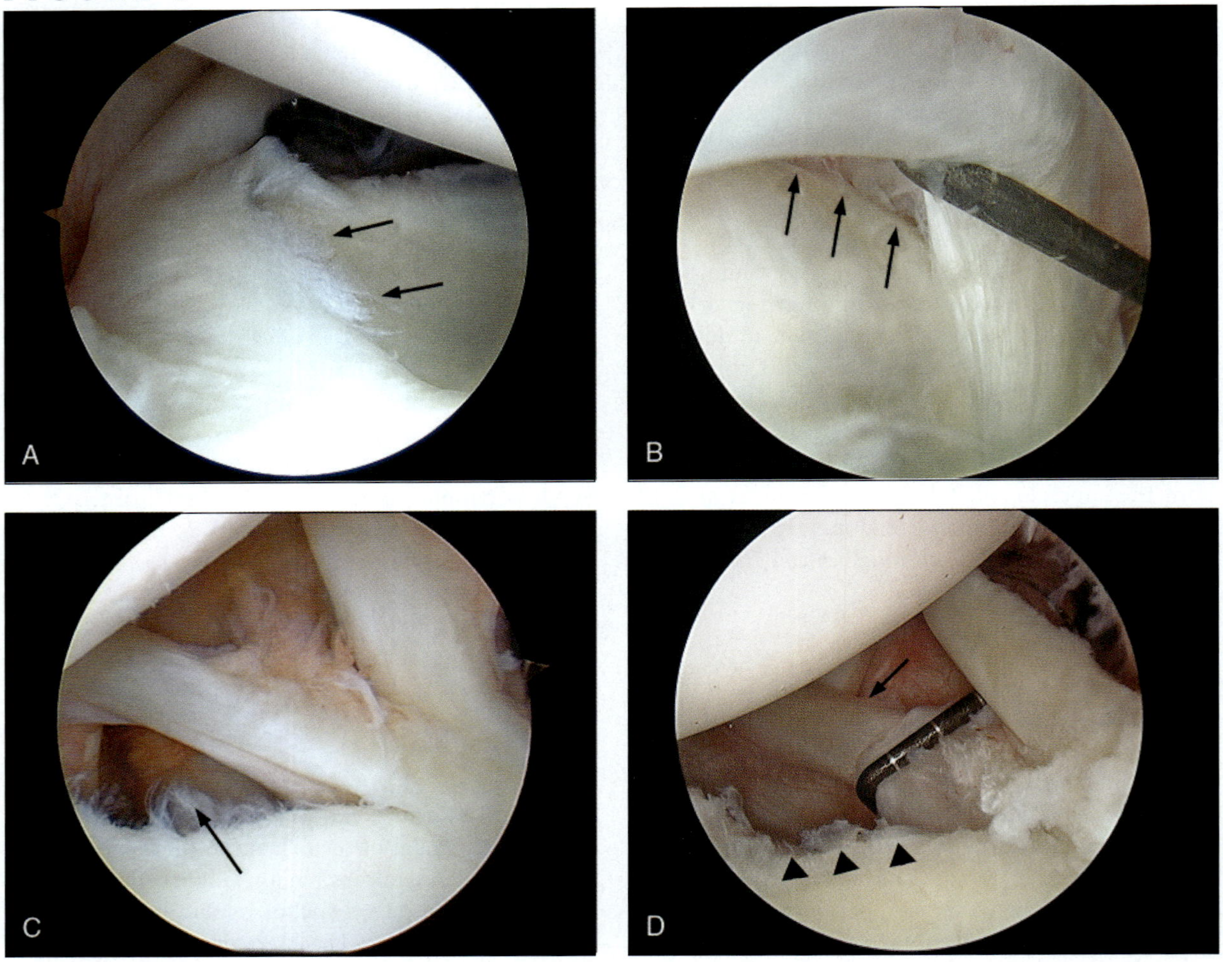

Arthroscopic views of normal anatomic variants. **A,** The meniscoid superior labrum (arrows) overlies the articular cartilage and can be confused with a SLAP tear. **B,** The sublabral recess (arrows) is present in up to 73% of patients and can be confused with a type II SLAP tear. **C,** The sublabral foramen (arrow) is a hole in the sublabral region between the 12 o'clock and the 3 o'clock positions (for a right shoulder). **D,** The Buford complex (arrow) is an absent anterosuperior labrum (arrowheads) with an associated cord-like glenohumeral ligament. Inadvertent repair of this normal anatomic variant can cause shoulder pain and loss of motion.

probing of the biceps anchor and superior labrum that results in a freely mobile detached region indicates a type II lesion. Additionally, applying traction to the biceps anchor results in the tendon and the labrum arching at least 5 mm away from the glenoid.[11,30] Associated hemorrhagic or granulation tissue may be appreciated around the biceps anchor or superior labrum. In a shoulder with a Buford complex, traction applied to the MGHL causes separation of the biceps anchor from the glenoid, which suggests a type II SLAP tear.

A positive result for the peel-back sign suggests a posterior SLAP lesion, as first described by Burkhart and Morgan.[14] The arm must be released from traction and placed in abduction and 90° of external rotation while directly visualizing the biceps tendon anchor at the superior labrum. A positive sign is defined as medial-

FIGURE 6

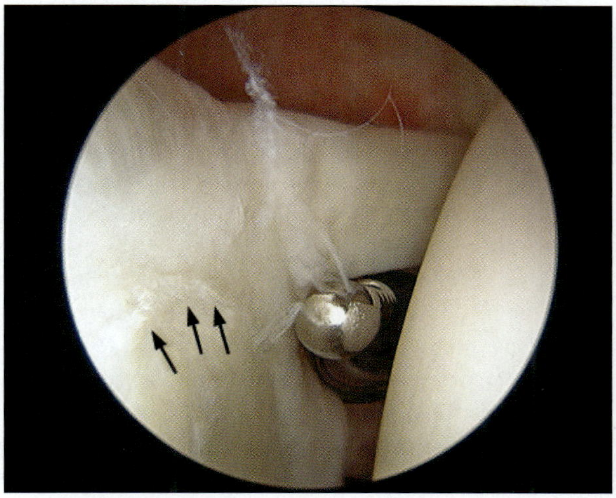

Arthroscopic view of a type I SLAP tear with a frayed superior labrum (arrows).

FIGURE 7

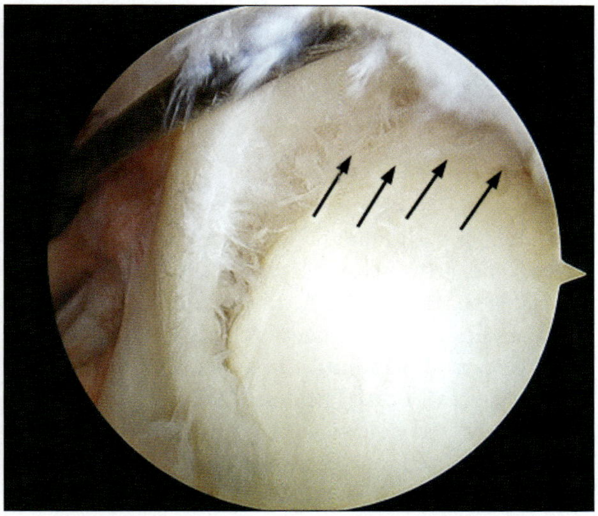

Arthroscopic view of a type II SLAP tear with a frayed superior labrum and associated separation of the biceps root from the glenoid (arrows).

ization of the biceps anchor, with the labrum peeling off the posterosuperior glenoid rim. A cadaver study showed that the peel-back sign was associated with a labral disruption to at least the 2 o'clock position and does not occur with biceps anchor disruption alone.[43]

The drive-through sign is often used as another indicator of a posterior or combined anterior-posterior lesion. The drive-through sign is determined by whether the arthroscope can easily traverse between the glenoid and humeral head at the level of the anterior band of the inferior glenohumeral ligament. A posterior SLAP lesion is thought to cause anteroinferior pseudolaxity, allowing the arthroscope to "drive through" this space.[11,30,44] Morgan et al[5] demonstrated that repairing a posterior lesion eliminates the drive-through sign. However, controversy exists on this subject. McFarland et al[45] found no correlation between a positive drive-through sign and SLAP tears.

Type III SLAP Tear

A Type III SLAP tear consists of a bucket-handle tear of the superior labrum with an intact biceps tendon and can be seen during arthroscopy as a central fragment of the labrum that is displaceable into the joint.[2] Careful probing of the LHB tendon confirms that it remains intact, differentiating this lesion from a type IV lesion. Any labral extension should also be explored. Although uncommon, significant anterior and posterior extension of the labral tear has been described for type III tears.[46]

Type IV SLAP Tear

A type IV tear is a bucket-handle tear that extends into the biceps tendon. As with a type III lesion, a fragment of the labral tear can be displaced into the joint with a potentially displaceable root of the LHB tendon.[2] The LHB tendon should be probed carefully to assess for involvement of the MGHL, which can occur with type III and type IV tears.[47]

Type V, VI, and VII SLAP Tears

Type V, VI, and VII SLAP tears were originally described by Maffet et al[3] after it was noted that 38% of patients with SLAP lesions could not be classified using the method developed by Snyder et al.[2] A type V tear is a Bankart lesion with superior extension in the biceps tendon; type VI, a labral flap with separation of the biceps tendon; and type VII, a lesion with anterior extension under the MGHL.

Type VIII, IX, and X SLAP Tears

Few reports describe arthroscopic findings for type VIII, XI, and X SLAP tears, which are type II lesions with posterior, circumferential, and posteroinferior extension, respectively.

Conclusion

The method of diagnosing SLAP tears continues to evolve as physical examination findings, radiologic adjuncts, and arthroscopic experience build on current knowledge of the lesions. A combination of patient history, physical examination, and radiographic findings helps discern these injuries in patients. However, even with advances in diagnostic modalities, the identification of SLAP tears is challenging, and arthroscopy is the gold standard. The surgeon should be able to recognize normal anatomic variants of the region in which SLAP tears occur because high-level imaging studies may not accurately portray the presence of a SLAP tear. Appropriate management of SLAP tears is firmly grounded on the recognition of pathology, and thus, proper arthroscopic identification continues to be essential. Types I through IV have been well described in the literature; however, many of the more recently recognized types (types V through X) need additional research to better understand their pathology, outcomes, and treatment options.

References

1. Andrews JR, Carson WG Jr, McLeod WD: Glenoid labrum tears related to the long head of the biceps. *Am J Sports Med* 1985;13(5):337-341.
2. Snyder SJ, Karzel RP, Del Pizzo W, Ferkel RD, Friedman MJ: SLAP lesions of the shoulder. *Arthroscopy* 1990;6(4):274-279.
3. Maffet MW, Gartsman GM, Moseley B: Superior labrum-biceps tendon complex lesions of the shoulder. *Am J Sports Med* 1995;23(1):93-98.
4. Barber A, Field LD, Ryu R: Biceps tendon and superior labrum injuries: Decision-marking. *J Bone Joint Surg Am* 2007;89(8):1844-1855.
5. Morgan CD, Burkhart SS, Palmeri M, Gillespie M: Type II SLAP lesions: Three subtypes and their relationships to superior instability and rotator cuff tears. *Arthroscopy* 1998;14(6):553-565.
6. Choi NH, Kim SJ: Avulsion of the superior labrum. *Arthroscopy* 2004;20(8):872-874.
7. Mileski RA, Snyder SJ: Superior labral lesions in the shoulder: Pathoanatomy and surgical management. *J Am Acad Orthop Surg* 1998;6(2):121-131.
8. Bey MJ, Elders GJ, Huston LJ, Kuhn JE, Blasier RB, Soslowsky LJ: The mechanism of creation of superior labrum, anterior, and posterior lesions in a dynamic biomechanical model of the shoulder: The role of inferior subluxation. *J Shoulder Elbow Surg* 1998;7(4): 397-401.
9. Clavert P, Bonnomet F, Kempf JF, Boutemy P, Braun M, Kahn JL: Contribution to the study of the pathogenesis of type II superior labrum anterior-posterior lesions: A cadaveric model of a fall on the outstretched hand. *J Shoulder Elbow Surg* 2004;13(1):45-50.
10. Pradhan RL, Itoi E, Hatakeyama Y, Urayama M, Sato K: Superior labral strain during the throwing motion: A cadaveric study. *Am J Sports Med* 2001;29(4):488-492.
11. Burkhart SS, Morgan CD, Kibler WB: The disabled throwing shoulder: Spectrum of pathology. Part II: Evaluation and treatment of SLAP lesions in throwers. *Arthroscopy* 2003;19(5):531-539.
12. Kuhn JE, Lindholm SR, Huston LJ, Soslowsky LJ, Blasier RB: Failure of the biceps superior labral complex: A cadaveric biomechanical investigation comparing the late cocking and early deceleration positions of throwing. *Arthroscopy* 2003;19(4):373-379.
13. Shepard MF, Dugas JR, Zeng N, Andrews JR: Differences in the ultimate strength of the biceps anchor and the generation of type II superior labral anterior posterior lesions in a cadaveric model. *Am J Sports Med* 2004;32(5):1197-1201.
14. Burkhart SS, Morgan CD: The peel-back mechanism: Its role in producing and extending posterior type II SLAP lesions and its effect on SLAP repair rehabilitation. *Arthroscopy* 1998;14(6):637-640.
15. Grossman MG, Tibone JE, McGarry MH, Schneider DJ, Veneziani S, Lee TQ: A cadaveric model of the throwing shoulder: A possible etiology of superior labrum anterior-to-posterior lesions. *J Bone Joint Surg Am* 2005;87(4):824-831.
16. Yergason RM: Supination sign. *J Bone and Joint Surg Br* 1931;13(1):160.
17. O'Brien SJ, Pagnani MJ, Fealy S, McGlynn SR, Wilson JB: The active compression test: A new and effective test for diagnosing labral tears and acromioclavicular joint abnormality. *Am J Sports Med* 1998;26(5):610-613.

18. Crenshaw AH, Kilgore WE: Surgical treatment of bicipital tenosynovitis. *J Bone Joint Surg Am* 1966;48(8):1496-1502.
19. Kibler WB: Specificity and sensitivity of the anterior slide test in throwing athletes with superior glenoid labral tears. *Arthroscopy* 1995;11(3):296-300.
20. Liu SH, Henry MH, Nuccion SL: A prospective evaluation of a new physical examination in predicting glenoid labral tears. *Am J Sports Med* 1996;24(6):721-725.
21. Hegedus EJ, Goode AP, Cook CE, et al: Which physical examination tests provide clinicians with the most value when examining the shoulder? Update of a systematic review with meta-analysis of individual tests. *Br J Sports Med* 2012;46(14):964-978.
22. Jia X, Yokota A, McCarty EC, et al: Reproducibility and reliability of the Snyder classification of superior labral anterior posterior lesions among shoulder surgeons. *Am J Sports Med* 2011;39(5):986-991.
23. Gobezie R, Zurakowski D, Lavery K, Millett PJ, Cole BJ, Warner JJ: Analysis of interobserver and intraobserver variability in the diagnosis and treatment of SLAP tears using the Snyder classification. *Am J Sports Med* 2008;36(7):1373-1379.
24. McFarland EG, Tanaka MJ, Garzon-Muvdi J, Jia X, Petersen SA: Clinical and imaging assessment for superior labrum anterior and posterior lesions. *Curr Sports Med Rep* 2009;8(5):234-239.
25. Iqbal HJ, Rani S, Mahmood A, Brownson P, Aniq H: Diagnostic value of MR arthrogram in SLAP lesions of the shoulder. *Surgeon* 2010;8(6):303-309.
26. Chandnani VP, Yeager TD, DeBerardino T, et al: Glenoid labral tears: Prospective evaluation with MRI imaging, MR arthrography, and CT arthrography. *AJR Am J Roentgenol* 1993;161(6):1229-1235.
27. Mohana-Borges AV, Chung CB, Resnick D: Superior labral anteroposterior tear: Classification and diagnosis on MRI and MR arthrography. *AJR Am J Roentgenol* 2003;181(6):1449-1462.
28. Huber WP, Putz RV: Periarticular fiber system of the shoulder joint. *Arthroscopy* 1997;13(6):680-691.
29. Rockwood CA: *The Shoulder*, ed 3. Philadelphia, PA, Saunders, 2004.
30. Snyder SJ: *Shoulder Arthroscopy*. Philadelphia, PA, Lippincott William & Wilkins, 2003.
31. Ghalayini SR, Board TN, Srinivasan MS: Anatomic variations in the long head of biceps: Contribution to shoulder dysfunction. *Arthroscopy* 2007;23(9):1012-1018.
32. Rao AG, Kim TK, Chronopoulos E, McFarland EG: Anatomical variants in the anterosuperior aspect of the glenoid labrum: A statistical analysis of seventy-three cases. *J Bone Joint Surg Am* 2003;85-A(4):653-659.
33. Ilahi OA, Cosculluela PE, Ho DM: Classification of anterosuperior glenoid labrum variants and their association with shoulder pathology. *Orthopedics* 2008;31(3):226.
34. Jazrawi LM, McCluskey GM III, Andrews JR: Superior labral anterior and posterior lesions and internal impingement in the overhead athlete. *Instr Course Lect* 2003;52:43-63.
35. Vangsness CT Jr, Jorgenson SS, Watson T, Johnson DL: The origin of the long head of the biceps from the scapula and glenoid labrum: An anatomical study of 100 shoulders. *J Bone Joint Surg Br* 1994;76(6):951-954.
36. Smith DK, Chopp TM, Aufdemorte TB, Witkowski EG, Jones RC: Sublabral recess of the superior glenoid labrum: Study of cadavers with conventional nonenhanced MR imaging, MR arthrography, anatomic dissection, and limited histologic examination. *Radiology* 1996;201(1):251-256.
37. Fealy S, Rodeo SA, Dicarlo EF, O'Brien SJ: The developmental anatomy of the neonatal glenohumeral joint. *J Shoulder Elbow Surg* 2000;9(3):217-222.
38. Prodromos CC, Ferry JA, Schiller AL, Zarins B: Histological studies of the glenoid labrum from fetal life to old age. *J Bone Joint Surg Am* 1990;72(9):1344-1348.
39. Ilahi OA, Labbe MR, Cosculluela P: Variants of the anterosuperior glenoid labrum and associated pathology. *Arthroscopy* 2002;18(8):882-886.
40. Tischer T, Vogt S, Kreuz PC, Imhoff AB: Arthroscopic anatomy, variants, and pathologic findings in shoulder instability. *Arthroscopy* 2011;27(10):1434-1443.
41. Williams MM, Snyder SJ, Buford D Jr: The Buford complex—the "cord-like" middle glenohumeral ligament and absent anterosuperior labrum complex: A normal anatomic capsulolabral variant. *Arthroscopy* 1994;10(3):241-247.
42. Kim TK, Queale WS, Cosgarea AJ, McFarland EG: Clinical features of the different types of SLAP lesions: An analysis of one hundred and thirty-nine cases. *J Bone Joint Surg Am* 2003;85-A(1):66-71.

43. Seneviratne A, Montgomery K, Bevilacqua B, Zikria B: Quantifying the extent of a type II SLAP lesion required to cause peel-back of the glenoid labrum—a cadaveric study. *Arthroscopy* 2006;22(11):e1-e6, e6.
44. Abrams GD, Safran MR: Diagnosis and management of superior labrum anterior posterior lesions in overhead athletes. *Br J Sports Med* 2010;44(5):311-318.
45. McFarland EG, Neira CA, Gutierrez MI, Cosgarea AJ, Magee M: Clinical significance of the arthroscopic drive-through sign in shoulder surgery. *Arthroscopy* 2001;17(1):38-43.
46. Rizio L: Type 3 SLAP tear with anterior and posterior extension. *Orthopedics* 2006;29(10):882-883.
47. D'Alessandro DF, Fleischli JE, Connor PM: Superior labral lesions: Diagnosis and management. *J Athl Train* 2000;35(3):286-292.

CHAPTER 8

Arthroscopic Treatment of Superior Labrum Anterior to Posterior Lesions

Benjamin Bruce, MD
Frank McCormick, MD
Anil K. Gupta, MD, MBA
Nikhil N. Verma, MD
Anthony A. Romeo, MD

Introduction

Superior labrum anterior to posterior (SLAP) lesions were first recognized by Andrews et al[1] almost 30 years ago in throwing athletes, and classified into four types by Snyder et al.[2] SLAP tears are considered to be traumatic such as those resulting from traction or a compression mechanism, or degenerative such as those seen in overhead athletes.[3] Type I lesions are characterized by a frayed inner margin of the labrum, which is considered a normal part of aging.[4] Type II lesions are the most common variant and involve a separation of the glenoid-labral junction, often characterized by erythema at the chondrolabral junction and a minimum of 5 mm of increased excursion. Type II lesions are further subclassified as anterior, posterior, or combined.[5] Type III lesions are characterized by an intact biceps complex junction at the superior glenoid, but with a bucket-handle tear involving the superior labral complex. A type IV tear is a type III tear with a concomitant separation of the superior labrum from the glenoid with extension

Dr. Verma or an immediate family member has received royalties from Smith & Nephew; serves as a paid consultant to or is an employee of Smith & Nephew and Arthrex; has stock or stock options held in Omeros; has received research or institutional support from Arthrex, Smith & Nephew, Athletico, ConMed Linvatec, Miomed, and Mitek; and serves as a board member, owner, officer, or committee member of the Arthroscopy Association Learning Center Committee. Dr. Romeo or an immediate family member has received royalties from Arthrex; is a member of a speakers' bureau or has made paid presentations on behalf of Arthrex; serves as a paid consultant to or is an employee of Arthrex; has received research or institutional support from Arthrex, DJO Surgical, Smith & Nephew, and Össur; has received nonincome support (such as equipment or services), commercially derived honoraria, or other non–research-related funding (such as paid travel) from Arthrex, and DJO Surgical; and serves as a board member, owner, officer, or committee member of the American Orthopaedic Society for Sports Medicine, the American Shoulder and Elbow Surgeons, and the Arthroscopy Association of North America. None of the following authors nor any immediate family member has received anything of value from or has stock or stock options held in a commercial company or institution related directly or indirectly to the subject of this chapter: Dr. Bruce, Dr. McCormick, and Dr. Gupta.

FIGURE 1

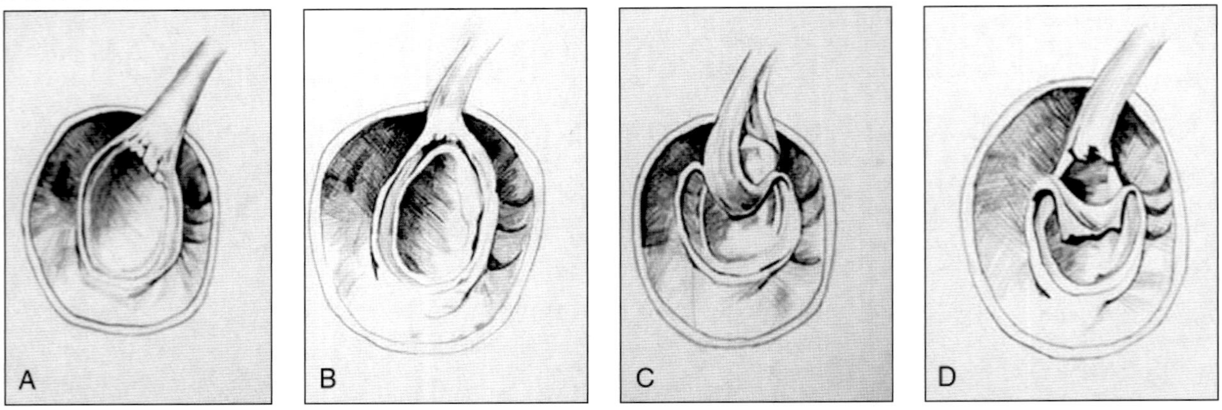

Snyder classification for types of SLAP lesions. **A,** type I; **B,** type II; **C,** type III; **D,** type IV. (Reproduced with permission from Snyder SJ, Karzel RP, Del Pizzo W, Ferkel RD, Friedman MJ: SLAP lesions of the shoulder. *Arthroscopy* 1990;6[4]:274-279.)

into the biceps anchor (**Figure 1**). Superior labral tears are further characterized into 10 subtypes based on concurrent instability and posterior extension.[6,7] These subtypes are not used in the literature as often as the original Snyder classification.

Imaging

No imaging test accurately diagnoses or excludes the presence of a SLAP lesion. Plain radiographs should be obtained to rule out coexisting shoulder pathologies. MRIs should be interpreted carefully and correlated with clinical findings because the specificity ranges from 50% to 85%.[8,9] Magnetic resonance arthrograms obtained with gadolinium improve accuracy, especially if interpreted by a fellowship-trained musculoskeletal radiologist.[10,11] In all cases, clinical correlation in conjunction with imaging and arthroscopy is the gold standard for diagnosis.

Indications

Controversy exists regarding the optimal treatment of patients with suspected SLAP tears. Most studies suggest that surgical intervention should not be considered until the patient has attempted at least 3 months of nonsurgical treatment, which begins with rest, activity modification, and anti-inflammatory medication. Physical therapy may be initiated to treat any scapular dyskinesis with open and closed kinetic chain exercises. In athletes with glenohumeral internal rotation deficit, posterior capsule stretching may be effective. The effectiveness of physical therapy in treating isolated SLAP tears, however, is unpredictable and poorly defined in the literature.[12]

When nonsurgical treatment is ineffective, surgical management should be considered. Currently, no absolute surgical indication exists for SLAP repair. Many patient-related factors must be considered when making this decision, including age, occupation, preinjury activity level, expected postoperative activity level, and worker's compensation status. Thus, a joint patient-physician decision is key to a successful outcome. However, weakness and atrophy in the supraspinatus and infraspinatus resulting from suprascapular nerve compression by a paralabral cyst may be a relative indication for early intervention.[13]

In general, type I tears should be treated using simple débridement. Type II lesion treatment depends on several factors. Older, more sedentary patients, or those with degenerative-appearing lesions, may have better results with simple débridement or biceps tenodesis. Younger, more active patients with a history and physical examination results consistent with a SLAP lesion should be considered for surgical repair. Preoperative evaluation may aid in decision making—patients with substantial preoperative findings that suggest biceps involvement should be considered for tenodesis. These findings may include positive tension test results (for example, the Speed and Yergason tests), bicipital groove or subpectoral tenderness, and anterior pain radiating into the biceps muscle belly. Intraoperatively, the shoulder is moved through abduction and external rotation to see if the biceps anchor has a peel-back injury. Type III lesions are treated with resection of the unstable portions of any bucket-handle tear of the labrum or repair if the residual biceps-labral complex is unstable. The treatment for type IV lesions depends on the extent of biceps involvement. Lesions that involve less than 30% of the biceps tendon should be considered for débridement. In most cases with substantial biceps involvement or preoperative evidence of biceps-related pain (positive tension test results, bicipital groove tenderness), biceps tenodesis should be considered.

Surgical Technique: Standard Suture Anchors

Unless contraindicated, all patients receive an interscalene block and general anesthesia. Although the beach chair position can be used, the authors of this chapter prefer to place patients in the lateral position because the fixed suspension in slight abduction reduces tension in the rotator cuff, providing more space above the glenoid (**Figures 2** and **3**). Further, the lateral position provides additional visualization of the inferior quadrant of the glenohumeral joint both anteriorly and posteriorly if the tear is found to extend inferiorly. With a concominant rotator cuff tear, glenohumeral arthritis, or an older patient (older than 40 years), the authors use the beach chair position to perform biceps tenodesis.[13]

An examination under anesthesia is performed to assess stability and range of motion of the surgical limb and compared with the opposite side. Glenohumeral diagnostic arthroscopy is performed via a posterior portal placed 2 cm inferior and 2 cm posterior to the posterolateral corner of the acromion. An anterosuperior portal is established just superior to the subscapularis and anterior to the biceps through the rotator interval using an outside-in technique (**Figure 4**). A spinal needle is placed parallel to the long head of the biceps to help with accurate placement of the portal, and an 8.25-mm cannula is inserted.

Because type II SLAP lesions may appear normal at first, a careful, standardized assessment of the labrum

FIGURE 2

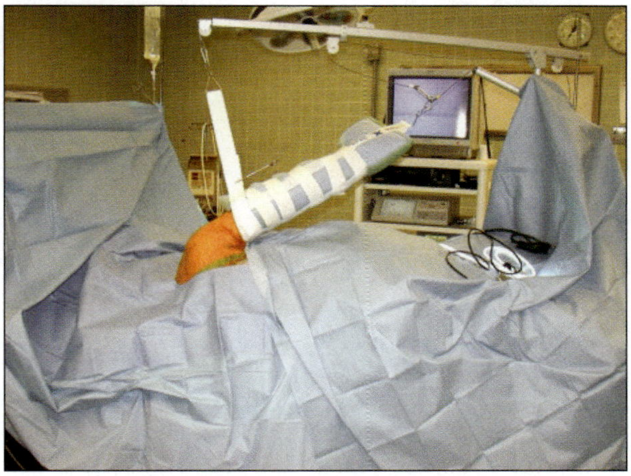

Photograph shows patient placed in the lateral position for a SLAP repair. Rolled towels may be placed in the axilla of the surgical extremity to increase glenohumeral distraction.

FIGURE 3

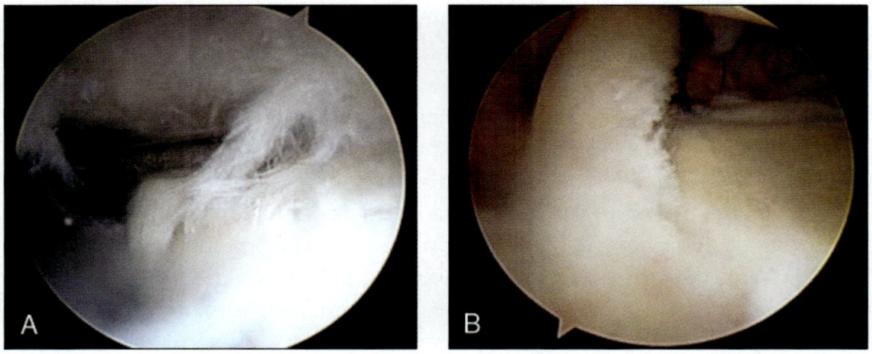

Arthroscopic views of a SLAP repair with the patient in the beach chair (**A**) and lateral (**B**) positions. The lateral position reduces rotator cuff tension, improving visualization of the superior labrum and associated structures.

FIGURE 4

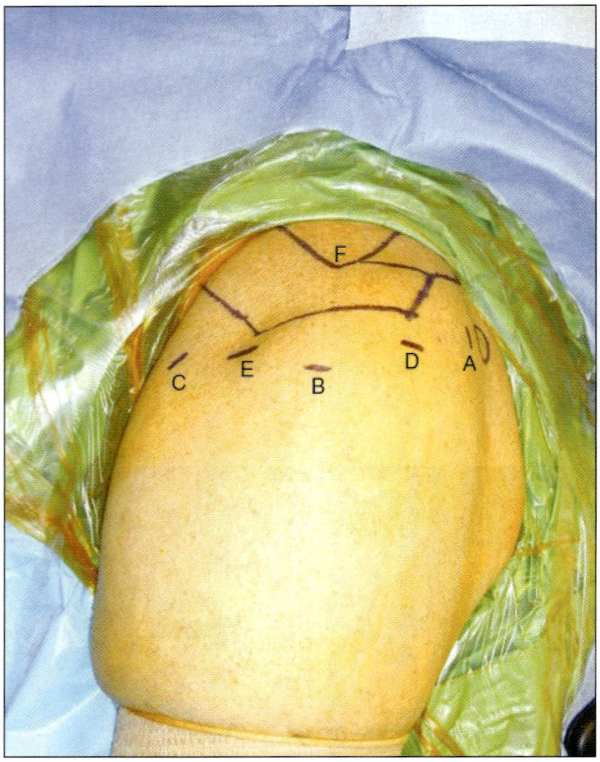

Photograph of a right shoulder shows standard anterior (**A**), lateral (**B**), and posterior (**C**) portals. Additional portals are the anterolateral (**D**), port of Wilmington (**E**), and Neviaser (**F**, not marked) portals.

FIGURE 5

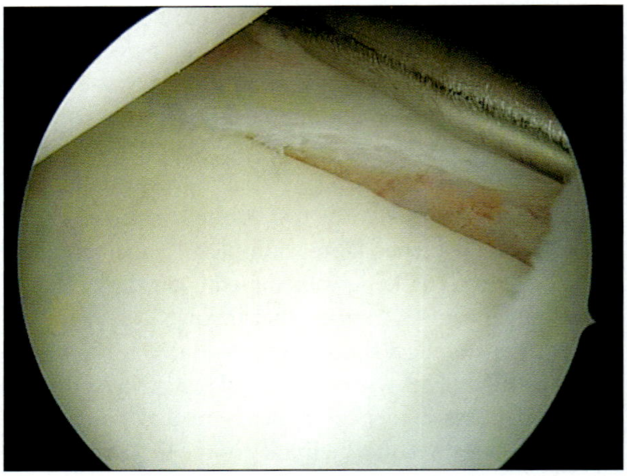

Arthroscopic view of a probe used to evaluate for the peel-back phenomenon, which demonstrates instability of the biceps anchor.

should be performed. The stability of the labral attachment to the glenoid is evaluated using a probe. Care must be taken to differentiate normal variations or degenerative findings from pathology that requires repair. Secondary findings that may indicate pathology include erythema or inflammation of the chondrolabral interface, and exposure of the underlying superior glenoid bone, which indicates pathologic detachment of the labrum. The probe can also be used to measure the length of the tear and/or glenolabral separation. In the overhead throwing athlete, damage can be further characterized by placing the arm in 90° of abduction and external rotation, simulating the throwing position, to evaluate for peel-back injury (**Figure 5**). With the arm in this position, the surgeon should assess for peeling back or pathologic displacement of the labrum off the glenoid rim, as well as abnormal contact and secondary tearing of the posterosuperior rotator cuff, which suggests internal impingement. The authors of this chapter perform this evaluation in the overhead athlete with a dry joint to reduce the influence of capsular distention.

The joint should be thoroughly inspected to identify associated pathology including labral tears, articular and bursal-side rotator cuff tears, capsular tears, and articular cartilage lesions.[2] Clinical studies have frequently reported concomitant pathology found during arthroscopy for SLAP repair, and that repair of the associated pathologies results in superior outcomes compared with SLAP repair alone.[14,15]

Arthroscopic visualization is established and pathologic tissue is removed by careful débridement of the detached labrum with a shaver via the anterosuperior portal. The authors of this chapter use a 4.0-mm shaver to minimize trauma to the adjacent structures. Aggressive débridement of labral tissue should be avoided because most failures occur at the labral-suture interface.[16-20] The labrum is then detached from the superior glenoid using a liberator. Care should be taken to avoid damaging the suprascapular nerve in the spinoglenoid notch by minimizing the medial excursion of any arthroscopic tool. The nerve lies approximately 2 cm medial to the glenoid rim. Decortication of the glenoid rim

FIGURE 6

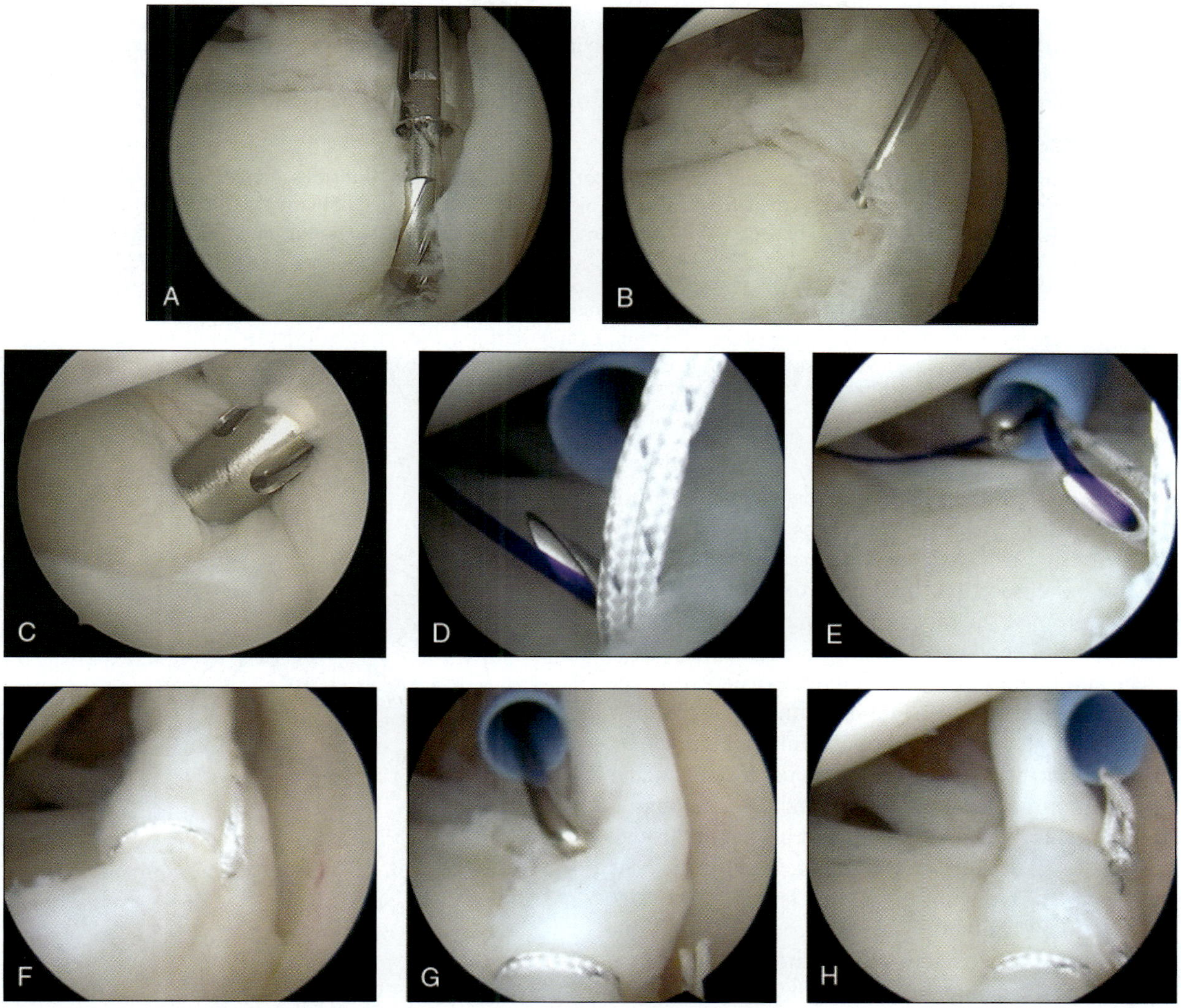

Images of a SLAP repair. **A,** Posterior arthroscopic view shows the arthroscopic shaver inserted via the anterior portal to prepare the superior rim of the labrum. The shaver blades should be oriented toward the bony surface to avoid aggressive labral resection. **B,** An 18-gauge spinal needle is used to localize the portal required for ideal trajectory and anchor placement. **C,** Arthroscopic view shows a small trocar placed through the posterosuperior portal onto the rim of the glenoid. **D,** A polydioxanone suture is passed through the labrum at the level of the anchor using a percutaneous 18-gauge spinal needle. **E,** The medial limb and polydioxanone suture are retrieved through the anterior portal and tied. The polydioxanone suture is withdrawn, shuttling the medial braided, long-chain polyethylene suture through the labral tissue. **F,** The initial half-hitch is placed posterior to the biceps. Knots should be tied away from the chondral surface to avoid irritation. **G,** The labrum is probed for stability. **H,** A second suture anchor is placed just posterior to the biceps, in a manner similar to that as in **E.**

TABLE 1 Arthroscopic Portals

Portal	Description
Anterolateral or Anterosuperior	Located 3–4 mm off the anterolateral corner of the acromion; used for anchor placement in the superior glenoid from the 11 o'clock to the 1 o'clock positions. Penetrate through the rotator interval or sharply through the rotator cuff muscle belly, parallel to the biceps.
Port of Wilmington	Located 1 cm lateral and 1 cm anterior to the posterolateral corner of the acromion; transmusculotendinous portal used for suture anchor placement of the posterior aspect of the biceps labral complex of SLAP injury types IIB, IIC, and IV. The shoulder should not be abducted beyond 30° to avoid tendon injury; a small metal, nondisposable cannula (<3 mm) should be used.
Neviaser	Located 1 cm medial to the medial border of the acromion, 1 cm posterior to the acromioclavicular joint, and 1 cm anterior to the scapular spine; used for suture passage from the 10 o'clock to the 2 o'clock positions.

is performed to elicit bleeding: bony surface healing is enhanced with the elution of marrow elements. This is performed either with the shaver operating in forward mode or using a 4.0-mm hooded burr (**Figure 6, A**). Aggressive bone resection should be avoided because this can compromise stability and loading mechanics in the glenohumeral joint.

The authors of this chapter prefer using an 18-gauge spinal needle with an outside-in technique to optimize the trajectory for suture anchor placement (**Figure 6, B**). The authors often use percutaneous suture anchor placement through the rotator cuff at the musculotendinous junction. A cannula should not be placed through the rotator cuff. Anchor placement is performed via the port of Wilmington portal just lateral to the edge of the acromion either posteriorly or anteriorly (**Table 1**), (**Figure 4**). Placement of the anchor anterior to the biceps tendon should be carefully evaluated because this may create tension on the anterior capsule and superior glenohumeral ligament (**Figure 7**). Studies have reported clinically significant loss of external rotation with anterior fixation of SLAP lesions.[21,22] A percutaneous portal is often used for posterior extension of labral injuries, placed directly adjacent to the lateral edge of the acromion, and 1 cm anterior to the posterolateral acromion corner (the port of Wilmington).

FIGURE 7

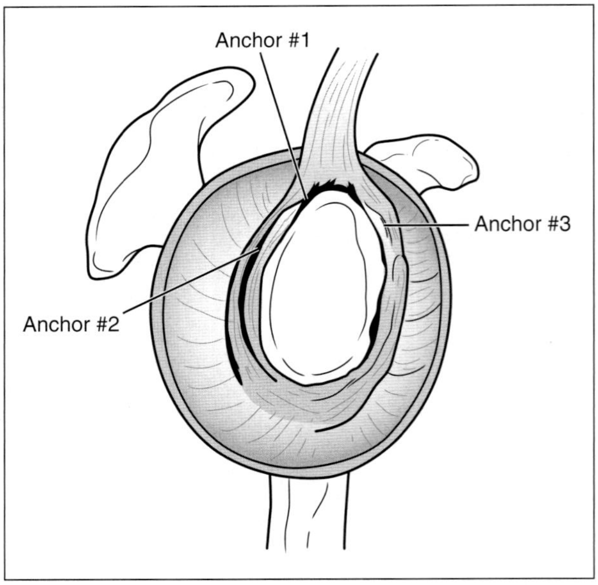

Illustration of optimal anchor placement for SLAP repairs. The surgeon should avoid placing suture anchors anterior to the biceps to prevent external rotation contractures. Note that if two anchors are required, the more posterior anchor should be placed first.

The suture anchors are placed through a drill trocar at approximately 30° to the articular surface, where the maximal medial-to-lateral bone stock is found.[23] When additional anchors are required posteriorly, the surgeon should be aware that significantly less bone stock is available and the angle of insertion may have to be decreased further to avoid blowout.[23]

SLAP repair suture anchors should be placed on the glenoid rim, not on the chondral surface, to restore the normal superior labral footprint, which lies approximately 4 mm medial to the articular surface. Chondral surface placement can result in overtightening of the biceps or impingement of the humerus on the implants in abduction. Special care should be taken to ensure that the drill holes and anchors do not skive off the glenoid, resulting in an unstable anchor or chondral damage.

After the holes have been drilled, a 3-mm bioabsorbable tack double-loaded with a high-strength braided suture is inserted through the drill sleeve (**Figure 6, C**). The drill sleeve should be held carefully in place on the superior glenoid rim during drilling and suture anchor insertion to avoid loss of the hole. The sutures are tensioned through the skin to ensure satisfactory anchor purchase. Visualization can be maximized throughout these steps by blocking fluid escape through the drill sleeve.

The medial limb from one of the sutures is retrieved via the anterior portal. A polydiaxonone suture is passed from medial to lateral through the superior labrum at the posterior aspect of the tear using either an 18-gauge needle via a Neviaser portal or a hook-type or lasso-type suture-passing device via the anterior portal (**Figure 6, D**). If a hook or lasso device is used, it is typically directed away from the surgical extremity (device angled 45° to the left for a right shoulder). The tip of the suture-passing device should emerge at the chondrolabral junction. The free limb of the polydioxanone suture is retrieved from the glenoid side via the anterior portal (**Figure 6, E**). If the polydioxanone suture is passed via the Nevaiser portal with an 18-guage spinal needle, the supralabral foramen should be cleared of synovium to ensure satisfactory visualization of the polydioxanone suture for later retrieval. The polydioxanone suture and anchor suture are tied outside the body and the polydioxanone is used as a relay to pull or shuttle the anchor suture retrograde through the labrum. The sutures are then tied through the anterior cannula in a simple knot with alternating half-hitches. Care must be taken to retrieve both sutures above the biceps to avoid trapping the tendon in the suture loop. The knots are tensioned parallel to the glenolabral surface to prevent pull-through. The knots must be tied medial to the glenoid to avoid irritating the chondral surface or biceps tendon (**Figure 6, F**). The labrum is probed for stability (**Figure 6, G**). With double-loaded anchor placement, both sutures are passed before tying the suture to help suture passage. For larger tears, a second, more anterior anchor may be placed in a manner similar to that of the first (**Figure 6, H**).

Key Surgical Pearls

(1) The posterior portal should be placed 2 cm lateral to the glenohumeral joint line to enable visualization and potential anchor placement. (2) The peel-back test should be performed with a dry joint to avoid the effect of capsular distention. (3) The suture anchors should be placed posterior to the biceps to avoid tightening the anterior ligaments and capsule. (4) The anchors should be placed at approximately 30° relative to the articular surface to maximize bony support. (5) The knots should be tied away from the articular surface to avoid suture irritation with abduction.

Knotless Suture Anchor Technique

Dines et al[24] described an arthroscopic knotless suture anchor technique for SLAP lesions. The knotless technique is thought to reduce the mechanical irritation of the surrounding soft tissue and re-create the normal meniscoid appearance of the superior labrum. An 18-gauge needle is used to identify a satisfactory trajectory for anchor placement. A 3-mm cannula is placed via the superior transtendinous accessory portal. A hook suture-passing device is used via the posterior portal to pass a polydiaxonone suture through the labrum posterior to the biceps. The polydioxanone suture is retrieved through the accessory portal and used to shuttle a nonabsorbable braided, long-chain polyethylene No. 2 suture through the labrum. The suture-passing device is used to pass a second polydioxanone suture approximately 5 mm posterior to the first suture. The suture is retrieved via the accessory portal and used to shuttle the other limb of the braided, long-chain polyethylene suture through the labrum, forming a horizontal mattress pattern. The sutures are retrieved via the posterior portal. A pilot hole is drilled posterior to the biceps at the superior glenoid rim using the transtendinous cannula. The sutures are subsequently retrieved through this cannula. Both limbs of the suture are passed through a bioabsorbable or plastic (polyether ether ketone) knotless anchor. The sutures are tensioned as the anchor is malleted into the pilot hole. The labrum should be probed for stability. For more extensive tears, other anchors may be placed in a similar manner as the first.

Postoperative Management

Postoperatively, patients are placed in a sling with an abduction pillow for 4 weeks. Formal physical therapy is initiated in postoperative week 2, beginning with passive range of motion in external rotation and the scapular plane with pendulum exercises, as well as active range of motion of the elbow, wrist, and fingers. Passive range of motion from 0° to 90° of forward elevation and external rotation is initiated at 3 weeks, with the goal of achieving full range of motion by 6 weeks. Strengthening exercises are initiated at 12 weeks and return to a throwing program is begun at 4 months. Full return to competitive throwing can be expected at 9 to 12 months. Rehabilitation protocols for associated pathology such as anterior instability or rotator cuff repair should be adopted, if necessary.

Current Areas of Study

Anchors

Various anchors have been successfully used to repair SLAP lesions. Recently, surgeons have shifted from using metallic screws to bioabsorbable or polyether ether ketone anchors to avoid potential anchor migration and interference with postoperative MRI.[24] Bioabsorbable poly-L-lactic acid sutures should be avoided because they have been associated with an increased risk of synovitis, osteolysis, chondrolysis, and reoperation rates.[25]

The number and type of suture anchors, along with the suture-passing method, have been studied using cadaver models. One double-loaded suture anchor has been found to be mechanically equivalent to two single-loaded anchors in load-to-failure testing.[26] Knotless suture anchors versus knotted suture anchors have also been evaluated.[16] The theoretical advantages of knotless repairs include avoiding technical difficulties associated with knot tying, potentially faster surgical times, and the absence of potentially symptomatic knots, which may result in soft-tissue irritation or chondral abrasion during range of motion. Uggen et al[20] reported no difference between knotless and knotted suture anchors for type II SLAP repairs in stiffness, yield load, or ultimate failure. Furthermore, no evidence was reported of initial overtightening of the glenohumeral joint with either anchor type. Another study, however, demonstrated that repair performed with a knotless anchor was weaker than with knotted anchors in longitudinal cyclic loading of the biceps.[16] Nonetheless, successful outcomes have been reported with knotless anchors, and the potential drawbacks of knotted anchors should be weighed when selecting the type of anchor to use. If knotted anchors are selected, all knots should be tied away from the articular surface to avoid humeral head abrasion and stress to the repair site as the arm is moved into the throwing position.

In general, the authors of this chapter try to minimize the number of implants used to preserve bone, limit the cost, and avoid suture anchor–associated complications. Usually, a double-loaded anchor placed posterior to the biceps in a simple configuration is sufficient for a type II SLAP lesion. The authors prefer a double-loaded anchor because anchor failure is much less common than suture pullout, and double-loaded implants provide two points of fixation with only one implant.[26] However, additional suture anchors may be required, depending on the tear pattern. If the tear extends posteriorly to the 9 o'clock position with a peel-back injury, an additional single-loaded anchor is added posteriorly. The most critical component of fixation is placing the anchor beneath the biceps root and passing the suture loop posterior to it. This allows two simple sutures from a double-loaded anchor to be placed posteriorly to the biceps root to restore labral stability and prevent further peel back from occurring. The repair should proceed from posterior to anterior because the anterior working portal is used for suture passage; placing the anterior suture anchor first limits access to the more posterior aspects of the labrum. Placing the anchor anterior to the biceps tendon should be avoided because this may place tension on the anterior capsule and superior glenohumeral ligament. Morgan et al[27] showed that two suture anchors placed posterior to the biceps were biomechanically equivalent to two anchors placed on either side of the biceps.[28] Domb et al[18] also found that when using longitudinal traction, anterior suture anchors did not improve initial strength under cyclic loading compared with an anchor placed inferior to the biceps insertion. Furthermore, a single anchor with a single suture placed posterior to the biceps was found to be at least equivalent to either a single anchor with a mattress suture pattern or two anchors with simple suture patterns placed posterior to the biceps.[17] If an anterior suture anchor is considered necessary, care should be taken to repair the labral tissue only and to avoid overtensioning the superior and middle glenohumeral ligament complex.

Suture Configuration

Compared with a mattress suture configuration, simple sutures have been shown to have a higher load to failure,[17,27] although using mattress sutures significantly increased the labral height. Biomechanical analysis comparing both suture types has demonstrated similar properties.[27] A prospective double-blind randomized clinical trial comparing horizontal with simple sutures found no difference between the two configurations in postoperative range of motion or outcome scores.[29] Suture configuration should be selected according to surgeon discretion to provide optimal labral stability.

Management of Spinoglenoid Cysts

The intraoperative management of spinoglenoid cysts associated with labral tears is controversial. Some authors suggest that arthroscopic decompression of these cysts results in greater gains in external rotation strength compared with patients who undergo isolated SLAP repairs.[13,15] Cyst decompression is performed before SLAP repair by inserting a blunt instrument through the posterosuperior aspect of the SLAP tear. The labrum is débrided and the glenoid bone is prepared. Working through the anterior portal, a Bankart elevator or switching stick can be used to gently penetrate below the labrum into the expected location of the cyst based on preoperative MRIs. Successful decompression is evidenced by the release of a viscous material into the glenohumeral joint. Limited débridement of the cyst can be completed using a shaver, although care should be taken to avoid injury to the suprascapular nerve, which is 2 cm medial to the glenoid rim. After cyst decompression is completed, a standard labral repair is performed. However, Schroder et al[30] demonstrated that 88% of spinoglenoid cysts associated with labral tears resolved with overall excellent shoulder outcome scores after labral repair without formal cyst decompression. Therefore, the indication for cyst decompression remains unclear. Because the authors of this chapter consider decompression of the cyst to be simple and to add little time or complexity to the labral repair, it is performed in all cases.

COMPLICATIONS

Surgeons reported a complication rate for SLAP repairs of 4.7%.[31] Postoperative stiffness is the most common complication. The inappropriate repair of normal anatomic variants such as a Buford complex or sublabral recess results in an overtightened shoulder and unsatisfactory outcomes.[32] In addition, scarring of the rotator interval and superior labral recess may result in a restricted range of motion postoperatively. Most cases are managed nonsurgically with aggressive stretching, oral medication, and glenohumeral cortisone injection. When adequate motion is not restored by 6 to 12 months postoperatively, arthroscopic capsular release and manipulation should be considered.

Pain or tenosynovitis in the long head of the biceps is the second most common complication following SLAP repair. Byram et al[33] identified a group of patients who demonstrated humeral head abrasion under the biceps tendon in patients with failed SLAP repairs. These patients were significantly older and the authors theorized that older patients with bicipital tendinitis may experience increased friction under the biceps, which may increase the contact pressure on the humeral head. In addition, overconstraint of the biceps altered the biceps tracking, which resulted in secondary tenosynovitis. Initially, nonsurgical management is undertaken, including NSAIDs and potential biceps sheath injection. In cases of persistent pain localized to the long head of the biceps tendon, tenodesis may be considered.

Prominent hardware following SLAP repair can result in catastrophic chondromalacia. One series of 24 failed SLAP repairs demonstrated 2 shoulders with severe iatrogenic arthritis and 14 shoulders with articular damage.[34] Caution should be exercised when treating a SLAP tear in older patients because the patients may have better results with a tenotomy or tenodesis. In addition, to minimize the risk of subsequent chondral injury, careful attention to detail during hardware placement is imperative at the time of the index surgery. The treatment of young patients in whom significant postoperative chondromalacia develops postoperatively is difficult, and only limited salvage surgical options are available.

Iatrogenic injury to the suprascapular nerve has been reported with anchor placement, with the distal tip protruding beyond the medial cortical bone of the glenoid.[35] In a cadaver study, all 12 suture anchors placed arthroscopically violated the medial glenoid neck, and 4 anchors came into direct contact with the suprascapular nerve directly.[33,36] Patients with decreased acromiohumeral distances were at increased risk for medial perforation of the glenoid. The low acromion prevented a satisfactory trajectory for anchor placement. Careful attention to preoperative radiographs can help with portal selection and placement. Koh et al[36] also suggested using a shorter drill bit and associated anchor to minimize suprascapular nerve compromise. Lehtinen et al[23] showed that an anchor trajectory of 30° from the articular surface maximizes bone support.

Outcomes

Studies evaluating primary repair have demonstrated relatively unpredictable results. To date, most studies have been retrospective cases series with a heterogeneous patient population frequently undergoing adjunctive procedures. Results have also varied, depending on different patient demographics including age and activity level. Many of the current outcome measures that are commonly used do not capture outcomes regarding return to high-level sports, which is often the indication for SLAP repair in the younger population.

In patients with type II SLAP repair, Denard et al[37] reported a 91% patient satisfaction rate and 82% return to his or her previous athletic level. The authors reported worse outcomes in workers' compensation cases and older patients. Friel et al[38] showed that 76% of patients had good or excellent outcomes after type II SLAP repair. Other studies, however, have demonstrated less successful results. Coleman et al[14] demonstrated that only 65% of patients who underwent isolated type II SLAP repair had good or excellent outcomes. Verma et al[39] showed that although pain scores improved after SLAP repair, all patients maintained significant postoperative pain scores. Furthermore, only 37% of workers' compensation patients who underwent type II SLAP repair were able to return to his or her previous level of work. Alpert et al[40] showed that 14% of young patients who underwent isolated SLAP repair would not undergo the same surgery again. Kim et al[34] showed that overhead athletes had significantly lower shoulder and function scores compared with nonoverhead athletes. Boileau et al[41] reported low patient satisfaction (40%) and return to previous level of sport (20%), suggesting that primary tenodesis is appropriate, especially in the older population.

Conclusion

Multiple techniques have been described to address SLAP lesions. Successful treatment is predicated on the correlation of history, physical examination, imaging, and intraoperative findings. A thorough workup should exclude other causes of pain or dysfunction. An understanding of pathology, anatomy, and surgical implants should be used to minimize complications. Appropriately selected patients can realize excellent outcomes after surgical intervention.

References

1. Andrews JR, Carson WG Jr, McLeod WD: Glenoid labrum tears related to the long head of the biceps. *Am J Sports Med* 1985;13(5):337-341.
2. Snyder SJ, Karzel RP, Del Pizzo W, Ferkel RD, Friedman MJ: SLAP lesions of the shoulder. *Arthroscopy* 1990;6(4):274-279.
3. Keener JD, Brophy RH: Superior labral tears of the shoulder: Pathogenesis, evaluation, and treatment. *J Am Acad Orthop Surg* 2009;17(10):627-637.
4. Schulz CU, Anetzberger H, Maier M, Pfahler M, Refior HJ: The sublabral foramen. Congenital or an acquired variance? *Unfallchirurg* 2002;105(12):1088-1091.
5. Morgan CD, Burkhart SS, Palmeri M, Gillespie M: Type II SLAP lesions: Three subtypes and their relationships to superior instability and rotator cuff tears. *Arthroscopy* 1998;14(6):553-565.
6. Powell SE, Nord KD, Ryu RK: The diagnosis, classification, and treatment of SLAP lesions. *Oper Tech Sports Med* 2004;12:99-110.
7. Maffet MW, Gartsman GM, Moseley B: Superior labrum-biceps tendon complex lesions of the shoulder. *Am J Sports Med* 1995;23(1):93-98.
8. Amin MF, Youssef AO: The diagnostic value of magnetic resonance arthrography of the shoulder in detection and grading of SLAP lesions: Comparison with arthroscopic findings. *Eur J Radiol* 2012;81(9): 2343-2347.

9. Iqbal HJ, Rani S, Mahmood A, Brownson P, Aniq H: Diagnostic value of MR arthrogram in SLAP lesions of the shoulder. *Surgeon* 2010;8(6):303-309.
10. Jee WH, McCauley TR, Katz LD, Matheny JM, Ruwe PA, Daigneault JP: Superior labral anterior posterior (SLAP) lesions of the glenoid labrum: Reliability and accuracy of MR arthrography for diagnosis. *Radiology* 2001;218(1):127-132.
11. Reuss BL, Schwartzberg R, Zlatkin MB, Cooperman A, Dixon JR: Magnetic resonance imaging accuracy for the diagnosis of superior labrum anterior-posterior lesions in the community setting: Eighty-three arthroscopically confirmed cases. *J Shoulder Elbow Surg* 2006;15(5): 580-585.
12. Edwards SL, Lee JA, Bell JE, et al: Nonoperative treatment of superior labrum anterior posterior tears: Improvements in pain, function, and quality of life. *Am J Sports Med* 2010;38(7):1456-1461.
13. Pillai G, Baynes JR, Gladstone J, Flatow EL: Greater strength increase with cyst decompression and SLAP repair than SLAP repair alone. *Clin Orthop Relat Res* 2011;469(4):1056-1060.
14. Coleman SH, Cohen DB, Drakos MC, et al: Arthroscopic repair of type II superior labral anterior posterior lesions with and without acromioplasty: A clinical analysis of 50 patients. *Am J Sports Med* 2007;35(5): 749-753.
15. Enad JG, Gaines RJ, White SM, Kurtz CA: Arthroscopic superior labrum anterior-posterior repair in military patients. *J Shoulder Elbow Surg* 2007;16(3):300-305.
16. Sileo MJ, Lee SJ, Kremenic IJ, et al: Biomechanical comparison of a knotless suture anchor with standard suture anchor in the repair of type II SLAP tears. *Arthroscopy* 2009;25(4):348-354.
17. Yoo JC, Ahn JH, Lee SH, et al: A biomechanical comparison of repair techniques in posterior type II superior labral anterior and posterior (SLAP) lesions. *J Shoulder Elbow Surg* 2008;17(1):144-149.
18. Domb BG, Ehteshami JR, Shindle MK, et al: Biomechanical comparison of 3 suture anchor configurations for repair of type II SLAP lesions. *Arthroscopy* 2007;23(2):135-140.
19. DiRaimondo CA, Alexander JW, Noble PC, Lowe WR, Lintner DM: A biomechanical comparison of repair techniques for type II SLAP lesions. *Am J Sports Med* 2004;32(3):727-733.
20. Uggen C, Wei A, Glousman RE, et al: Biomechanical comparison of knotless anchor repair versus simple suture repair for type II SLAP lesions. *Arthroscopy* 2009;25(10):1085-1092.
21. Yoneda M, Hirooka A, Saito S, Yamamoto T, Ochi T, Shino K: Arthroscopic stapling for detached superior glenoid labrum. *J Bone Joint Surg Br* 1991;73(5): 746-750.
22. Kartus J, Kartus C, Brownlow H, Burrow G, Perko M: Repair of type-2 SLAP lesions using Corkscrew anchors: A preliminary report of the clinical results. *Knee Surg Sports Traumatol Arthrosc* 2004;12(3):229-234.
23. Lehtinen JT, Tingart MJ, Apreleva M, Ticker JB, Warner JJ: Anatomy of the superior glenoid rim: Repair of superior labral anterior to posterior tears. *Am J Sports Med* 2003;31(2):257-260.
24. Dines JS, Elattrache NS: Horizontal mattress with a knotless anchor to better recreate the normal superior labrum anatomy. *Arthroscopy* 2008;24(12):1422-1425.
25. Ozbaydar M, Elhassan B, Warner JJ: The use of anchors in shoulder surgery: A shift from metallic to bioabsorbable anchors. *Arthroscopy* 2007;23(10):1124-1126.
26. Park MJ, Hsu JE, Harper C, Sennett BJ, Huffman GR: Poly-L/D-lactic acid anchors are associated with reoperation and failure of SLAP repairs. *Arthroscopy* 2011;27(10):1335-1340.
27. Morgan RJ, Kuremsky MA, Peindl RD, Fleischli JE: A biomechanical comparison of two suture anchor configurations for the repair of type II SLAP lesions subjected to a peel-back mechanism of failure. *Arthroscopy* 2008;24(4):383-388.
28. Baldini T, Snyder RL, Peacher G, Bach J, McCarty E: Strength of single- versus double-anchor repair of type II SLAP lesions: A cadaveric study. *Arthroscopy* 2009;25(11):1257-1260.
29. Boddula MR, Adamson GJ, Gupta A, McGarry MH, Lee TQ: Restoration of labral anatomy and biomechanics after superior labral anterior-posterior repair: Comparison of mattress versus simple technique. *Am J Sports Med* 2012;40(4):875-881.
30. Schroder CP, Skare O, Stiris M, Gjengedal E, Uppheim G, Brox JI: Treatment of labral tears with associated spinoglenoid cysts without cyst decompression. *J Bone Joint Surg Am* 2008;90(3):523-530.
31. Weber SC, Martin DF, Seiler JG III, Harrast JJ: Superior labrum anterior and posterior lesions of the shoulder:

Incidence rates, complications, and outcomes as reported by American Board of Orthopedic Surgery: Part II candidates. *Am J Sports Med* 2012;40(7):1538-1543.

32. Silberberg JM, Moya-Angeler J, Martín E, Leyes M, Forriol F: Vertical versus horizontal suture configuration for the repair of isolated type II SLAP lesion through a single anterior portal: A randomized controlled trial. *Arthroscopy* 2011;27(12):1605-1613.
33. Byram IR, Dunn WR, Kuhn JE: Humeral head abrasion: An association with failed superior labrum anterior posterior repairs. *J Shoulder Elbow Surg* 2011;20(1):92-97.
34. Kim S-H, Koh Y-G, Sung C-H, Moon H-K, Park Y-S: Iatrogenic suprascapular nerve injury after repair of type II SLAP lesion. *Arthroscopy* 2010;26(7):1005-1008.
35. Modarresi S, Motamedi D, Jude CM: Superior labral anteroposterior lesions of the shoulder: Part 1. Anatomy and anatomic variants. *AJR Am J Roentgenol* 2011;197(3):596-603.
36. Koh KH, Park WH, Lim TK, Yoo JC: Medial perforation of the glenoid neck following SLAP repair places the suprascapular nerve at risk: A cadaveric study. *J Shoulder Elbow Surg* 2011;20(2):245-250.
37. Denard PJ, Lädermann A, Burkhart SS: Long-term outcome after arthroscopic repair of type II SLAP lesions: Results according to age and workers' compensation status. *Arthroscopy* 2012;28(4):451-457.
38. Friel NA, Karas V, Slabaugh MA, Cole BJ: Outcomes of type II superior labrum, anterior to posterior (SLAP) repair: Prospective evaluation at a minimum two-year follow-up. *J Shoulder Elbow Surg* 2010;19(6):859-867.
39. Verma NN, Garretson R, Romeo AA: Outcome of arthroscopic repair of type II SLAP lesions in worker's compensation patients. *HSS J* 2007;3(1):58-62.
40. Alpert JM, Verma N, Wysocki R, Yanke AB, Romeo AA: Arthroscopic treatment of multidirectional shoulder instability with minimum 270 degrees labral repair: Minimum 2-year follow-up. *Arthroscopy* 2008;24(6):704-711.
41. Boileau P, Parratte S, Chuinard C, Roussanne Y, Shia D, Bicknell R: Arthroscopic treatment of isolated type II SLAP lesions: Biceps tenodesis as an alternative to reinsertion. *Am J Sports Med* 2009;37(5):929-936.

CHAPTER 9

Injuries to the Biceps Pulley

Arnaud Godenèche, MD
Laurent Nové-Josserand, MD
Stéphane Audebert, MD
Bruno Toussaint, MD
Allan Young, MBBS, MSpMed, PhD, FRACS
Gilles Walch, MD

Introduction

Walch et al[1] demonstrated the clinical importance of the biceps reflection pulley system, which stabilizes the long head of the biceps (LHB) tendon as it exits the joint. The LHB tendon travels intra-articularly, and the shape of the bony bicipital groove contributes to the stability of the LHB tendon. However, the biceps reflection pulley, a soft-tissue sling, is fundamental to the stabilization of the course of the tendon. This chapter describes the anatomy of the biceps pulley, the functional anatomy and the pathomechanics of injury, pulley lesions seen both at arthroscopy and with imaging, and how to treat these lesions. A personal prospective series of patients who underwent arthroscopic shoulder surgery in cases of subscapularis tendon tears was analyzed to determine the prevalence of pulley lesions.

Anatomy

The biceps reflection pulley is composed of fibers of the superior glenohumeral ligament (SGHL), the coracohumeral ligament (CHL), and partially of fibers from the subscapularis and supraspinatus tendons. The anatomy of this biceps pulley is intimately linked to the anatomy of the rotator interval, and therefore related to stability of the LHB.

Jost et al[2] described the anatomy of the rotator interval as follows: The lateral part consists of four layers, from superficial to deep. Layer 1 consists of the superficial fibers of the CHL that cover the rotator interval and extend to the insertion points of the subscapularis and supraspinatus tendons. Layer 2 consists of the fibers of the supraspinatus and subscapularis tendons that crisscross the rotator interval to blend into each other and

---

Dr. Godenèche or an immediate family member has received royalties from Tornier; and serves as a paid consultant to or is an employee of Mitek. Dr. Toussaint or an immediate family member has received royalties from Total Shoulder Prosthesis; is a member of a speakers' bureau or has made paid presentations on behalf of Smith & Nephew; and serves as a paid consultant to or is an employee of Arthrex, Smith & Nephew, Biomet Sports & Medicine, Zimmer, and DePuy. Dr. Young or an immediate family member serves as a paid consultant to or is an employee of Rotation Medical; and has received nonincome support (such as equipment or services), commercially derived honoraria, or other non–research-related funding (such as paid travel) from Tornier. Dr. Walch or an immediate family member has received royalties from Tornier; has received nonincome support (such as equipment or services), commercially derived honoraria, or other non–research-related funding (such as paid travel) from Tornier. Neither of the following authors nor any immediate family member has received anything of value from or has stock or stock options held in a commercial company or institution related directly or indirectly to the subject of this chapter: Dr. Nové-Josserand and Dr. Audebert.

FIGURE 1

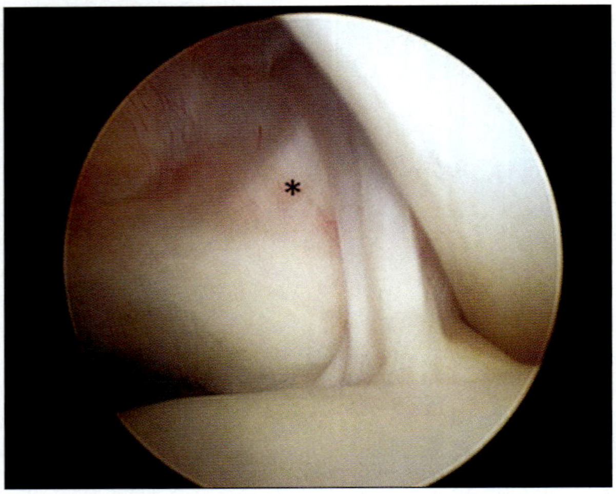

Arthroscopic view shows the normal anatomy of the subscapularis tendon and the biceps pulley. The asterisk indicates where fibers of the superior glenohumeral ligament and coracohumeral ligament complex insert onto the subscapularis tendon.

with parts of the CHL. Layer 3 consists of the deep fibers of the CHL; the main part inserts at the greater tuberosity and the smaller part inserts at the lesser tuberosity. Layer 4 consists of the SGHL and the joint capsule. The three superficial layers form a fibrous plate that fills the lateral rotator interval region.

The medial part of the rotator interval consists of two layers, superficial and deep. Layer 1 consists of the CHL. Layer 2 consists of the SGHL and the joint capsule. The CHL and the SGHL form a band that covers the LHB tendon anteriorly (superficially and deep, respectively) and ends at the lesser tuberosity.

A histologic, anatomic study by Boon et al[3] showed that a posterolateral extension of the subscapularis tendon interdigitates with the supraspinatus tendon. The biceps tendon is unsheathed by interwoven fibers that may be derived from the subscapularis and supraspinatus tendons at the proximal end of the bicipital groove.

Lo and Burkhart[4] were the first to describe the arthroscopic comma sign, an arc formed by a portion of the superior of the SGHL/CHL complex, a useful marker of the superolateral corner of a torn, retracted subscapularis tendon. The SGHL/CHL complex and the subscapularis tendon are intimately associated at their insertions onto the lesser tuberosity; classically, the SGHL inserts proximal to the subscapularis insertion on the lesser tuberosity (**Figure 1**). This close association is likely the reason that these structures can simultaneously tear away from the humerus but remain attached to one another.

Functional Anatomy

Cadaver studies have shown the CHL as the key ligament responsible for maintaining LHB alignment within the bicipital groove.[5,6] Furthermore, Werner et al[7] and Habermeyer et al[8] found that the orientation of the SGHL fibers toward the LHB seemed to withstand anterior shearing forces in the lateral rotator interval, indicating that the primary function of the SGHL stabilized the LHB in its intra-articular course. SGHL tears have been shown to result in instability and medial subluxation of the LHB.

Other authors have suggested that the SGHL and CHL act as a pulley system for the LHB. Walch et al[1] and Kolts et al[9] showed that the SGHL can be separate from the CHL medially, but they are united at the lateral rotator interval (**Figure 2**). However, Boardman et al[10] reported that meticulous blunt dissection allowed complete separation of the CHL from the SGHL. Gambill et al[11] reported a unique case of a dislocated LHB tendon over intact subscapularis and supraspinatus tendons in a patient with traumatic posterior instability of the shoulder. This dislocation probably resulted from injury to the CHL, SGHL, and other soft-tissue structures contained within the rotator interval and shows the importance of the rotator interval as a restraint to biceps subluxation.

However, many studies have shown that the subscapularis tendon is a key structure in the LHB pulley system and plays a crucial role in stabilization. Sakurai et al[12] performed an anatomic, clinical, and MRI-based study showing that most of the pathologic changes of the subscapularis tendon occurred on the articular side of the subscapularis tendon. In the cadaver specimens with an articular-side incomplete tear, the height of the medial wall of the bicipital groove was decreased, potentially causing medial subluxation or dislocation of the LHB. Arai et al[13] described how the superiormost part of the subscapularis tendon attaches to the upper margin of the lesser tuberosity and extends to the fovea capitis of the humerus (a distinct depression, such as found on the femur) as a thin, tendinous "slip." The SGHL runs spirally along the biceps tendon and histologically attaches to the tendinous slip. The SGHL attaches to the tendinous slip of the subscapularis insertion as a fold of loose connective tissue and directly supports the LHB. The CHL, which is also a part of the same loose connective tissue, provides tension to the SGHL. The superiormost insertion point of the subscapularis tendon supports the LHB from behind the SGHL. Bennett[14] confirmed this with an arthroscopic study showing that the outer surface of the subscapularis tendon is intimately associated with the CHL and the SGHL with interdigitating fibers. This pulley system protects the biceps tendon from subluxation. Except in very rare cases of LHB tendon dislocation with an intact subscapularis tendon,[1,11] LHB instability is always associated with a subscapularis tendon tear.[15,16]

Pathophysiology

Le Huec et al[17] described a series of traumatic rotator interval or pulley lesions. Most lesions resulted from trauma sustained with the arm in internal rotation; however, pulley lesions can also result from a fall onto an outstretched arm (in either full internal or external rotation) or a fall backward onto the hand or elbow. Furthermore, a forcefully stopped overhead throwing motion may result in a pulley lesion.[8] Eccentric contraction of the biceps muscle slows elbow extension in the deceleration and follow-through phases of the throwing motion and the strain in the LHB tendon increases during deceleration, which provokes maximum LHB contraction and can cause tears in the rotator interval capsule.

Degenerative causes have also been proposed for pulley lesions. Gerber and Sebesta[18] described intra-articular impingement that was responsible for painful structural disease of the shoulder. With the arm in a position of horizontal adduction and internal rotation, the undersurface of the reflection pulley and the subscapularis tendon impinge against the anterosuperior glenoid rim. This appears to be a possible cause of pulley lesions and subscapularis tendon lesions. With the arm in more than 90° of elevation, the zone of mechanical contact occurs between the LHB and the pulley region and superiormost aspect of the labrum. With a decrease in elevation, impingement occurs between the tendinous insertion of the subscapularis and the anterior glenoid labrum and rim.

FIGURE 2

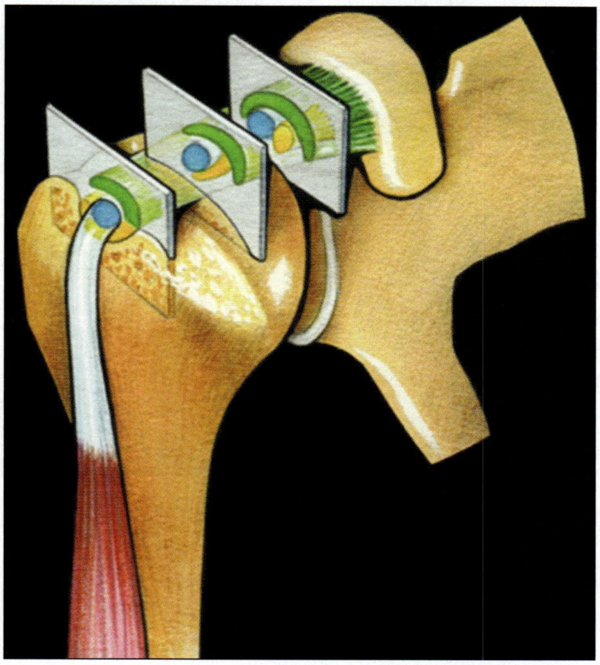

Illustration of the supeior glenohumeral ligament/coracohumeral ligament (SGHL/CHL) complex (green) shows the relationship of the CHL, SGHL, and long head of the biceps (blue) from medial to lateral. (Reproduced with permission from Walch G, Nové-Josserand L, Boileau P, Levigne C: Subluxations and dislocations of the tendon of the long head of the biceps. *J Shoulder Elbow Surg* 1998;7[2]:100-108.)

Habermeyer et al[8] described internal anterosuperior impingement of the shoulder associated with lesions of the biceps pulley and the rotator cuff. The authors determined that a progressive lesion of the pulley system, which may include a partial tear of the subscapularis and supraspinatus tendons, contributes significantly to the development of anterosuperior impingement. A pulley lesion can result in LHB instability, causing increased passive anterior translation and an upward migration of the humeral head, resulting in anterosuperior impingement. In addition, a partial articular-side tear of the subscapularis and supraspinatus reinforces anterosuperior impingement.

FIGURE 3

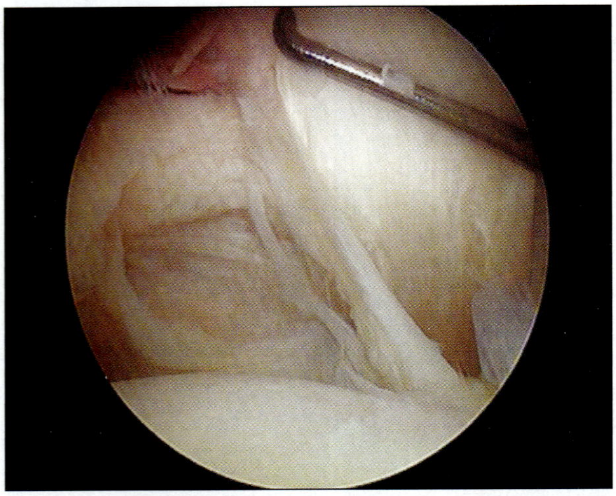

Arthroscopic view shows an intact but stretched biceps pulley with a torn subscapularis tendon and a pathologic long head of the biceps tendon.

Braun et al[19] performed a biomechanical study that evaluated the shear force vectors resulting in injury of the biceps reflection pulley. The authors showed that the increased shear load in forward flexion with internal or neutral rotation and in neutral flexion with internal rotation may cause direct injury to the biceps reflection pulley during high loads. The authors suggested that the mechanisms could result in wear and failure of the biceps reflection pulley in common working positions, particularly when working and/or lifting overhead, or when lifting heavy weights with the arms in front of the body (for example, when performing biceps curls).

Arthroscopic Evaluation

Braun et al[20] analyzed the pathoanatomy of the biceps pulley in 229 consecutive patients who underwent shoulder arthroscopy. The authors showed a significant association between pathologic abnormalities of the LHB and tears of the pulley system. Furthermore, superior labrum anterior to posterior tears showed a significant association with biceps pulley tears.

The prevalence of biceps pulley tears increased with the presence of a torn rotator cuff. Pulley tears had a significant association with rotator cuff lesions, particularly for lesions of the supraspinatus and subscapularis tendons. Lafosse et al[21] also reported that partial lesions of the subscapularis tendon were significantly more frequent in patients with anterior dislocation of the LHB tendon than in patients with anterior subluxation. Moreover, pulley tears were more common in older patients, which may indicate a degenerative process. Finally, the width of the LHB tendon was substantially greater when a pulley tear was present. This supports the theory by Boileau et al[22] that hourglass deformities of the LHB can cause injury to the pulley.

Personal Series

In association with the French Arthroscopic Society, the authors of this chapter prospectively collected data on 218 consecutive patients who underwent arthroscopic treatment for a subscapularis tear between March, 2010 and January, 2011.[23] All patients had severe impairment and pain, especially at night. Four senior surgeons analyzed the video data of all 218 procedures. Each patient had subscapularis tendon involvement, either isolated or in association with a partial or small nonretracted supraspinatus tear. The SGHL/CHL lesions (normal, stretched, absent) were analyzed (**Figure 3**). The LHB was assessed for stability (centered, subluxated, dislocated, torn) and tendinosis (normal, pathologic, torn). Distal to the SGHL/CHL complex, the soft-tissue medial wall of the bicipital sheath (normal, partially torn, completely torn) in the bicipital groove was analyzed.

Of 218 patients, the SGHL/CHL complex was normal in 54 patients (25%), stretched in 84 (39%), absent in 77 (35%), and not documented in 3 (1%). The data regarding the relationships between the SGHL/CHL complex and the LHB lesions are summarized in **Tables 1** and **2**. In the bicipital groove distal to the SGHL/CHL complex, the medial wall of the LHB tendon sheath was normal in 25% of patients, partially torn in 39%, completely torn in 35%, and not documented in 1%. A pathologic LHB with an intact SGHL/CHL complex was observed in 25 patients. Of these, 92% had a torn medial wall of the bicipital sheath (**Figure 4**).

This study showed that with a subscapularis tear and an intact SGHL/CHL complex, the LHB was usually centered. Nevertheless, tendinosis or a tear of the LHB was observed for at least one half of all occurrences because of a lesion in the medial wall of the bicipital sheath distal to the SGHL/CHL complex. These data

TABLE 1 **Stability of the Long Head of the Biceps**

Stability	SHGL/CHL Complex Normal (n = 54)	 Stretched (n = 84)	 Absent (n = 77)
Centered	87%	18%	16%
Subluxated	4%	64%	38%
Dislocated	0%	4%	23%
Completely torn	2%	10%	19%
Not documented	7%	5%	4%

CHL = coracohumeral ligament, LHB = long head of the biceps, SGHL = superior glenohumeral ligament.

TABLE 2 **Diagnosis of the Long Head of the Biceps**

Diagnosis	SHGL/CHL Complex Normal (n = 54)	 Stretched (n = 84)	 Absent (n = 77)
Normal	41%	17%	12%
Tendinosis	46%	68%	66%
Completely torn	2%	9%	19%
Not documented	11%	6%	3%

FIGURE 4

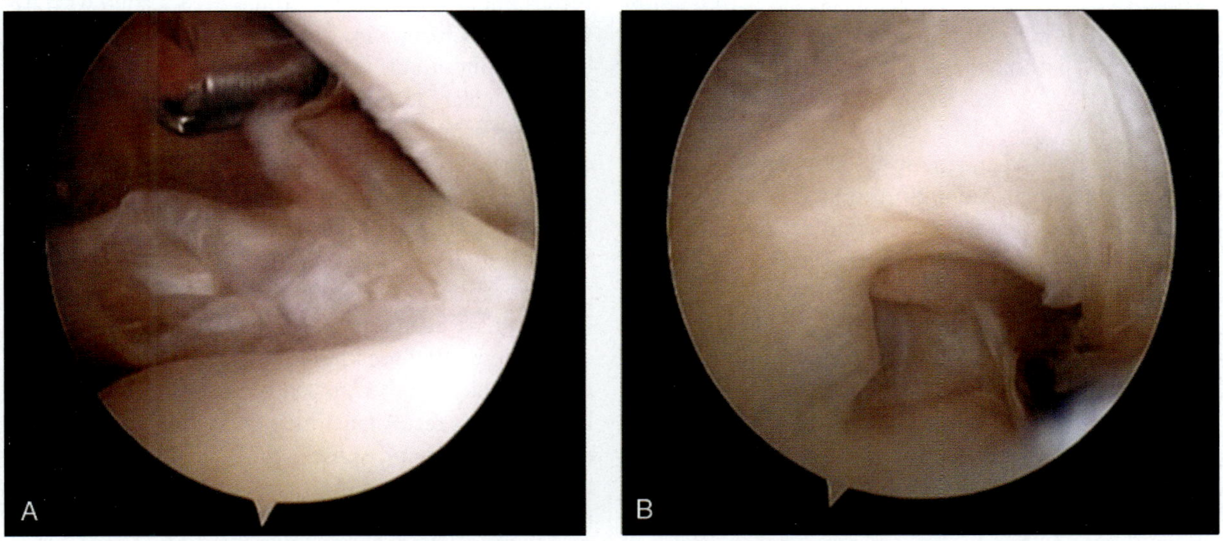

Arthroscopic views show an intact supeior glenohumeral ligament/coracohumeral ligament complex and a partial deep subscapularis tear (**A**), and an intra-articular lesion of the medial wall of the intertubercular groove with a tear in contact with the subscapularis footprint (**B**).

FIGURE 5

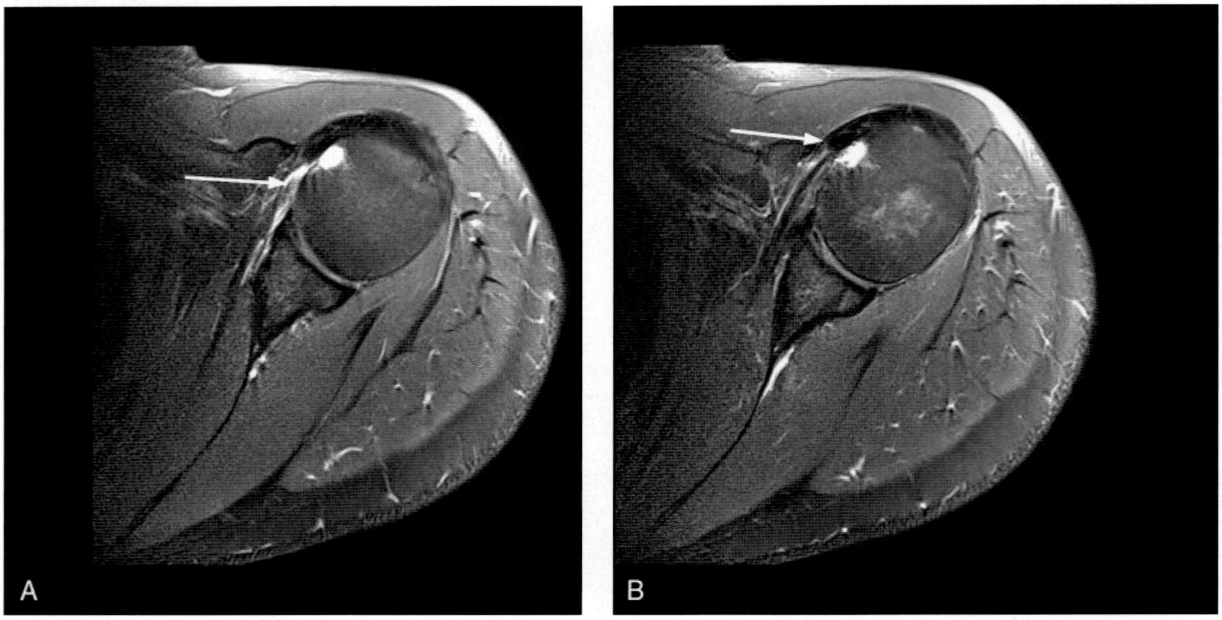

MRI shows a pulley lesion (arrow) with a partial tear of the proximal subscapularis (**A**) and subluxation (arrow) of the long head of the biceps (**B**).

confirmed that the subscapularis tendon is important for LHB stability and should be included in the pulley system. When a subscapularis tear occurs with a lesion of the SGHL/CHL complex, the LHB is almost always unstable and pathologic.

Imaging

Nakata et al[24] used magnetic resonance arthrography with intra-articular gadolinium injection to help analyze the biceps pulley and the surrounding musculotendinous structures (the LHB, labrum, and rotator cuff). The authors of this chapter also use MRI (**Figure 5**). Magnetic resonance arthrography clearly demonstrates the normal anatomy and pathologic conditions of this area, as well as any associated findings. Oblique sagittal and axial images should be obtained for the evaluation of pulley lesions. Injury to the anterosuperior aspect of the shoulder is better understood as part of a spectrum of pathology than simply as an isolated lesion. When an abnormality of one component of the system is suspected, a thorough imaging assessment of the entire system is especially important.

Treatment of Biceps Pulley Lesions

Biceps pulley lesions are commonly associated with pathology and instability of the LHB tendon, usually in cases of rotator cuff tears. Medical treatment involving intra-articular steroid injection, usually performed under fluoroscopic or ultrasonographic guidance, can be effective for pain relief.

The pain likely results from the windshield wiper effect, and standard surgical treatment includes either biceps tenodesis or tenotomy. However, residual discomfort and muscle spasm, in addition to cosmetic deformity, have been reported following both procedures, and the potential for functional impairment is controversial. Maier et al[25] reported the results of open stabilization with reconstruction of the pulley system and repair of traumatic subscapularis tears with unstable but structurally intact LHB tendons. The procedure was performed in the acute phase following injury. The authors obtained good functional outcomes and recommended this procedure as an alternative to tenodesis or tenotomy, particularly for young patients.

FIGURE 6

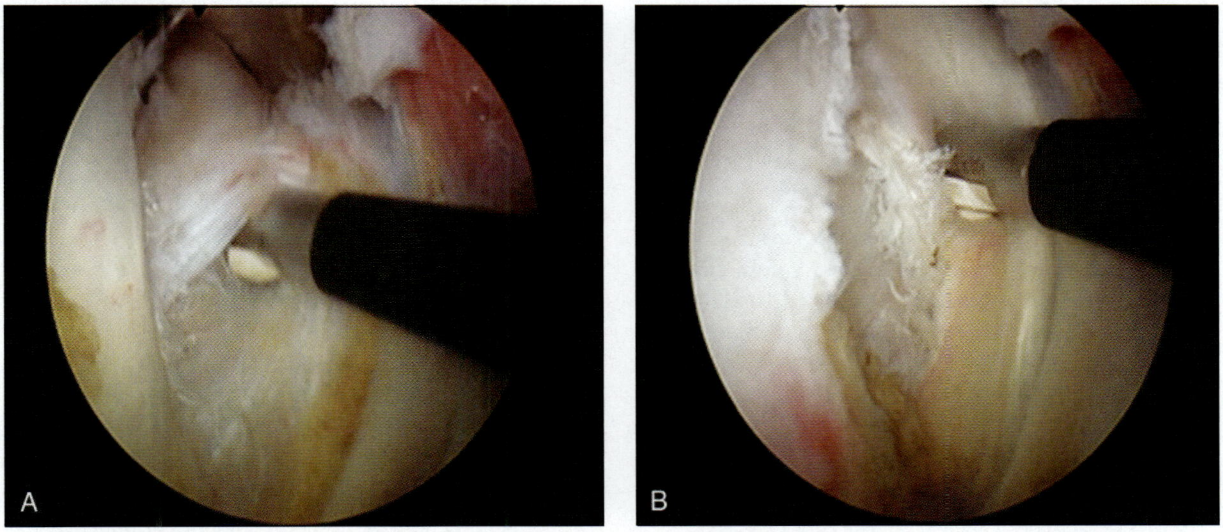

Arthroscopic views show an extra-articular lesion of the medial wall of the bicipital groove with a partial subscapularis tear (**A**), and instability and severe tendinosis of the long head of the biceps, with a normal supeior glenohumeral ligament/coracohumeral ligament complex and a normal intra-articular subscapularis tendon (**B**).

Walch et al,[26] Edwards et al,[27] and Boileau et al[28] have all shown that both arthroscopic biceps tenotomy and tenodesis can effectively treat severe pain or dysfunction in selected patients with rotator cuff tears associated with a biceps lesion. Arthroscopic biceps tenotomy does not appear to alter the natural progressive radiographic changes occurring with long-standing rotator cuff tears.

Conclusion

The biceps pulley system, including the SGHL/CHL complex and subscapularis tendon, merits recognition as an important anatomic structure, and lesions in this area contribute to shoulder pathology. In either traumatic cases or degenerative situations, biceps pulley lesions are usually associated with an LHB lesion and/or a subscapularis tear. When a subscapularis tear is suspected and the SGHL/CHL complex appears normal during arthroscopy, the LHB must be examined in the bicipital groove and the medial wall of the groove must be assessed. This assessment can be performed either intra-articularly or after opening the transverse ligament with an anterolateral extra-articular inspection (**Figure 6**). Further clinical studies are needed to confirm whether isolated LHB tenotomy or tenodesis is sufficient for surgical management of biceps pulley system tears or if additional subscapularis repair is required.

References

1. Walch G, Nové-Josserand L, Boileau P, Levigne C: Subluxations and dislocations of the tendon of the long head of the biceps. *J Shoulder Elbow Surg* 1998;7(2):100-108.
2. Jost B, Koch PP, Gerber C: Anatomy and functional aspects of the rotator interval. *J Shoulder Elbow Surg* 2000;9(4):336-341.
3. Boon JM, de Beer MA, Botha D, Maritz NG, Fouche AA: The anatomy of the subscapularis tendon insertion as applied to rotator cuff repair. *J Shoulder Elbow Surg* 2004;13(2):165-169.
4. Lo IK, Burkhart SS: The comma sign: An arthroscopic guide to the torn subscapularis tendon. *Arthroscopy* 2003;19(3):334-337.
5. Slätis P, Aalto K: Medial dislocation of the tendon of the long head of the biceps brachii. *Acta Orthop Scand* 1979;50(1):73-77.

6. Ferrari DA: Capsular ligaments of the shoulder: Anatomical and functional study of the anterior superior capsule. *Am J Sports Med* 1990;18(1):20-24.
7. Werner A, Mueller T, Boehm D, Gohlke F: The stabilizing sling for the long head of the biceps tendon in the rotator cuff interval: A histoanatomic study. *Am J Sports Med* 2000;28(1):28-31.
8. Habermeyer P, Magosch P, Pritsch M, Scheibel MT, Lichtenberg S: Anterosuperior impingement of the shoulder as a result of pulley lesions: A prospective arthroscopic study. *J Shoulder Elbow Surg* 2004;13(1):5-12.
9. Kolts I, Busch LC, Tomusk H, et al: Anatomical composition of the anterior shoulder joint capsule: A cadaver study on 12 glenohumeral joints. *Ann Anat* 2001;183(1):53-59.
10. Boardman ND, Debski RE, Warner JJ, et al: Tensile properties of the superior glenohumeral and coracohumeral ligaments. *J Shoulder Elbow Surg* 1996;5(4):249-254.
11. Gambill ML, Mologne TS, Provencher MT: Dislocation of the long head of the biceps tendon with intact subscapularis and supraspinatus tendons. *J Shoulder Elbow Surg* 2006;15(6):e20-e22.
12. Sakurai G, Ozaki J, Tomita Y, Kondo T, Tamai S: Incomplete tears of the subscapularis tendon associated with tears of the supraspinatus tendon: Cadaveric and clinical studies. *J Shoulder Elbow Surg* 1998;7(5):510-515.
13. Arai R, Mochizuki T, Yamaguchi K, et al: Functional anatomy of the superior glenohumeral and coracohumeral ligaments and the subscapularis tendon in view of stabilization of the long head of the biceps tendon. *J Shoulder Elbow Surg* 2010;19(1):58-64.
14. Bennett WF: Visualization of the anatomy of the rotator interval and bicipital sheath. *Arthroscopy* 2001;17(1):107-111.
15. Arai R, Sugaya H, Mochizuki T, Nimura A, Moriishi J, Akita K: Subscapularis tendon tear: An anatomic and clinical investigation. *Arthroscopy* 2008;24(9):997-1004.
16. Sethi N, Wright R, Yamaguchi K: Disorders of the long head of the biceps tendon. *J Shoulder Elbow Surg* 1999;8(6):644-654.
17. Le Huec JC, Schaeverbeke T, Moinard M, et al: Traumatic tear of the rotator interval. *J Shoulder Elbow Surg* 1996;5(1):41-46.
18. Gerber C, Sebesta A: Impingement of the deep surface of the subscapularis tendon and the reflection pulley on the anterosuperior glenoid rim: A preliminary report. *J Shoulder Elbow Surg* 2000;9(6):483-490.
19. Braun S, Millett PJ, Yongpravat C, et al: Biomechanical evaluation of shear force vectors leading to injury of the biceps reflection pulley: A biplane fluoroscopy study on cadaveric shoulders. *Am J Sports Med* 2010;38(5):1015-1024.
20. Braun S, Horan MP, Elser F, Millett PJ: Lesions of the biceps pulley. *Am J Sports Med* 2011;39(4):790-795.
21. Lafosse L, Reiland Y, Baier GP, Toussaint B, Jost B: Anterior and posterior instability of the long head of the biceps tendon in rotator cuff tears: A new classification based on arthroscopic observations. *Arthroscopy* 2007;23(1):73-80.
22. Boileau P, Ahrens PM, Hatzidakis AM: Entrapment of the long head of the biceps tendon: The hourglass biceps—a cause of pain and locking of the shoulder. *J Shoulder Elbow Surg* 2004;13(3):249-257.
23. Toussaint B, Audebert S, Barth J, et al: Arthroscopic repair of subscapularis tears: Preliminary data from a prospective multicentre study. *Orthop Traumatol Surg Res* 2012;98(Suppl 8):S193-S200.
24. Nakata W, Katou S, Fujita A, Nakata M, Lefor AT, Sugimoto H: Biceps pulley: Normal anatomy and associated lesions at MR arthrography. *Radiographics* 2011;31(3):791-810.
25. Maier D, Jaeger M, Suedkamp NP, Koestler W: Stabilization of the long head of the biceps tendon in the context of early repair of traumatic subscapularis tendon tears. *J Bone Joint Surg Am* 2007;89(8):1763-1769.
26. Walch G, Edwards TB, Boulahia A, Nové-Josserand L, Neyton L, Szabo I: Arthroscopic tenotomy of the long head of the biceps in the treatment of rotator cuff tears: Clinical and radiographic results of 307 cases. *J Shoulder Elbow Surg* 2005;14(3):238-246.
27. Edwards TB, Walch G, Nové-Josserand L, et al: Arthroscopic debridement in the treatment of patients with isolated tears of the subscapularis. *Arthroscopy* 2006;22(9):941-946.
28. Boileau P, Baqué F, Valerio L, Ahrens P, Chuinard C, Trojani C: Isolated arthroscopic biceps tenotomy or tenodesis improves symptoms in patients with massive irreparable rotator cuff tears. *J Bone Joint Surg Am* 2007;89(4):747-757.

CHAPTER 10

Biceps Tenotomy Versus Tenodesis

Eugene T.H. Ek, MBBS, PhD, FRACS
Lewis L. Shi, MD
Jon J.P. Warner, MD

Introduction

Pathology of the long head of the biceps (LHB) tendon often represents a significant source of shoulder pain and dysfunction.[1,2] Interestingly, the contribution of the LHB as a key pain generator is in stark contradiction to its perceived lack of importance in overall shoulder function of individuals who do not participate in overhead throwing sports. Nevertheless, the LHB is one of the most commonly treated structures within the shoulder because it is frequently associated with other conditions such as chronic rotator cuff tears, impingement, and glenohumeral arthritis.[3-5]

LHB disease comprises a spectrum of pathologic processes that include degenerative tendinosis, inflammatory tendinitis, partial tendon tears, and tendon instability.[6,7] LHB disease commonly manifests as anterior shoulder pain and tenderness over the bicipital groove, and positive results for several clinical tests such as the Speed, Yergason, O'Brien, and the dynamic labral shear tests.[8,9] The pathogenesis of LHB pathology is likely to be secondary to a combination of inflammatory, degenerative, and traumatic processes, as well as overuse conditions.[6] Therefore, LHB disease almost universally has concomitant pathologies such as rotator cuff tears, glenohumeral arthritis, biceps pulley lesions, impingement, superior labral tears, and acromioclavicular joint degeneration.[7] Isolated biceps tendinitis does occur, but with a reported incidence of approximately 5%.[10]

When nonsurgical measures fail, the surgical treatment of LHB pathology, irrespective of the underlying cause, most commonly involves simple biceps tenotomy at its superior labral insertion with or without tenodesis. Both tenotomy and tenodesis have proved extremely effective in relieving pain and restoring shoulder function.[11-14] However, no consensus exists as to whether tenotomy or tenodesis is the ideal treatment method. This chapter discusses and compares the rationale for and clinical results of both surgical techniques and suggests relative indications for using either for the treatment of LHB pathology.

Biceps Tenotomy

In recent years, biceps tenotomy has become an increasingly more common and reliable method of treating patients with LHB pathology. Tenotomy is a technically simple operation, has low morbidity, and requires minimal postoperative rehabilitation. However, the potential disadvantages include potential cosmetic deformity (**Figure 1**) and functional weakness in elbow flexion and forearm supination.[14-16] As a result, biceps tenotomy has been generally advocated in physiologically older patients with lower physical demands.[17,18]

Dr. Warner or an immediate family member has received nonincome support (such as equipment or services), commercially derived honoraria, or other non–research-related funding (such as paid travel) from Arthrocare, DJ Orthopaedics, Arthrex, Mitek, Breg, and Smith & Nephew. Neither of the following authors nor any immediate family member has received anything of value from or has stock or stock options held in a commercial company or institution related directly or indirectly to the subject of this chapter: Dr. Ek and Dr. Shi.

FIGURE 1

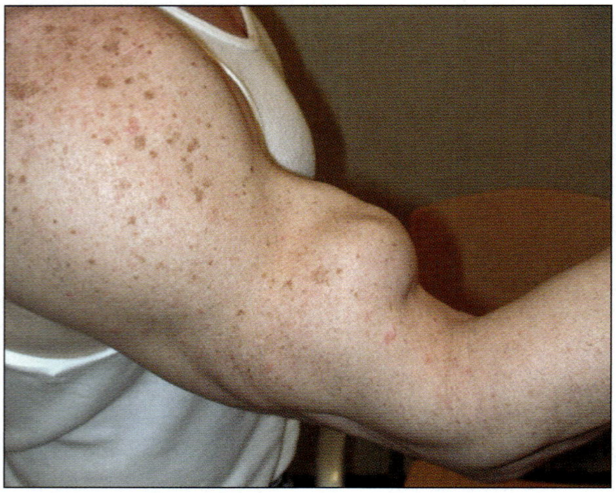

Clinical photograph demonstrates the Popeye cosmetic deformity following biceps tenotomy.

Rationale

The concept of releasing the biceps tendon at the superior labral insertion and allowing it to distally retract within the bicipital groove has been popularized by Walch et al since the late 1980s.[4,17] The authors noted that many patients with chronic rotator cuff tears achieve spontaneous symptomatic relief shortly following rupture of the biceps tendon.In 2005, Walch et al[4] reported on arthroscopic biceps tenotomy performed in 307 patients for the treatment of rotator cuff tears and demonstrated significant improvement in functional outcome with high satisfaction rates. Boileau et al[5] showed that, in patients with massive irreparable rotator cuff tears, isolated arthroscopic biceps tenotomy or tenodesis can effectively relieve severe shoulder pain and improve shoulder function.

One early concern with biceps tenotomy was potential proximal humeral head migration. Several biomechanical studies have shown that the LHB acts as a humeral head depressor and glenohumeral stabilizer.[19-21] Warner and McMahon[21] observed superior humeral head migration with various degrees of shoulder abduction on plain radiographs in seven patients following biceps tenotomy. In contrast, Yamaguchi et al[22] used electromyography to demonstrate that the LHB does not actively contract during shoulder range of motion. Furthermore, Walch et al[4] reported in a large series that early proximal humeral migration was not observed following biceps tenotomy, and Nové-Josserand et al[23] showed that LHB tendon rupture did not influence the acromiohumeral interval in 264 patients with chronic rotator cuff tears.

Indications, Technique, and Results

The primary objective of biceps tenotomy is pain relief—cosmesis and strength are less important considerations. Tenotomy is also appropriate in patients who cannot adhere to the postoperative immobilization associated with biceps tenodesis. Biceps tenotomy is usually performed arthroscopically and the tendon is cut at its superior labral insertion and allowed to retract into the bicipital groove (**Figure 2**). Tenotomy can be performed using either electrocautery or an arthroscopic cutting device. As an isolated procedure, tenotomy requires no postoperative restrictions, and the patient may wear a sling for comfort for 1 to 2 days.

The adverse effects of biceps tenotomy include the potential for biceps muscle cramping and pain, weakness with elbow flexion or supination, and cosmetic deformity.[4,14,18,24] Boileau et al[5] noted that biceps cramping occurred in 21% of patients who underwent tenotomy and 9% of patients who underwent tenodesis. In most individuals, biceps pain and cramping are associated with exertional activities; hence, in lower demand patients, this may be less problematic.[24,25] The loss of strength in elbow flexion and forearm supination in the setting of biceps tenotomy is a potential concern. With distal migration of the proximal LHB, supination strength decreased by 20% and flexion strength decreased by 8% to 20%.[26,27] In addition, distal retraction of the LHB tendon commonly results in loss of the normal biceps muscle contour, resulting in a prominent muscle belly and a cosmetic deformity called the Popeye sign (**Figure 1**). The prevalence of this deformity varies after biceps tenotomy, ranging between 3% and 70% in the literature.[18,24,28]

Duff and Campbell[16] recently compared the results of biceps tenotomy in younger, physically active patients with those of older, sedentary patients and found no significant difference in biceps cramping, weakness, or subjective appreciation of deformity. Furthermore, ob-

FIGURE 2

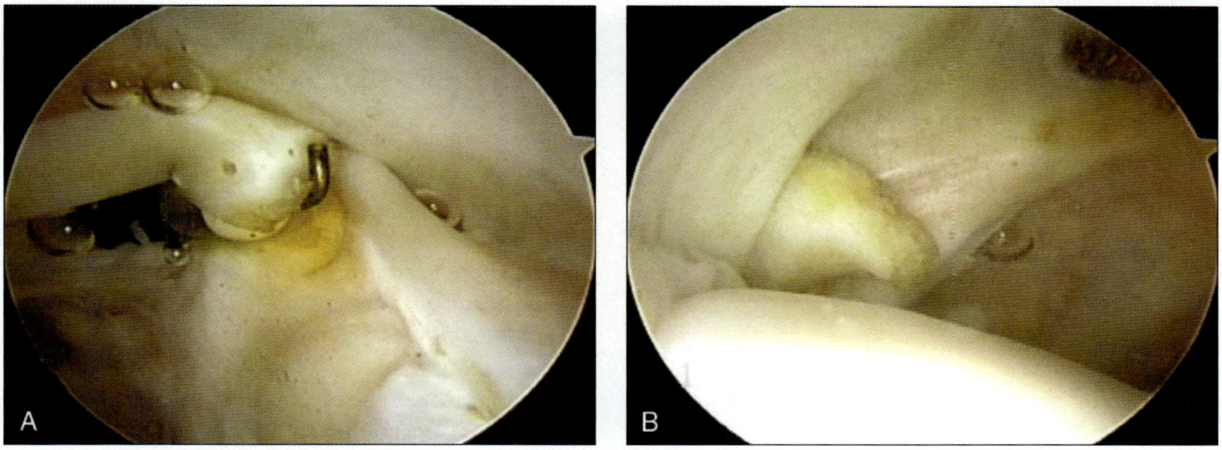

Arthroscopic views of a biceps tenotomy. **A,** The long head of the biceps tendon is divided at its insertion onto the superior labrum. **B,** Following tenotomy, the biceps tendon retracts distally into the bicipital groove.

jective strength testing revealed no significant difference in elbow flexion or forearm supination between surgical and nonsurgical sides.

The outcome of biceps tenotomy is generally good. Walch et al[4] reported on biceps tenotomy performed in 307 patients with irreparable rotator cuff tears at a mean follow-up of 57 months. The mean Constant score improved from 48.4 to 67.6 and 87% of patients reported being satisfied or very satisfied with their results. Kelly et al[25] conducted a retrospective review of 40 patients who underwent arthroscopic biceps tenotomy (9 as an isolated procedure, 31 as a combined procedure), with a minimum follow-up of 2 years. At the latest follow-up, 70% of all patients had a cosmetic deformity; men had a significantly higher incidence than women (83% vs 37%). Thirty-eight percent reported fatigue with resisted elbow flexion; however, 95% described a significant decrease in pain and no residual bicipital tenderness. Boileau et al[5] retrospectively reviewed 72 cases of irreparable rotator cuff tears that were treated with biceps tenotomy or tenodesis and found that cosmetic deformity was clinically apparent in 62% of patients in the tenotomy group. No patients were concerned or bothered by it; one third of these patients did not notice the deformity.

Biceps Tenodesis

The principal tenets of biceps tenodesis are to release the tendon at its superior labral attachment and distal reattachment either to soft tissue or bone while the normal length-tension relationship of the biceps muscle is maintained. Therefore, biceps tenodesis has the theoretical advantage of achieving a better cosmetic result and preserving strength in elbow flexion and supination. The clinical relevance of this issue is debatable. The disadvantages of tenodesis are the increased complexity and surgical time of the procedure; it often involves expensive implants, and the rehabilitation is prolonged, with a period of immobilization necessary.

Historical Perspective

In 1925, Gilcreest[29] first reported on biceps tenodesis for LHB rupture, and described transferring the biceps tendon to the base of the coracoid and suturing it to the conjoint tendon. In 1944, Lippman[30] recognized the importance of tendon–to–tendon sheath gliding as a significant contributor of pain and showed that patients achieved significant symptom relief after spontaneous adhesion of the biceps tendon to the groove. Based on this observation, Lippman[30] and Hitchcock and Bechtol[31] described techniques of securing the

TABLE 1 Options for Biceps Tenodesis

Site of tenodesis
Rotator interval
Rotator cuff tendons
Bicipital groove (proximal, mid, distal)
Subpectoral
Conjoint tendon
Mode of fixation
Sutures
Suture anchors
Knotless anchors
Keyhole tenodesis
Interference screws

tenotomized LHB into the bicipital groove using transosseous nonabsorbable sutures[30] or by placing the tendon under an osteoperiosteal sleeve raised from the floor of the bicipital groove.[31] In 1975, Froimson and O[32] popularized the keyhole technique, which involves placing a knotted biceps tendon into a keyhole-shaped cut made in the bicipital groove without needing supplemental suture fixation. Since then, the technique has gradually evolved, with multiple different methods described in the literature. Furthermore, with the advent of arthroscopy, most biceps tenodesis procedures can be performed completely arthroscopically or with arthroscopic-assisted methods using mini-open incisions.

Biceps tenodesis can be performed open, arthroscopically, or with arthroscopic assistance, and the tendon can be placed in the suprapectoral region (above the pectoralis major tendon insertion),[33] the subpectoral region (below the pectoralis major tendon insertion),[34] or on the conjoint tendon. Moreover, a range of tendon fixation methods exist including the use of interference screws,[34] suture anchors,[35] sutures to the adjacent soft tissue,[36] and keyhole fixation into the bone[32] (**Table 1**). However, given the numerous options, no single technique has demonstrated clearly superior results, and very few comparative studies have been performed to date.

Tenodesis Site

With tenodesis, the biceps can be reattached to three main regions: suprapectoral, subpectoral, and to the conjoint tendon. Within the suprapectoral region, the tenotomized tendon can be secured to the soft tissues in the rotator interval,[36,37] to the rotator cuff tendons,[38] or into the bone at various sites along the bicipital groove.[32,33,37,39] One advantage of suprapectoral tenodesis is that it can be performed completely arthroscopically using modern instrumentation that enables insertion of suture anchors or interference screws to secure the tendon.[39-41] However, the disadvantage is that suprapectoral tenodesis may be technically more challenging, resulting in increased surgical time. Subpectoral tenodesis is most commonly performed via a small incision, which can be placed in the axilla for cosmesis (**Figure 3**). With this approach, the LHB tendon is identified after retracting the pectoralis major tendon proximally and laterally, and tenodesis is performed most commonly using suture anchors or interference screws.[35,42]

Currently, most biceps tenodesis procedures are performed either in the suprapectoral or subpectoral region. However, Verma et al[43] described arthroscopic transfer of the LHB tendon to the conjoint tendon, with reported results that were comparable with other techniques.[44] The main advantage of transfer to the conjoint tendon is that no implants are required.

Two level III studies compared clinical results based on the site of tenodesis. Lutton et al[33] conducted a study of 17 patients who underwent suprapectoral tenodesis and reported that tenodesis distal to the bicipital groove (10 patients) resulted in a significantly lower incidence of postoperative anterior shoulder pain (0%) compared with tenodesis more proximally along the groove (7 patients; incidence of pain, 28.6%). Sanders et al[45] conducted a study of 127 patients and reported that the revision rate for bicipital groove pain was significantly lower for subpectoral tenodesis (7.7%) compared with suprapectoral tenodesis (23.3%). In addition, the authors noted that when the transverse humeral ligament was released in conjunction with biceps tenodesis, the revision rate was 6.8% compared with 30.4% when not released.

Tendon Fixation

With the transition from routinely open procedures to predominantly minimally invasive or arthroscopic

FIGURE 3

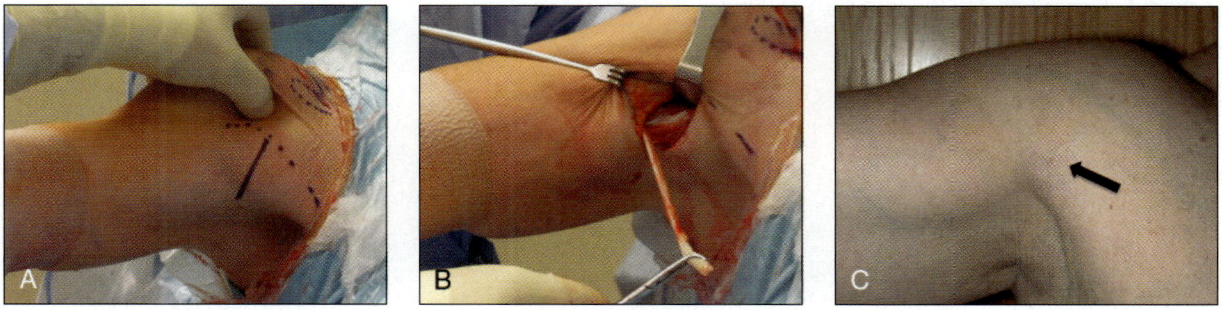

Clinical photographs of a subpectoral tenodesis. **A,** A 3- to 4-cm incision is made in the axillary crease over the inferior aspect of the pectoralis major tendon. **B,** The diseased proximal biceps tendon is retrieved and delivered out of the incision. The humeral shaft is exposed and the tendon is secured to bone using either suture anchors or interference screw fixation. The pathologic proximal biceps tendon is excised following fixation. **C,** The incision (arrow) is well healed and barely visible.

procedures, tendon fixation techniques have evolved substantially. However, the use of modern implants invariably increases the cost and complexity. Whether this improves patient outcome is unclear. Biomechanically, several studies have shown that interference screw fixation has a higher maximum load to failure when compared with suture anchors or keyhole tenodesis.[46-49] Although Lopez-Vidriero et al[48] demonstrated no significant difference in the in vitro strength between percutaneous soft-tissue tenodesis and suture anchor fixation, Scheibel et al[50] reported that 74.9% of soft-tissue tenodesis procedures resulted in tendon migration to the distal bicipital groove on MRI, compared with 35% in the suture anchor group. This finding correlated with a higher incidence of cosmetic deformity and reduced elbow flexion strength; however, no difference was observed in functional outcome scores. Millett et al[35] compared the use of suture anchors with interference screws for subpectoral tenodesis and reported no functional difference between patients in the two groups.

Irrespective of the method of fixation and the site of tendon reattachment, the overall results of biceps tenodesis are good to excellent for most patients, with numerous studies reporting reliable relief of biceps-related symptoms and improved shoulder function in up to 90%.[11,34,35,37,38,51] The authors of this chapter prefer to perform subpectoral biceps tenodesis with suture anchor fixation in young, active individuals or older patients with thin arms, for whom cosmesis may be a concern. However, given the lack of high-level evidence studies comparing these different techniques, further randomized controlled studies are needed to determine the optimal method of biceps tenodesis.

Biceps Tenotomy Versus Tenodesis

Considerable debate has been ongoing as to whether biceps tenotomy or tenodesis is the optimal method for the treatment of biceps tendon pathology. Each technique has pros and cons (**Table 2**), and relative indications (**Table 3**). Biceps tenotomy is advantageous because it is a quick, simple procedure that does not require any specific immobilization. However, this needs to be weighed against the potential for residual bicipital pain and spasm, cosmetic deformity, and elbow weakness during flexion and supination. Although biceps tenodesis can help treat issues of strength and deformity, it invariably results in a longer surgical time and a technically more demanding procedure, often requiring the use of implants and a period of immobilization while the tendon heals. As such, various factors should be considered in the decision-making process, and treatment should be individualized based on patient characteristics such as age, activity level, and concern for cosmesis.

A recent systematic review by Slenker et al[14] compared the clinical results of 16 studies that reported on 699 biceps tenotomy and 433 biceps tenodesis procedures.

TABLE 2 **Comparison of Biceps Tenotomy With Tenodesis**

Procedure	Advantages	Disadvantages
Biceps tenotomy	Quick and simple operation	Cosmetic deformity
	Short rehabilitation	Weakness[a]
	Does not require immobilization	Biceps cramping[a]
Biceps tenodesis	Preservation of strength[a]	Technically demanding
	Reduced risk of cosmetic deformity	Longer surgical time
		Cost of implants
		Longer rehabilitation
		Need for immobilization
		Higher complication rate

[a]Level II studies have shown no significant difference between tenotomy and tenodesis.[11,12]

Of note, only one level II study was used; the remaining studies were level IV evidence. For patients who underwent tenodesis, the authors reported good or excellent results in 74% of patients, an 8% incidence of cosmetic deformity, and residual bicipital pain in 24%. For patients who underwent tenotomy, the authors reported good or excellent results in 77%, a 43% incidence of cosmetic deformity, and residual bicipital pain in 19%. Furthermore, similar functional results and failure rates were observed in patients who underwent either tenotomy or tenodesis in the setting of a concomitant rotator cuff tear. The only main difference between the two groups was in the significantly higher incidence of cosmetic deformity with biceps tenotomy. Interestingly, Osbahr et al[18] specifically compared cosmetic results after biceps tenotomy and tenodesis and found no significant difference in patient subjective assessment of biceps appearance; similar results were also observed in both men and women.

Although proponents of biceps tenodesis claim that biceps tenotomy results in loss of strength, few data in the literature support this claim. Shank et al[15] compared the loss of supination and elbow flexion strength between biceps tenotomy and tenodesis and showed no significant difference on isokinetic strength test results at various degrees of flexion. Sentürk et al[52] also showed no difference between tenotomy and tenodesis in manual strength test results.

To date, only two level II prospective randomized studies have compared the clinical outcomes of biceps tenotomy and tenodesis. Koh et al[11] demonstrated no clinical difference in functional outcomes, strength, and biceps cramping between biceps tenotomy and tenodesis; however, patients in the tenotomy group had a higher incidence of subjective cosmetic deformity. De Carli et al[12] also showed comparable clinical and functional results between tenotomy and tenodesis; again, the only difference was a higher incidence of Popeye deformity.

Biceps tenodesis was performed in the suprapectoral region in both studies. Koh et al[11] used suture anchor fixation in the bicipital groove, and De Carli et al[12] only used sutures to secure the tenotomized biceps tendon to the rotator cuff. The results of biceps tenodesis can vary with the site of tenodesis and the method of fixation. Therefore, further high-quality studies are necessary to compare the outcomes of biceps tenotomy with those of various types of tenodesis before any difference between the two can be determined.

Conclusion

Biceps tenotomy and tenodesis are both reliable, effective methods for the treatment of LHB tendon pa-

TABLE 3 Relative Indications for Biceps Tenotomy and Tenodesis

Biceps tenotomy
Older patients
Low physical demands
Obese patients with large arms
Patients with no concerns about cosmesis
Patients who cannot tolerate postoperative immobilization
Biceps tenodesis
Younger patients
Physically active patients
Patients with thin arms
Patients with concerns about cosmetic deformity

thology. Each technique clearly has advantages and disadvantages, with the main clinical difference being the development of postoperative cosmetic deformity. Therefore, biceps tenotomy or tenodesis should be chosen based on the patient's age, activity level, ability to comply with the postoperative regime, expectations, and cosmetic concerns.

With biceps tenodesis, the surgeon must be aware that not all procedures are the same, with increasing evidence indicating better results and lower residual bicipital groove pain with more distal or subpectoral reattachment and fixation to the bone using either suture anchors or interference screws. However, given the lack of high-quality level I or II studies, further comparative studies are needed.

Based on the current available data, the authors of this chapter prefer to perform biceps tenotomy in physiologically older, low-demand patients or in those who are obese and have large arms, where a prominent biceps muscle belly can be concealed. The authors reserve biceps tenodesis for younger, more active patients or those with thinner arms and for whom cosmesis may be of concern, and prefer subpectoral tenodesis with suture anchor fixation.[1]

REFERENCES

1. Friedman DJ, Dunn JC, Higgins LD, Warner JJ: Proximal biceps tendon: Injuries and management. *Sports Med Arthrosc* 2008;16(3):162-169.
2. Murthi AM, Vosburgh CL, Neviaser TJ: The incidence of pathologic changes of the long head of the biceps tendon. *J Shoulder Elbow Surg* 2000;9(5):382-385.
3. Lafosse L, Reiland Y, Baier GP, Toussaint B, Jost B: Anterior and posterior instability of the long head of the biceps tendon in rotator cuff tears: A new classification based on arthroscopic observations. *Arthroscopy* 2007;23(1):73-80.
4. Walch G, Edwards TB, Boulahia A, Nové-Josserand L, Neyton L, Szabo I: Arthroscopic tenotomy of the long head of the biceps in the treatment of rotator cuff tears: Clinical and radiographic results of 307 cases. *J Shoulder Elbow Surg* 2005;14(3):238-246.
5. Boileau P, Baqué F, Valerio L, Ahrens P, Chuinard C, Trojani C: Isolated arthroscopic biceps tenotomy or tenodesis improves symptoms in patients with massive irreparable rotator cuff tears. *J Bone Joint Surg Am* 2007;89(4):747-757.
6. Sethi N, Wright R, Yamaguchi K: Disorders of the long head of the biceps tendon. *J Shoulder Elbow Surg* 1999;8(6):644-654.
7. Khazzam M, George MS, Churchill RS, Kuhn JE: Disorders of the long head of biceps tendon. *J Shoulder Elbow Surg* 2012;21(1):136-145.
8. Holtby R, Razmjou H: Accuracy of the Speed's and Yergason's tests in detecting biceps pathology and SLAP lesions: Comparison with arthroscopic findings. *Arthroscopy* 2004;20(3):231-236.
9. Ben Kibler W, Sciascia AD, Hester P, Dome D, Jacobs C: Clinical utility of traditional and new tests in the diagnosis of biceps tendon injuries and superior labrum anterior and posterior lesions in the shoulder. *Am J Sports Med* 2009;37(9):1840-1847.
10. Favorito PJ, Harding WG III, Heidt RS Jr: Complete arthroscopic examination of the long head of the biceps tendon. *Arthroscopy* 2001;17(4):430-432.
11. Koh KH, Ahn JH, Kim SM, Yoo JC: Treatment of biceps tendon lesions in the setting of rotator cuff tears: Prospective cohort study of tenotomy versus tenodesis. *Am J Sports Med* 2010;38(8):1584-1590.

12. De Carli A, Vadalà A, Zanzotto E, et al: Reparable rotator cuff tears with concomitant long-head biceps lesions: Tenotomy or tenotomy/tenodesis? *Knee Surg Sports Traumatol Arthrosc* 2012;20(12):2553-2558.
13. Nho SJ, Frank RM, Reiff SN, Verma NN, Romeo AA: Arthroscopic repair of anterosuperior rotator cuff tears combined with open biceps tenodesis. *Arthroscopy* 2010;26(12):1667-1674.
14. Slenker NR, Lawson K, Ciccotti MG, Dodson CC, Cohen SB: Biceps tenotomy versus tenodesis: Clinical outcomes. *Arthroscopy* 2012;28(4):576-582.
15. Shank JR, Singleton SB, Braun S, et al: A comparison of forearm supination and elbow flexion strength in patients with long head of the biceps tenotomy or tenodesis. *Arthroscopy* 2011;27(1):9-16.
16. Duff SJ, Campbell PT: Patient acceptance of long head of biceps brachii tenotomy. *J Shoulder Elbow Surg* 2012;21(1):61-65.
17. Walch G, Nové-Josserand L, Boileau P, Levigne C: Subluxations and dislocations of the tendon of the long head of the biceps. *J Shoulder Elbow Surg* 1998;7(2):100-108.
18. Osbahr DC, Diamond AB, Speer KP: The cosmetic appearance of the biceps muscle after long-head tenotomy versus tenodesis. *Arthroscopy* 2002;18(5):483-487.
19. Itoi E, Kuechle DK, Newman SR, Morrey BF, An KN: Stabilising function of the biceps in stable and unstable shoulders. *J Bone Joint Surg Br* 1993;75(4):546-550.
20. Kumar VP, Satku K, Balasubramaniam P: The role of the long head of biceps brachii in the stabilization of the head of the humerus. *Clin Orthop Relat Res* 1989;(244):172-175.
21. Warner JJ, McMahon PJ: The role of the long head of the biceps brachii in superior stability of the glenohumeral joint. *J Bone Joint Surg Am* 1995;77(3):366-372.
22. Yamaguchi K, Riew KD, Galatz LM, Syme JA, Neviaser RJ: Biceps activity during shoulder motion: An electromyographic analysis. *Clin Orthop Relat Res* 1997;(336):122-129.
23. Nové-Josserand LL, Lévigne C, Noël E, Walch G: The acromio-humeral interval: A study of the factors influencing its height. *Rev Chir Orthop Reparatrice Appar Mot* 1996;82(5):379-385.
24. Gill TJ, McIrvin E, Mair SD, Hawkins RJ: Results of biceps tenotomy for treatment of pathology of the long head of the biceps brachii. *J Shoulder Elbow Surg* 2001;10(3):247-249.
25. Kelly AM, Drakos MC, Fealy S, Taylor SA, O'Brien SJ: Arthroscopic release of the long head of the biceps tendon: Functional outcome and clinical results. *Am J Sports Med* 2005;33(2):208-213.
26. Mariani EM, Cofield RH, Askew LJ, Li GP, Chao EY: Rupture of the tendon of the long head of the biceps brachii: Surgical versus nonsurgical treatment. *Clin Orthop Relat Res* 1988;(228):233-239.
27. Soto-Hall RS: Treatment of ruptures of the long head of biceps brachii. *Am J Orthop* 1960;2:192-193.
28. Frost A, Zafar MS, Maffulli N: Tenotomy versus tenodesis in the management of pathologic lesions of the tendon of the long head of the biceps brachii. *Am J Sports Med* 2009;37(4):828-833.
29. Gilcreest E: Rupture of muscles and tendons: Particularly subcutaneous rupture biceps flexor cubiti. *JAMA* 1925;84(24):1819-1822.
30. Lippman R: Bicipital tenosynovitis. *N Y State J Med* 1944;90:2235-2241.
31. Hitchcock HH, Bechtol CO: Painful shoulder; observations on the role of the tendon of the long head of the biceps brachii in its causation. *J Bone Joint Surg Am* 1948;30-A(2):263-273.
32. Froimson AI, O I: Keyhole tenodesis of biceps origin at the shoulder. *Clin Orthop Relat Res* 1975;(112):245-249.
33. Lutton DM, Gruson KI, Harrison AK, Gladstone JN, Flatow EL: Where to tenodese the biceps: Proximal or distal? *Clin Orthop Relat Res* 2011;469(4):1050-1055.
34. Mazzocca AD, Cote MP, Arciero CL, Romeo AA, Arciero RA: Clinical outcomes after subpectoral biceps tenodesis with an interference screw. *Am J Sports Med* 2008;36(10):1922-1929.
35. Millett PJ, Sanders B, Gobezie R, Braun S, Warner JJ: Interference screw vs. suture anchor fixation for open subpectoral biceps tenodesis: Does it matter? *BMC Musculoskelet Disord* 2008;9:121.
36. Sekiya JK, Elkousy HA, Rodosky MW: Arthroscopic biceps tenodesis using the percutaneous intra-articular transtendon technique. *Arthroscopy* 2003;19(10): 1137-1141.
37. Elkousy HA, Fluhme DJ, O'Connor DP, Rodosky MW: Arthroscopic biceps tenodesis using the percutaneous, intra-articular trans-tendon technique: Preliminary results. *Orthopedics* 2005;28(11):1316-1319.
38. Checchia SL, Doneux PS, Miyazaki AN, et al: Biceps tenodesis associated with arthroscopic repair of

rotator cuff tears. *J Shoulder Elbow Surg* 2005;14(2): 138-144.

39. Boileau P, Parratte S, Chuinard C, Roussanne Y, Shia D, Bicknell R: Arthroscopic treatment of isolated type II SLAP lesions: Biceps tenodesis as an alternative to reinsertion. *Am J Sports Med* 2009;37(5):929-936.
40. Lo IK, Burkhart SS: Arthroscopic biceps tenodesis using a bioabsorbable interference screw. *Arthroscopy* 2004;20(1):85-95.
41. Ahmad CS, ElAttrache NS: Arthroscopic biceps tenodesis. *Orthop Clin North Am* 2003;34(4):499-506.
42. Provencher MT, LeClere LE, Romeo AA: Subpectoral biceps tenodesis. *Sports Med Arthrosc* 2008;16(3): 170-176.
43. Verma NN, Drakos M, O'Brien SJ: Arthroscopic transfer of the long head biceps to the conjoint tendon. *Arthroscopy* 2005;21(6):764.
44. Drakos MC, Verma NN, Gulotta LV, et al: Arthroscopic transfer of the long head of the biceps tendon: Functional outcome and clinical results. *Arthroscopy* 2008;24(2):217-223.
45. Sanders B, Lavery KP, Pennington S, Warner JJ: Clinical success of biceps tenodesis with and without release of the transverse humeral ligament. *J Shoulder Elbow Surg* 2012;21(1):66-71.
46. Golish SR, Caldwell PE III, Miller MD, et al: Interference screw versus suture anchor fixation for subpectoral tenodesis of the proximal biceps tendon: A cadaveric study. *Arthroscopy* 2008;24(10):1103-1108.
47. Kusma M, Dienst M, Eckert J, Steimer O, Kohn D: Tenodesis of the long head of biceps brachii: Cyclic testing of five methods of fixation in a porcine model. *J Shoulder Elbow Surg* 2008;17(6):967-973.
48. Lopez-Vidriero E, Costic RS, Fu FH, Rodosky MW: Biomechanical evaluation of 2 arthroscopic biceps tenodeses: Double-anchor versus percutaneous intra-articular transtendon (PITT) techniques. *Am J Sports Med* 2010;38(1):146-152.
49. Mazzocca AD, Bicos J, Santangelo S, Romeo AA, Arciero RA: The biomechanical evaluation of four fixation techniques for proximal biceps tenodesis. *Arthroscopy* 2005;21(11):1296-1306.
50. Scheibel M, Schröder R-J, Chen J, Bartsch M: Arthroscopic soft tissue tenodesis versus bony fixation anchor tenodesis of the long head of the biceps tendon. *Am J Sports Med* 2011;39(5):1046-1052.
51. Nord KD, Smith GB, Mauck BM: Arthroscopic biceps tenodesis using suture anchors through the subclavian portal. *Arthroscopy* 2005;21(2):248-252.
52. Sentürk I, Ozalay M, Akpınar S, Leblebici B, Cınar BM, Tuncay C: Clinical and isokinetic comparison between tenotomy and tenodesis in biceps pathologies. *Acta Orthop Traumatol Turc* 2011;45(1):41-46.

CHAPTER 11

Arthroscopic Treatment of Biceps Tendon Injuries: Interference Screw Technique

Clay Riley, MD
T. Bradley Edwards, MD

Introduction

The long head of the biceps tendon has long been identified as a source of pain and dysfunction in the shoulder. Although biceps tendon disease can occur as an isolated pathology, it most commonly is associated with concomitant shoulder problems, usually involving the rotator cuff. Many techniques have been described for biceps tenodesis, including the keyhole technique,[1] those using transosseous sutures[2] or suture anchors,[3] suturing the biceps to the rotator cuff,[4] and those using an interference screw.[5-7] Historically, each has been performed as an open procedure, but as surgeons gain more experience with arthroscopy, some techniques have been adapted to be performed arthroscopically.

Many studies on biceps tenodesis have found it to be a reliable method of treating anterior shoulder pain. Most of these studies were clinical, but some biomechanical studies have investigated various methods of fixation used in biceps tenodesis. Although some instances have been reported in which the interference screw technique was considered biomechanically equivalent, it typically had better results than all other types of fixation tested.[8-11]

Indications

Once nonsurgical treatment has failed, the indications for biceps tenodesis include clinically identifiable bicipital tendinitis pain, partial biceps tears, superior labrum anterior to posterior (SLAP) lesions in older patients, biceps subluxation or dislocation, and biceps entrapment. Additionally, the authors of this chapter perform biceps tenodesis in almost all cases of repair of a rotator cuff tear involving the subscapularis or the anterior aspect of the supraspinatus.

Not many contraindications exist for biceps tenodesis. The authors of this chapter try to avoid performing tenodesis in young throwing athletes with dominant-side rotator cuff tears in which the biceps appears completely normal. Although not a contraindication, some patients may respond better to biceps tenotomy. Many studies have shown tenotomy to be reliable for pain relief, but the risk of cosmetic deformity is increased.[12] Tenotomy can be considered in older patients, obese patients, and those who can accept a potential cosmetic deformity. Tenotomy should also be considered for a tendon that is severely damaged where the interference screw will be placed because obtaining secure fixation

Dr. Edwards or an immediate family member has received royalties from Tornier and Orthohelix; is a member of a speakers' bureau or has made paid presentations on behalf of Tornier; serves as a paid consultant to or is an employee of Kinamed and Tornier; serves as an unpaid consultant to Gulf Coast Surgical Services; has received research or institutional support from Tornier; has received nonincome support (such as equipment or services), commercially derived honoraria, or other non–research-related funding (such as paid travel) from Tornier; and serves as a board member, owner, officer, or committee member of the American Shoulder and Elbow Surgeons. Neither Dr. Riley nor any immediate family member has received anything of value from or has stock or stock options held in a commercial company or institution related directly or indirectly to the subject of this chapter.

FIGURE 1

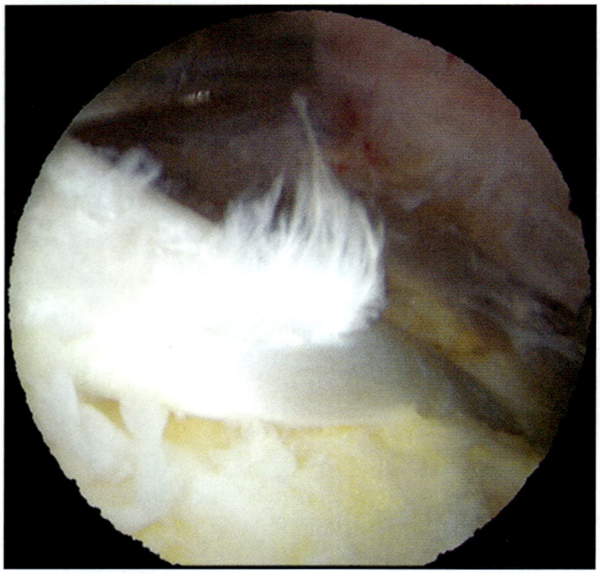

Arthroscopic view of a biceps tendon freed from the bicipital groove. Note the frayed extra-articular portion.

FIGURE 2

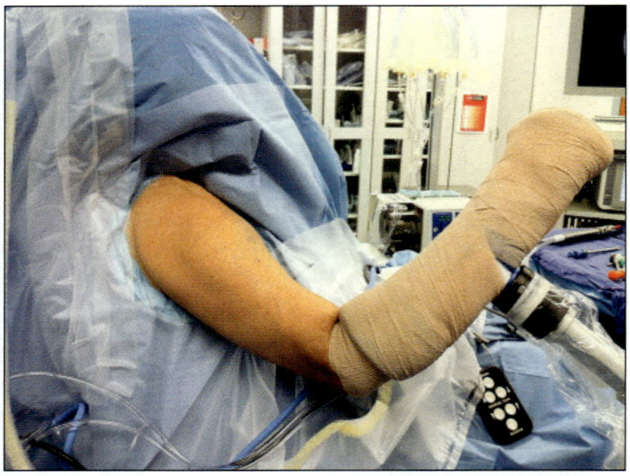

Photograph shows the arm held in flexion and external rotation by the arm positioner.

FIGURE 3

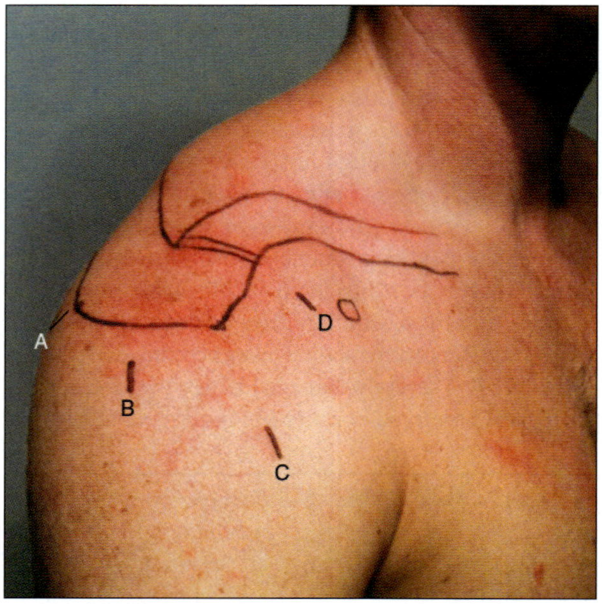

Photograph of anatomic landmarks with portal positions. *A* = posterior, *B* = lateral, *C* = anterolateral, *D* = anterior.

may be difficult to implement. These damaged tendons are usually large, flat, and have shredded fibers.

Surgical Technique

The authors of this chapter perform all arthroscopic procedures with the patient in the beach chair position and under general anesthesia, and typically with an interscalene block. An adjustable arm positioner is used to hold the arm in the preferred position. A standard arthroscopic camera and equipment are used.

Diagnostic Arthroscopy and Biceps Tenotomy

A standard posterior portal is created and diagnostic arthroscopy is performed. An anterior portal is created and the biceps is pulled into the joint with a probe to visualize the extra-articular portion. Even if the tendon initially appears normal, any extra-articular tendon fraying is revealed at this point (**Figure 1**). The arm can also be elevated to check for entrapment, and an hourglass appearance of the biceps may be observed in some instances.[13] Once the decision to perform a biceps tenodesis is made, the biceps is released from its junction with the superior labrum using arthroscopic scissors or electrocautery. Any other necessary glenohumeral procedure should be performed at this time, and the ar-

FIGURE 4

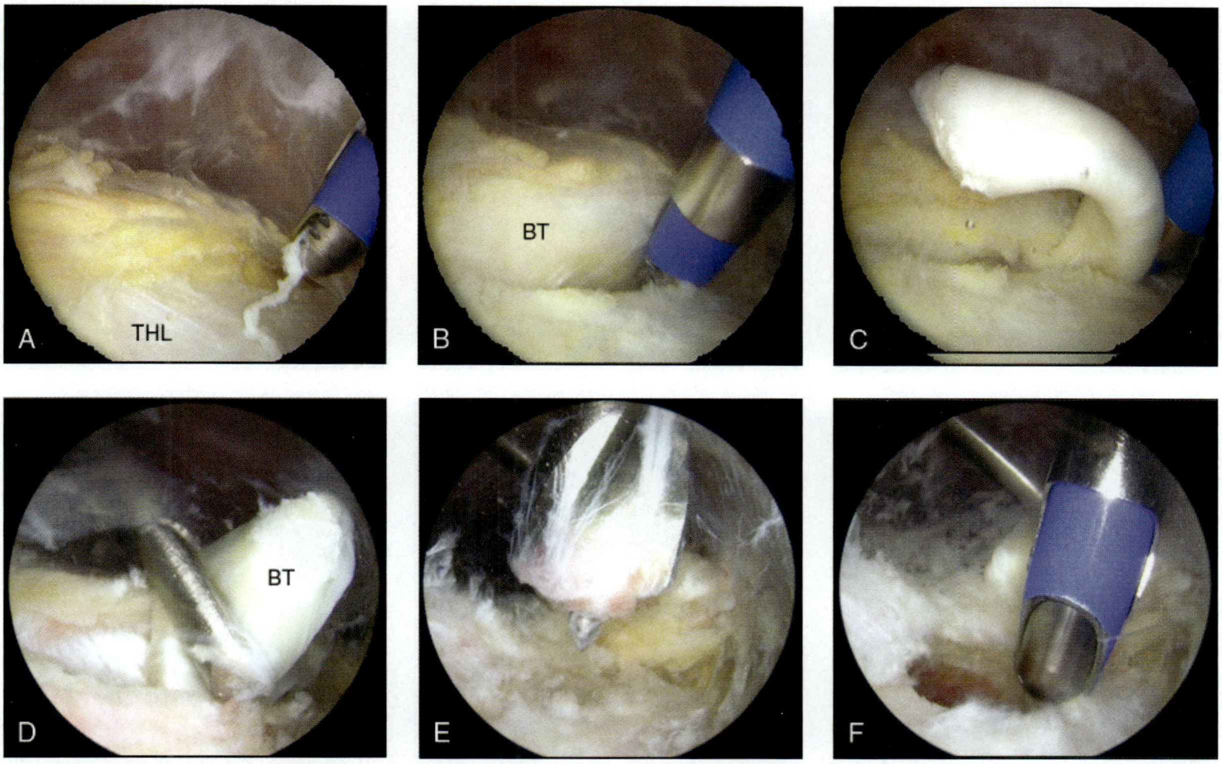

Arthroscopic views of a biceps tenotomy. **A,** Fibers of the transverse humeral ligament (THL). **B,** The biceps tendon (BT) is released from its sheath. **C,** Spontaneous extrusion of the biceps tendon from the groove after adequate release. **D,** Removal of the biceps tendon from the groove with the locking grasper. **E,** The trochar-tipped drill is placed in line with the bicipital groove for humeral socket drilling. **F,** Humeral socket after drilling and debris removal.

throscope is withdrawn in preparation for entering the subacromial space.

Bursectomy and Locating the Bicipital Groove

The arthroscope is introduced into the subacromial space and a standard lateral portal is created. A routine subacromial bursectomy is performed along with any further diagnostic exploration. For biceps tenodesis performed with a rotator cuff repair, the tenodesis should be performed first. After performing the subacromial bursectomy, the arthroscope is placed in the lateral portal. The arm is elevated and placed in external rotation to allow additional anterior bursectomy and identification of the bicipital groove (**Figure 2**). A rotator cuff tear, if present, makes identification of the groove easier. An accessory anterolateral portal is created as the main working portal for the tenodesis. This portal is created in line with the scapular spine, approximately 4 cm from the anterior corner of the acromion (**Figure 3**). Sometimes the white fibers of the transverse humeral ligament can be visualized (**Figure 4, A**), but more often, the location of the bicipital groove is confirmed using instruments to palpate either the transition from the tuberosities to the groove or the soft, mobile biceps tendon.

Once the biceps and bicipital groove are identified, the sheath is released using a shaver and electrocautery (**Figure 4, B**). This area is highly vascular, so blood pressure control and electrocautery are essential for visualization. Attention to hemostasis also minimizes postoperative ecchymosis along the anterior aspect of the arm, which may be of concern to some patients. The biceps

FIGURE 5

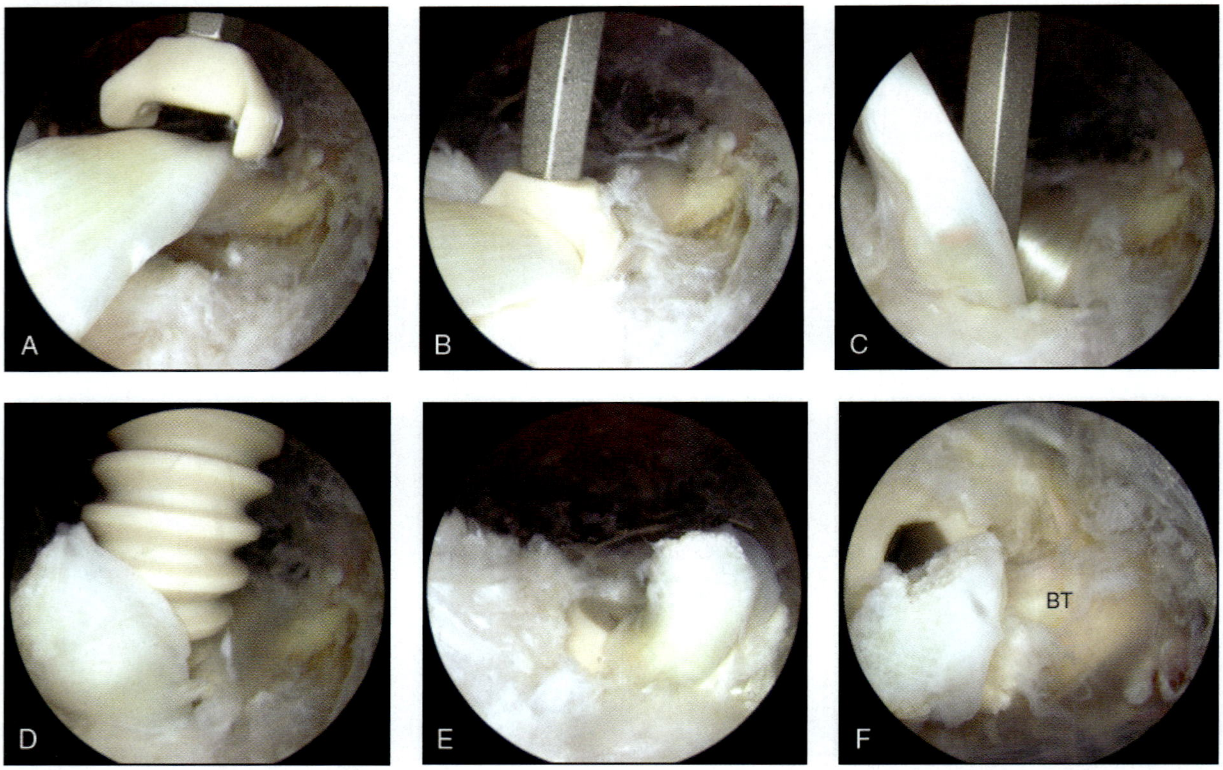

Arthroscopic views of screw insertion for biceps tenodesis **A,** The end piece is used to guide the tendon into the drilled hole and keep it centered during screw insertion. **B,** The biceps tendon is engaged. **C,** The biceps tendon is held at the bottom of the socket using the inserter. **D,** The tenodesis screw is advanced. **E,** The tenodesis screw is used to secure the residual biceps tendon stump in the bicipital groove. **F,** The biceps tendon (BT) is fixed using the tenodesis screw.

should extrude from the groove once it is adequately released from its sheath; if not, it can be removed with a locking grasper (**Figure 4, C**). The biceps is secured with the grasper via the anterior portal and retracted medially below the pectoralis major (**Figure 4, D**). Any residual tissue in the bicipital groove should be resected at this time.

Humeral Drilling

A trochar-tipped drill is introduced via the accessory anterolateral portal and the humeral socket is drilled (**Figure 4, E**). The authors of this chapter typically use an 8.5-mm drill for an 8-mm screw. The screw and drill size selection vary depending on tendon size and quality as well as bone density. After drilling, the shaver is reintroduced to clear debris from the hole (**Figure 4, F**). The hole must be deep enough to fully seat the screw—the appropriate depth is marked on the drill bit.

Interference Screw Placement

The grasper holding the biceps tendon is now stretched back in line with the groove and the drilled hole. An interference screw with a U-shaped endpiece is used to help center the tendon while guiding it into the hole. The tendon is pushed into the bottom of the socket and held in place with this inserter (**Figure 5, A** through **D**). The screw is advanced until it is secure and flush with the bone (**Figure 5, E** and **F**). The endpiece helps prevent the tendon from wrapping around the screw during insertion. After adequate fixation is confirmed, any excess tendon stump can be resected with a shaver or a grasper and scissors. Any additional arthroscopic procedures that are necessary can be performed at this time.

Postoperative Management

The postoperative management and rehabilitation protocol is usually determined by other procedures performed in conjunction with the biceps tenodesis, typically a rotator cuff repair. If tenodesis is performed in isolation, an arm sling is worn for 6 weeks. Activity is usually restricted by pain and can progress slowly. Eccentric loading of the biceps should be avoided for at least 6 months postoperatively.

Conclusion

This arthroscopic biceps tenodesis technique is a reliable method for the treatment of proximal biceps tendon pathology. It is reproducible and can be performed relatively quickly, allowing ample time to treat other concomitant shoulder pathologies arthroscopically.

References

1. Froimson AI, O I: Keyhole tenodesis of biceps origin at the shoulder. *Clin Orthop Relat Res* 1975;112:245-249.
2. Post M, Benca P: Primary tendinitis of the long head of the biceps. *Clin Orthop Relat Res* 1989;246:117-125.
3. Gartsman GM, Hammerman SM: Arthroscopic biceps tenodesis: Operative technique. *Arthroscopy* 2000;16(5):550-552.
4. Elkousy HA, Fluhme DJ, O'Connor DP, Rodosky MW: Arthroscopic biceps tenodesis using the percutaneous, intra-articular trans-tendon technique: Preliminary results. *Orthopedics* 2005;28(11):1316-1319.
5. Edwards TB, Walch G: Open biceps tenodesis: The interference screw technique. *Tech Shoulder Elbow Surg* 2003;4(4):195-198.
6. Boileau P, Krishnan SG, Coste JS, Walch G: Arthroscopic biceps tenodesis: A new technique using bioabsorbable interference screw fixation. *Arthroscopy* 2002;18(9):1002-1012.
7. Lo IK, Burkhart SS: Arthroscopic biceps tenodesis using a bioabsorbable interference screw. *Arthroscopy* 2004;20(1):85-95.
8. Ozalay M, Akpinar S, Karaeminogullari O, et al: Mechanical strength of four different biceps tenodesis techniques. *Arthroscopy* 2005;21(8):992-998.
9. Mazzocca AD, Bicos J, Santangelo S, Romeo AA, Arciero RA: The biomechanical evaluation of four fixation techniques for proximal biceps tenodesis. *Arthroscopy* 2005;21(11):1296-1306.
10. Golish SR, Caldwell PE III, Miller MD, et al: Interference screw versus suture anchor fixation for subpectoral tenodesis of the proximal biceps tendon: A cadaveric study. *Arthroscopy* 2008;24(10):1103-1108.
11. Kusma M, Dienst M, Eckert J, Steimer O, Kohn D: Tenodesis of the long head of biceps brachii: Cyclic testing of five methods of fixation in a porcine model. *J Shoulder Elbow Surg* 2008;17(6):967-973.
12. Slenker NR, Lawson K, Ciccotti MG, Dodson CC, Cohen SB: Biceps tenotomy versus tenodesis: Clinical outcomes. *Arthroscopy* 2012;28(4):576-582.
13. Boileau P, Ahrens PM, Hatzidakis AM: Entrapment of the long head of the biceps tendon: The hourglass biceps—a cause of pain and locking of the shoulder. *J Shoulder Elbow Surg* 2004;13(3):249-257.

CHAPTER *12*

Arthroscopic Treatment of Biceps Tendon Injuries: Biceps Transfer to the Conjoint Tendon

Samuel A. Taylor, MD
Nikolas J. Baret
Stephen J. O'Brien, MD, MBA

Introduction

The long head of the biceps (LHB) tendon is recognized by orthopaedic surgeons as a source of anterior shoulder symptoms. Alpantaki et al[1] demonstrated a network of thinly myelinated sensory neurons within the LBH tendon with a proximal predominance. Treatment and surgical techniques, however, are still widely debated among many experts. This debate is due, at least in part, to the incomplete knowledge regarding the function of the LHB tendon with respect to overall glenohumeral mechanics. Kumar et al[2] reported on the function of the LHB tendon as a humeral head depressor. Kuhn et al[3] determined that the LHB tendon is also active during external rotation as a restraint to the abducted shoulder. Other authors consider the LHB tendon to have limited functional significance, even considering it to be vestigial structure.[4,5] Disparate views of LHB tendon function have resulted in an array of treatment algorithms ranging from highly conservative to very aggressive.

Pathology can occur in the biceps-labral complex either in isolation or in conjunction with other shoulder injuries. Accurate management relies on an accurate diagnosis. First-line therapy consists of nonsurgical measures such as oral NSAIDs, activity modification, local steroid injection, and physical therapy. However, when nonsurgical therapies fail, surgical options may be considered, including tenodesis, tenotomy, and tendon transfer. This chapter presents indications, surgical technique, postoperative rehabilitation protocols, and results for subdeltoid transfer of the LHB tendon to the conjoint tendon

Indications

Multiple pathologies can affect the LHB tendon, including tendinopathy, synovitis, instability, loose bodies and stenosis in the bicipital groove, and partial or complete tears. Initial management is expectant and focused on the resolution of presenting symptoms. Nonsurgical approaches include activity modification, NSAIDs, local steroid injections, and physical therapy.

A thorough physical examination is critical to help make an accurate diagnosis of LHB tendon and concomitant pathologies. Historically, several tests have been described to examine the biceps-labral complex including the Speed, Yergason, and O'Brien tests.[6] During the past 2 decades, the senior author (SJO), has used

None of the following authors nor any immediate family member has received anything of value from or has stock or stock options held in a commercial company or institution related directly or indirectly to the subject of this chapter: Dr. Taylor, Mr. Baret, and Dr. O'Brien.

FIGURE 1

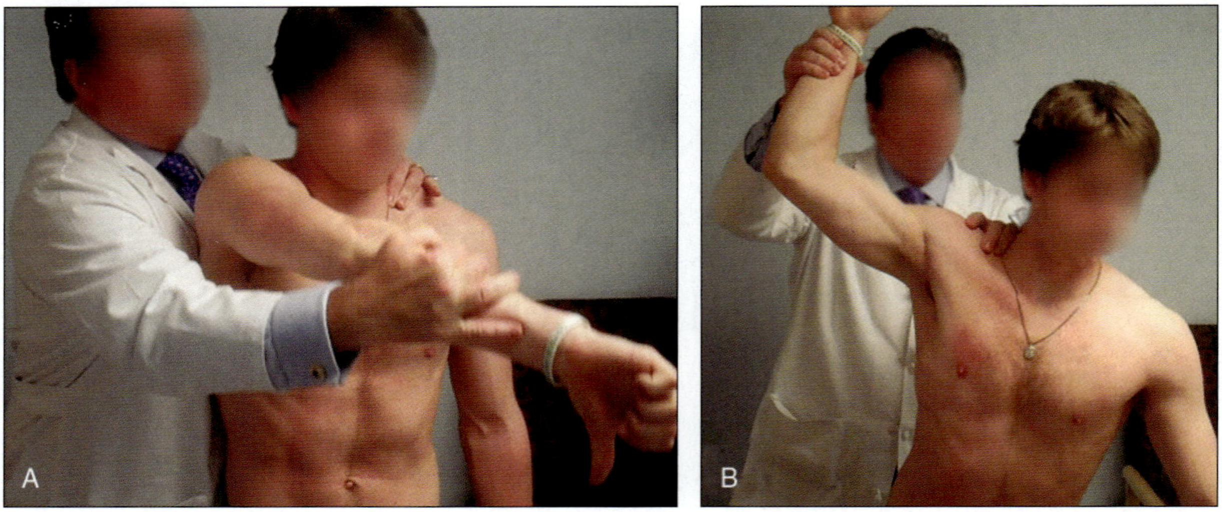

Photographs show the active compression test (**A**) and the thrower test (**B**).

the results of three examination techniques to identify and localize LHB tendon pathology in symptomatic patients: tenderness to palpation in the bicipital groove, a positive result for the active compression test, and a positive result for the thrower test.

During examination, the bicipital groove is palpated with the arm in neutral and again with the arm in passive internal and external rotation. If palpation reproduces the patient's symptoms, the examination result is considered positive. The active compression test, also called the O'Brien test (**Figure 1, A**), is performed by having the patient place the affected shoulder in 90° of forward flexion, 15° to 30° of adduction, and the humerus in internal rotation with the thumb pointing down. The examiner exerts a downward force, which the patient resists. If pain that was reproduced deep within the shoulder improves or disappears with the humerus in external rotation, a SLAP lesion or proximal LHB tendon pathology is indicated. The thrower test (**Figure 1, B**) is performed with the arm in 90° of abduction, 90° of elbow flexion, and moved through a simulated throwing motion while the examiner provides resistance. The test is considered positive when the patient's symptoms are reproduced. These clinical examination tests are most effective in determining the specificity and sensitivity of LHB tendon pathology when used in combination. In a recent validation study, clinical examination data was compared with intraoperative arthroscopic findings.[7] The authors (SJO and SAT) reported high sensitivity and specificity for tenderness to palpation in the bicipital groove and high specificity for a positive throwing test result.

Treatment algorithms (**Figure 2**) focus first on nonsurgical measures including NSAIDs,[8,9] activity modification, and physical therapy. If symptoms persist, a corticosteroid injection of the bicipital sheath may be considered at 6 weeks, and again at 3 months, if necessary. In a randomized controlled trial, Hashiuchi et al[10] reported significantly improved accuracy of corticosteroid injection for ultrasonographic guidance compared with unguided injections. Nonsurgical measures should be attempted for a minimum of 6 months before surgical intervention is considered. Most patients respond to nonsurgical measures, obviating the need for surgery.

A small subset of patients, however, have recalcitrant LHB tendon–related symptoms for longer than 6 months, and may be considered for surgical intervention. Numerous procedures including tenotomy as well as bony and soft-tissue tenodesis techniques have been described. An earlier report suggested that tenotomy of

FIGURE 2

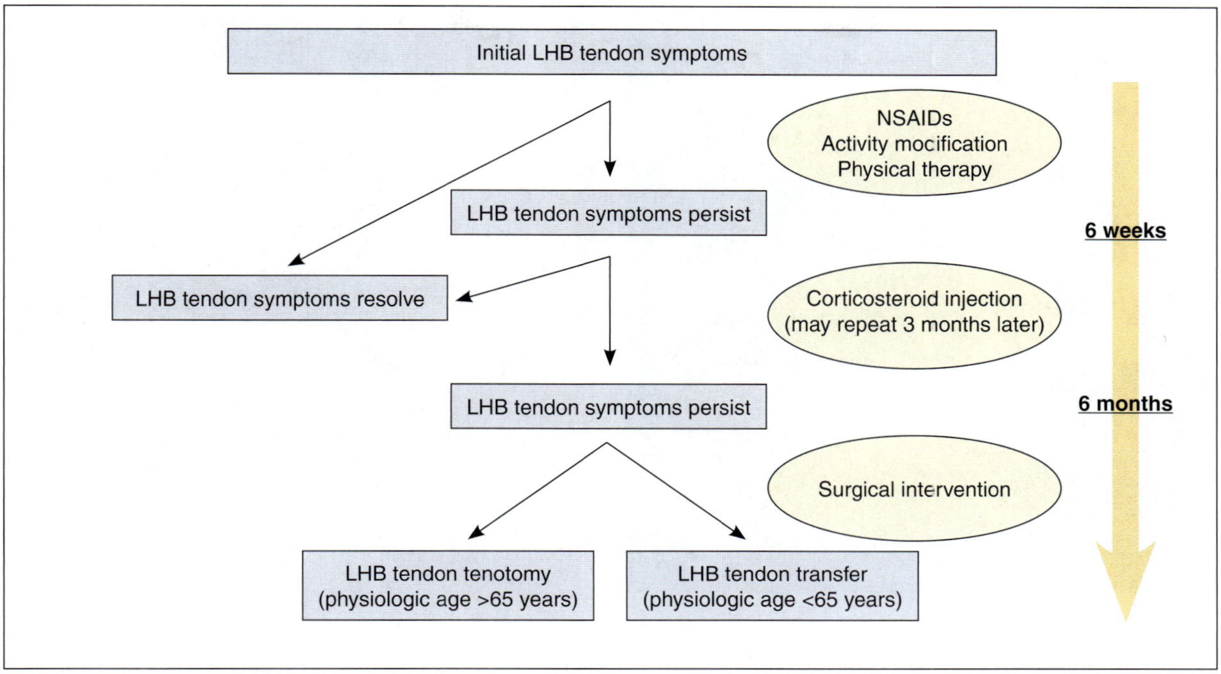

Algorithm for nonsurgical measures that result in symptom resolution for most patients. LHB = long head of the biceps.

the LHB tendon alone provided symptomatic relief in most patients.[11] Specifically, the authors found that patients older than 65 years had the best outcomes. In patients younger than 65 years, suboptimal outcomes were attributed to "fatigue and discomfort" and displeasing cosmesis related to the Popeye deformity. Therefore, transfer of the LHB tendon to the conjoint tendon is the preferred surgical approach of the authors for chronically symptomatic patients younger than 65 years. The senior author (SJO) has developed a subdeltoid transfer of the LHB tendon to the conjoint tendon, which has been reliably reproduced in more than 400 cases during the past 10 years.

Surgical Technique

All biceps tendon transfer procedures are performed with the patient in the beach chair position and as outpatient procedures, unless the patient has medical concerns requiring overnight observation. Following an examination under anesthesia, the arthroscope is introduced via a standard posterior portal. An anterior rotator cuff interval portal is established using direct needle localization. Diagnostic arthroscopy is performed by inspecting the LHB tendon from its insertion at the supraglenoid tubercle to the most distally visualized portion of the tendon for evidence of fraying, synovitis, hypertrophy, and tearing. The surgeon must be cognizant of signs of dynamic pathology such as humeral head chondromalacia resulting from chronic abrasion of the humeral head by the LHB tendon. A positive result for the arthroscopic active compression test may also indicate subtle LHB tendon instability that can have clinical implications that are not as subtle.[12] Hart et al[13] reported that the LHB tendon is best visualized with the arm in 30° forward flexion, 40° of abduction, and 90° of elbow flexion. Taylor et al[14] reported that even with ideal arm positioning and traction on the tendon, only 78% of the LHB tendon relative to the inferior margin of the bony bicipital groove and 55% of the tendon relative to the proximal margin of the pectoralis major can be vi-

FIGURE 3

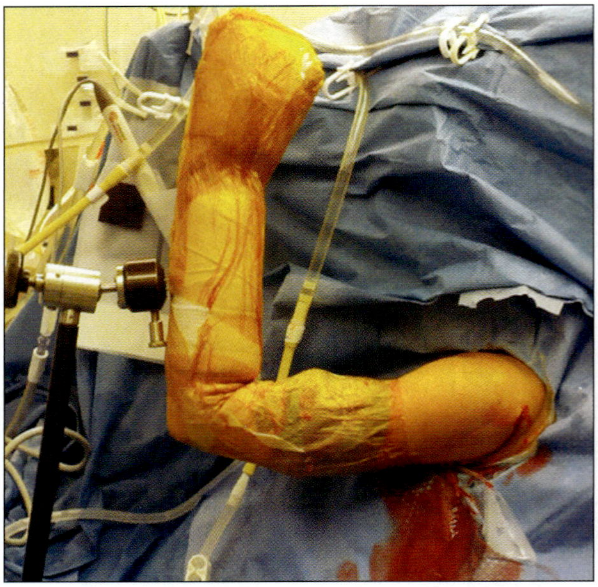

Photograph shows the 90-90-15 position used to facilitate exposure of the subdeltoid space. The shoulder is placed in 90° of forward flexion and 15° to 30° of adduction; the elbow is placed in 90° of flexion.

FIGURE 4

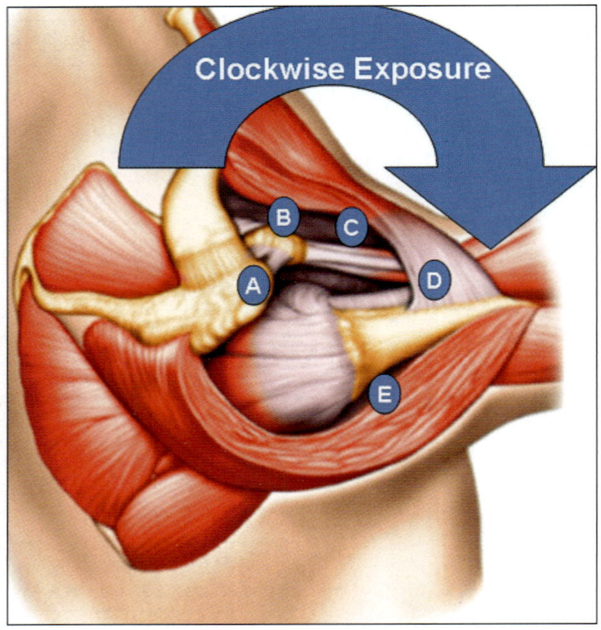

Illustration shows subdeltoid space exposure in a sequential clockwise fashion. The coracoacromial ligament (*A*) is identified and traced medially to the coracoid (*B*), and inferiorly along the conjoint tendon (*C*). The insertion of the pectoralis major tendon (*D*) marks the inferior border of the space and the lateral deltoid and humeral shaft mark the lateral border (*E*).

sualized during arthroscopy. Furthermore, the authors reported that 60 of 276 patients who underwent LHB tendon transfer to the conjoint tendon had a normal-appearing LHB tendon during diagnostic arthroscopy, but ultimately had pathology in the bicipital groove such as stenosis, loose bodies, synovitis, and partial tears.

All intra-articular pathology should be treated first. When tendon transfer is indicated, the LHB tendon is tagged with a suture and tenotomized using radiofrequency ablation. Tagging the LHB tendon facilitates its later retrieval and side-to-side tensioning. During tenotomy, care must be taken to preserve the intimately associated superior labrum.

The arthroscope is subsequently redirected into the subacromial space. Subacromial decompression is performed only when clinically indicated and is not necessary for exposure of the subdeltoid space.

For subdeltoid exposure,[15] the arm is repositioned in the 90-90-15 position (**Figure 3**): 70° to 90° of forward flexion, 90° of elbow flexion, and 15° to 30° of arm abduction. In this position, the humeral head falls posteriorly. The subdeltoid space is bordered superiorly by the anterior acromion and coracoacromial ligament, medially by the conjoint tendon, inferiorly by the superior border of the pectoralis major tendon, and laterally by the humerus and lateral deltoid. To expose the subdeltoid space, readily identifiable landmarks are cleared in a sequential, clockwise fashion (**Figure 4**). Radiofrequency ablation is used to trace the coracoacromial ligament medially to the coracoid process via an anterolateral working portal. The insertion of the conjoint tendon is visualized, traced distally to the musculotendinous portion of the pectoralis major tendon, and traced laterally to the humeral insertion. With all "safe" boundaries identified, the remaining subdeltoid bursa is ablated, yielding a spacious and relatively bloodless working field.

The pectoralis portal is placed near the humeral in-

FIGURE 5

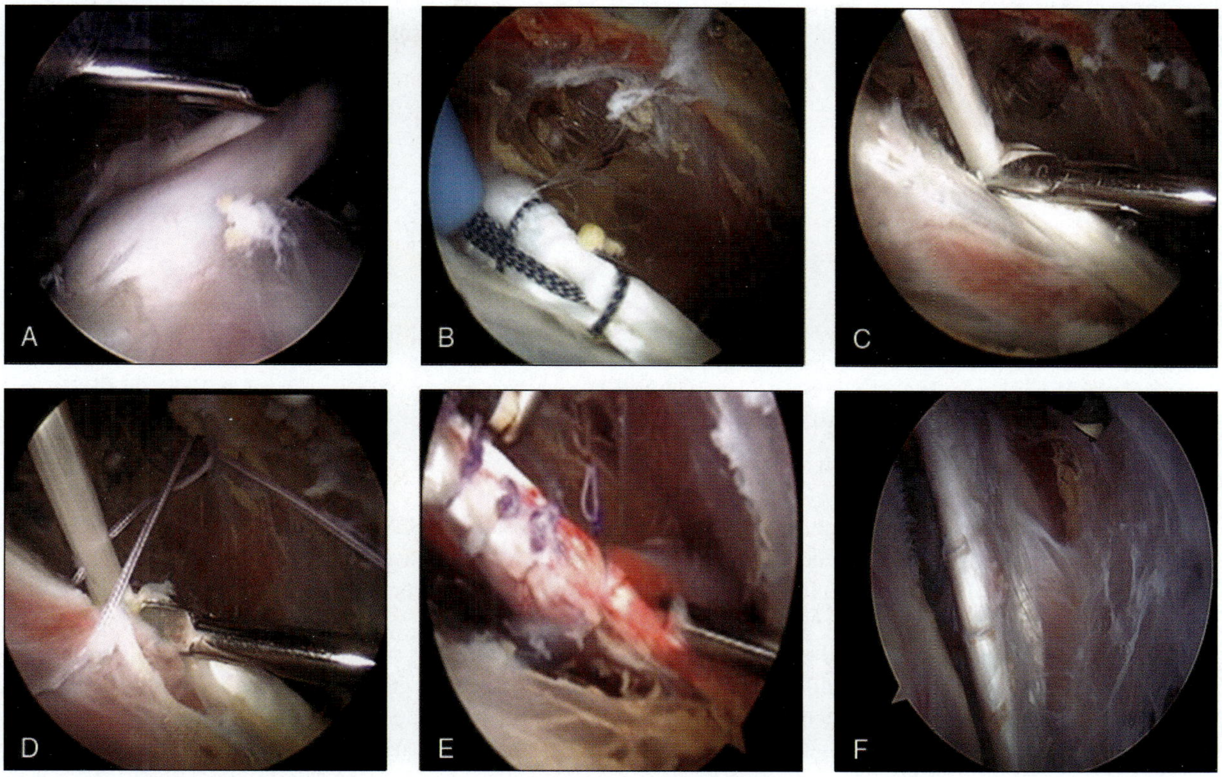

Arthroscopic views show full subdeltoid space exposure. **A,** An aperture is created in the bicipital hood and the long head of the biceps (LHB) tendon is pulled into the subdeltoid space. **B,** A traction suture is placed across the LHB tendon and pulled through a stab incision in line with the conjoint tendon proximally. After isometric tensioning, a grasper is used to maintain the LHB tendon parallel to the conjoint tendon (**C**) and sutures are passed through the LHB tendon and the anterolateral portion of the conjoint tendon (**D**) until three to four sutures are completed (**E**). **F,** Side-to-side healing as visualized at repeat subdeltoid arthroscopy 1 year postoperatively.

sertion of the pectoralis major tendon, and is important for clearing the subdeltoid space. The conjoint portal is placed 3 cm distal to the tip of the coracoid, in line with the conjoint tendon, and is later used for the side-to-side suturing of the LHB and conjoint tendons. Additional working portals may be created using spinal needle localization wherever they enable functional access. A skin-only incision is made, followed by blunt passage of a trochar through the deltoid muscle. This technique ensures simultaneous functional working vectors and safe introduction of trochars.

An aperture is made in the bicipital hood through which the tenotomized LHB tendon (**Figure 5, A**) is accessed. If the LHB tendon was not tagged before the tenotomy, it should be tagged with a No. 2 nonabsorbable traction stitch (**Figure 5, B**). A small stab incision is established anterior to the superior aspect of the coracoid through which the traction sutures are passed. This allows the LHB tendon to be placed parallel to the conjoint tendon and appropriately tensioned.

Traction is placed on the LHB tendon with the arm in the 90-90-15 position. Tension is considered appropriate when it appears isometric during flexion and extension of the elbow. A looped suture retriever is passed through one of the lateral portals to reduce the LHB tendon to the conjoint tendon (**Figure 5, C**). A suture-passing device is used to pass a nonabsorbable suture across both the LHB and conjoint tendons via the conjoint portal.

TABLE 1 Short-Term Results for Arthroscopic Subdeltoid LHB Tendon Transfer to the Conjoint Tendon

Parameter	Total Cohort (n = 40)	Isolated LHB Tendon Transfer (n = 25)
Popeye sign	5%	0%
Fatigue	12%	8%
L'Insalata score[a]	78.9 (35.7–100.0)	85.2
ASES score[a]	79.6 (30–100)	84.8
UCLA score[a]	27.8 (12–35)	29.5

ASES = American Shoulder and Elbow Surgeon, LHB = long head of the biceps, UCLA = UCLA Shoulder Rating Scale.
[a]Data are the mean; numbers in parentheses are the range.
Data adapted from Drakos MC, Verma NN, Gulotta LV, et al: Arthroscopic transfer of the long head of the biceps tendon: Functional outcome and clinical results. *Arthroscopy* 2008;24(2):217-223.

The suture is tied arthroscopically and the process repeated until the tendon transfer is secured with four or five sutures (**Figure 5, D** through **F**). It is imperative to suture the LHB tendon to the anterior portion of the lateral aspect of the conjoint tendon to avoid coracoid impingement or injury to the musculocutaneous nerve. All extraneous portions of the LHB tendon and tagging sutures are excised and discarded.

Results

Drakos et al[16] retrospectively investigated 40 patients who underwent transfer of the LHB tendon to the conjoint tendon (mean follow-up, 28 months; range, 24 to 53 months). Outcome measures (**Table 1**) included both subjective and objective measures. No significant side-to-side difference was identified during 10-lb biceps curls; 95% of patients reported relief of preoperative tenderness to palpation, and only 5% of patients with concomitant pathology had a Popeye deformity.

Recently, patient outcomes for this procedure were evaluated at a mean of 4.9 years postoperatively to provide more long-term follow-up data[17] (**Table 2**). In this study, 157 patients (25 women, 132 men; mean age, 50 years; mean follow-up, 4.9 years) were evaluated using the L'Insalata Shoulder Rating Scale, American Shoulder and Elbow Surgeons (ASES) score, and UCLA Shoulder Rating Scale questionnaires, which resulted in mean scores of 84.8, 83.4, and 29.8, respectively. In the 33 patients who underwent isolated LHB tendon transfer, the L'Insalata, ASES, and UCLA scores were 79.5, 84.0, and 27.6, respectively. Forty-three patients (7 women, 36 men; mean age, 50 years; mean follow-up, 5.1 years) underwent clinical examination by a physician other than the treating surgeon. No significant difference in side-to-side strength was reported using a 10-lb weight. No patient reported arm pain at rest regarding the biceps; 87.5% of patients reported no biceps tenderness with palpation of the bicipital groove and had a negative result for the throwing test; 94% of patients had a negative result for the active compression test; and the Speed and Yergason tests had negative results in 87.5% and 97.0% of patients, respectively. One patient (3.0%) reported fatigue discomfort (soreness) isolated to the biceps muscle following resisted elbow flexion, and 3 patients (9.3%) had a Popeye deformity. Among all patients, 88% self-rated as having good or excellent results and 12% self-rated as having fair or poor results.

Discussion

After nonsurgical management for LHB tendon–related pathology has failed, surgical intervention may be indicated. This can include biceps tenotomy, tenodesis, or transfer to the conjoint tendon.

LHB tenotomy provides reliable pain relief, but can result in cosmetic deformity (the Popeye sign), as well as fatigue and discomfort. Kelly et al[11] retrospectively reviewed 40 patients who underwent arthroscopic tenotomy with a mean follow-up of 2.7 years (range, 24

TABLE 2 Midterm Results for Arthroscopic Subdeltoid LHB Tendon Transfer to the Conjoint Tendon

Parameter	Total Cohort (n = 157)	Isolated LHB Tendon Transfer (n = 33)
Popeye sign	9.3%	0%
Fatigue	3%	0%
Mean L'Insalata score	84.8	79.5
Mean ASES score	83.4	84.0
Mean UCLA score	29.8	27.6

Data adapted from Taylor SA, Fabricant PD, Newman AM, Baret NJ, O'Brien SJ: e-poster: Arthroscopic transfer of the long head of the biceps tendon: 2-10 year functional outcome and clinical results. *AOSSM 2013 Annual Meeting.* Chicago, IL, July 11-14, 2013.

to 42 months). Tenderness with palpation of the bicipital groove was relieved in 96% of patients. Outcomes were positive including a mean L'Insalata score of 75.6 (range, 29.1 to 100), a mean UCLA score of 27.6 (range, 10 to 35), and a mean ASES score of 77.6 (range, 13.3 to 100). However, 38% of patients had fatigue and discomfort symptoms and 70% had a Popeye sign at rest or during active elbow flexion. Gill et al[18] surveyed 32 patients who underwent biceps tenotomy with a mean follow-up of 1.6 years. Although the mean ASES score (81.8) was similar to that of Kelly et al,[11] a complication rate of 13.3% was reported, including one occurrence of the Popeye sign.

Biceps tenodesis can be performed as an open or arthroscopic procedure, with either soft-tissue or bony fixation using anchors in or inferior to the bicipital groove, with varied results. Early tenodesis techniques reported on by Dines et al[19] had a 30% failure rate. In a retrospective case series, Becker et al[20] evaluated the results of 51 patients who underwent tenodesis with a mean follow-up of 7 years (range, 1 to 21 years). The authors reported that 26 patients (50%) continued to have moderate to severe pain. Post and Benca[21] reported on 17 patients at 42-month follow-up with 94% having good to excellent results.

Nho et al[22] reported a very low complication rate (7 of 535 patients) that included persistent bicipital pain and failure of fixation resulting in Popeye sign. Other authors reported postoperative fracture[23,24] and persistent bicipital groove symptoms following tenodesis.[11,18-20]

LHB tendon transfer to the conjoint tendon is a safe, effective alternative to tenodesis. LHB tendon transfer is performed in an avascular plane without the use of implants. Further, subdeltoid arthroscopic transfer allows direct visualization of both tendons, which enables appropriate tensioning of the LHB tendon. The LHB tendon is completely removed from the groove, isolating it from localized inflammatory or mechanical pathology. Cosmetic deformity and muscle cramping have improved results when compared with tenotomy because tendon transfer emulates the native axis of the pull of the biceps muscle and facilitates equal distribution of force between each head of the biceps. In addition, the soft-tissue healing is theorized to imitate the normal bungee effect of the biceps-labral complex.

Potential complications with LHB tendon transfer include incomplete release of the LHB tendon from the sheath, coracoid impingement, and neurovascular injury. When the LHB tendon is released from the bicipital groove, care must be taken to release the entire hood over the tendon—failure to do so results in an acute angle as the LHB tendon is transferred to the conjoint tendon. The LHB tendon should be placed laterally along the conjoint tendon to avoid coracoid impingement that can occur with posterior placement. Additionally, care must be taken to avoid injuring the musculocutaneous nerve, which usually enters the coracobrachialis a mean of 4.9 cm distal to the coracoid process, but may have a more proximal insertion site within 2 cm distal to the coracoid process in 5% of patients.[25]

Conclusion

Symptomatic pathology can occur along the entire biceps-labral complex. Most pathologies respond to nonsurgical measures. A small subset of patients may have recalcitrant pathology that requires surgical intervention. Arthroscopic subdeltoid transfer of the LHB tendon results in safe, reliable, and reproducible relief of symptoms in a manner comparable to that of tenotomy, and with a much lower risk of cosmetic deformity.

References

1. Alpantaki K, McLaughlin D, Karagogeos D, Hadjipavlou A, Kontakis G: Sympathetic and sensory neural elements in the tendon of the long head of the biceps. *J Bone Joint Surg Am* 2005;87(7):1580-1583.
2. Kumar VP, Satku K, Balasubramaniam P: The role of the long head of biceps brachii in the stabilization of the head of the humerus. *Clin Orthop Relat Res* 1989;244:172-175.
3. Kuhn JE, Huston LJ, Soslowsky LJ, Shyr Y, Blasier RB: External rotation of the glenohumeral joint: Ligament restraints and muscle effects in the neutral and abducted positions. *J Shoulder Elbow Surg* 2005;14(1, Suppl S): 39S-48S.
4. Levy AS, Kelly BT, Lintner SA, Osbahr DC, Speer KP: Function of the long head of the biceps at the shoulder: Electromyographic analysis. *J Shoulder Elbow Surg* 2001;10(3):250-255.
5. Yamaguchi K, Riew KD, Galatz LM, Syme JA, Neviaser RJ: Biceps activity during shoulder motion: An electromyographic analysis. *Clin Orthop Relat Res* 1997;336:122-129.
6. O'Brien SJ, Pagnani MJ, Fealy S, McGlynn SR, Wilson JB: The active compression test: A new and effective test for diagnosing labral tears and acromioclavicular joint abnormality. *Am J Sports Med* 1998;26(5):610-613.
7. O'Brien SJ, Newman AM, Taylor SA, et al: Presentation: Accurate diagnosis of biceps-labral complex lesions with MRI and "3-pack" physical examination—A retrospective analysis with prospective validation. *AOSSM 2013 Annual Meeting.* Chicago, IL, July 11-14, 2013, p 12.
8. Patton WC, McCluskey GM III: Biceps tendinitis and subluxation. *Clin Sports Med* 2001;20(3):505-529.
9. Eakin CL, Faber KJ, Hawkins RJ, Hovis WD: Biceps tendon disorders in athletes. *J Am Acad Orthop Surg* 1999;7(5):300-310.
10. Hashiuchi T, Sakurai G, Morimoto M, Komei T, Takakura Y, Tanaka Y: Accuracy of the biceps tendon sheath injection: Ultrasound-guided or unguided injection? A randomized controlled trial. *J Shoulder Elbow Surg* 2011;20(7):1069-1073.
11. Kelly AM, Drakos MC, Fealy S, Taylor SA, O'Brien SJ: Arthroscopic release of the long head of the biceps tendon: Functional outcome and clinical results. *Am J Sports Med* 2005;33(2):208-213.
12. Verma NN, Drakos M, O'Brien SJ: The arthroscopic active compression test. *Arthroscopy* 2005;21(5):634.
13. Hart ND, Golish SR, Dragoo JL: Effects of arm position on maximizing intra-articular visualization of the biceps tendon: A cadaveric study. *Arthroscopy* 2012;28(4): 481-485.
14. Taylor SA, Khair MM, Gulotta L, et al: Hidden lesions of the long head of the biceps tendon: A cadaveric analysis and case series. *AAOS 2013 Annual Meeting Proceedings.* CD-ROM. Rosemont, IL, American Academy of Orthopaedic Surgeons, 2013, pp 944-945.
15. Verma NN, Drakos M, O'Brien SJ: Arthroscopic transfer of the long head biceps to the conjoint tendon. *Arthroscopy* 2005;21(6):764.
16. Drakos MC, Verma NN, Gulotta LV, et al: Arthroscopic transfer of the long head of the biceps tendon: Functional outcome and clinical results. *Arthroscopy* 2008;24(2):217-223.
17. Taylor SA, Fabricant PD, Newman AM, Baret NJ, O'Brien SJ: e-poster: Arthroscopic transfer of the long head of the biceps tendon: 2-10 year functional outcome and clinical results. *AOSSM 2013 Annual Meeting.* Chicago, IL, July 11-14, 2013, p 22.
18. Gill TJ, McIrvin E, Mair SD, Hawkins RJ: Results of biceps tenotomy for treatment of pathology of the long head of the biceps brachii. *J Shoulder Elbow Surg* 2001;10(3):247-249.
19. Dines D, Warren RF, Inglis AE: Surgical treatment of lesions of the long head of the biceps. *Clin Orthop Relat Res* 1982;164:165-171.
20. Becker DA, Cofield RH: Tenodesis of the long head of the biceps brachii for chronic bicipital tendinitis: Long-term results. *J Bone Joint Surg Am* 1989;71(3):376-381.
21. Post M, Benca P: Primary tendinitis of the long head of the biceps. *Clin Orthop Relat Res* 1989;246:117-125.
22. Nho SJ, Reiff SN, Verma NN, Slabaugh MA, Mazzocca AD, Romeo AA: Complications associated with subpec-

toral biceps tenodesis: Low rates of incidence following surgery. *J Shoulder Elbow Surg* 2010;19(5):764-768.

23. Sears BW, Spencer EE, Getz CL: Humeral fracture following subpectoral biceps tenodesis in 2 active, healthy patients. *J Shoulder Elbow Surg* 2011;20(6):e7-e11.

24. Reiff SN, Nho SJ, Romeo AA: Proximal humerus fracture after keyhole biceps tenodesis. *Am J Orthop (Belle Mead NJ)* 2010;39(7):E61-E63.

25. Bach BR Jr, O'Brien SJ, Warren RF, Leighton M: An unusual neurological complication of the Bristow procedure: A case report. *J Bone Joint Surg Am* 1988;70(3):458-460.

CHAPTER 13

Arthroscopic Treatment of Biceps Tendon Injuries: An International Perspective

Knut Beitzel, MA, MD
Sepp Braun, MD
Andreas B. Imhoff, MD

Introduction

The anatomic position of the long head of the biceps (LHB) tendon near other critical structures of the glenohumeral joint is unique and makes it susceptible to specific biomechanical stress. Before entering the intertubercular groove, the tendon is guided by the structures of the biceps pulley system, which was first described by Walch et al.[1] The tendon is guided anteriorly by the superior glenohumeral ligament (SGHL) and subscapularis tendon, and posteriorly/laterally by the coracohumeral ligament (CHL) and the anterior fibers of the supraspinatus tendon. Other authors have already emphasized the importance of the SGHL and CHL for the stability of the tendon. Werner et al[2] demonstrated the complex histoanatomy of the pulley sling. Habermeyer et al[3] reported on the importance of the pulley sling for stabilization of the tendon and therefore introduced a classification for resulting instabilities.

Because of these anatomic and functional features, LHB tendon pathologies often occur in combination with additional glenohumeral joint lesions. Treating such pathologies arthroscopically often allows combined surgical treatment, which can be achieved directly and with reduced morbidity for the patient when compared with open procedures.

Rationale for Arthroscopic Treatment of the LHB

If nonsurgical treatment is unsuccessful (for example, the patient has persistent pain and cramping), the surgeon has many options for surgical treatment. Although wide controversy exists regarding various surgical techniques, objective data are scant.[4,5] In general, surgeons have two arthroscopic options: tenotomy and tenodesis, which fixes the stump at a more distal location. Arthroscopic tenotomy and tenodesis have been compared with varied results; neither technique has demonstrated clear clinical superiority.[4,5]

The rationale for performing both procedures arthroscopically is the fact that LHB lesions are often

---

Dr. Braun or an immediate family member is a member of a speakers' bureau or has made paid presentations on behalf of Arthrex; has received nonincome support (such as equipment or services), commercially derived honoraria, or other non–research-related funding (such as paid travel) from Arthrex; and serves as a board member, owner, officer, or committee member of the Society for Arthroscopy and Joint Surgery. Dr. Imhoff or an immediate family member has received royalties from Arthrex; serves as a paid consultant to or is an employee of Arthrex, Arthrosurface, and Medi Bayreuth; has received research or institutional support from Arthrex; and serves as a board member, owner, officer, or committee member of the International Society of Arthroscopy, Knee Surgery, and Orthopaedic Sports Medicine; the AGA; the DGOU; and the DGOOC. Neither Dr. Beitzel nor any immediate family member has received anything of value from or has stock or stock options held in a commercial company or institution related directly or indirectly to the subject of this chapter.

combined with additional intra-articular glenohumeral lesions. Performing all required procedures via the same surgical approach is more reasonable. It also minimizes the wound areas, and, if performed correctly, may reduce the risk of perioperative infection. Additionally, less invasive procedures may have cosmetic advantages. The advantages of open procedures include the potentially superior visualization of the surgical field and reduced surgical time, resulting in less soft-tissue swelling compared with arthroscopic procedures such as rotator cuff repair.

Patient Selection

The decision to treat biceps pathology should be based on the patient's age, activity level, arm dominance, history of symptoms, treatment goals, and willingness to participate in postoperative rehabilitation.[6] LHB tendon pathologies often occur in combination with instability, osteoarthritis, or other glenohumeral lesions such as rotator cuff lesions.[7] In these cases, treatment options should focus mainly on the concomitant pathology. However, biceps tenotomy or tenodesis alone have been shown to improve symptoms even with irreparable rotator cuff lesions.[8]

In general, LHB tenotomy should be considered for patients who are unwilling or unable to comply with the specific rehabilitation protocols, which are needed for tenodesis. Clinically relevant postoperative differences in elbow flexion strength have not been shown between tenotomy and tenodesis.[9] In contrast, significant differences have been found with cosmetic evaluation.[10] Tenotomy may result in a significant descent in the biceps muscle belly, also known as the Popeye sign. Therefore, biceps tenodesis is indicated in younger, active patients who have higher occupational or athletic demands and in patients who are concerned about cosmesis. However, given that no surgical procedure can be recommended over others,[11,12] treatment should be decided based on the situation and for each patient individually.

Surgical Technique

The patient may be placed in the beach chair or lateral decubitus position for all procedures. The authors of this chapter commonly place the patient in the beach chair position and use a standard posterior arthroscopic portal to inspect the glenohumeral joint. A thorough evaluation of the joint for any additional lesions of the intra-articular structures should always be performed because of the high incidence of combined lesions (for example, with rotator cuff tears or instability). The entire intra-articular length of the LHB is inspected. An additional anterior portal is established to evaluate the LHB tendon anchor for SLAP lesions, and the origin of the tendon and the superior labrum are probed. The tendon is pulled out of the sulcus and the stability of the pulley structures is tested.

Tenotomy

The surgical concept of tenotomy is based on the fact that although the role of the LHB tendon in the shoulder is controversial, its primary function is flexion and supination of the elbow.[11] Because of its undetermined function in the glenohumeral joint, some authors have even referred to it as the appendix of the shoulder.[7] Although the LHB may serve a more proprioceptive function, it has to be assumed that the biceps is stressed significantly when the rotator cuff is torn.

Currently, tenotomy is performed arthroscopically in almost all cases.[11] A standard working portal is used to cut the biceps at the insertion using either arthroscopic scissors or a radiofrequency cutter. Damage to the superior labrum should be avoided to maintain its function. After detaching the tendon, the surgeon should check that the tendon has slipped into the sulcus. This is important because thickening of the tendon (the "hourglass" biceps) or other degenerative lesions in the more distal parts and adhesions may make it susceptible to entrapment within the bicipital groove. After the tendon is detached, the proximal stump should be débrided just at the labrum. Damage to the labral structures should be avoided to preserve its function. If present, SLAP lesions may be débrided or fixed at this time.

Tenodesis

Biceps tenodesis was first described more than 60 years ago.[13] The LHB tendon is fixed distal to its origin because this allows a proper length-tension relationship of the biceps to be maintained, thereby minimizing muscle cramping, atrophy, and weakness that may be associated with LHB rupture or tenotomy.[6]

LHB tenodesis is the most common procedure for young, active patients. Many surgical techniques for

FIGURE 1

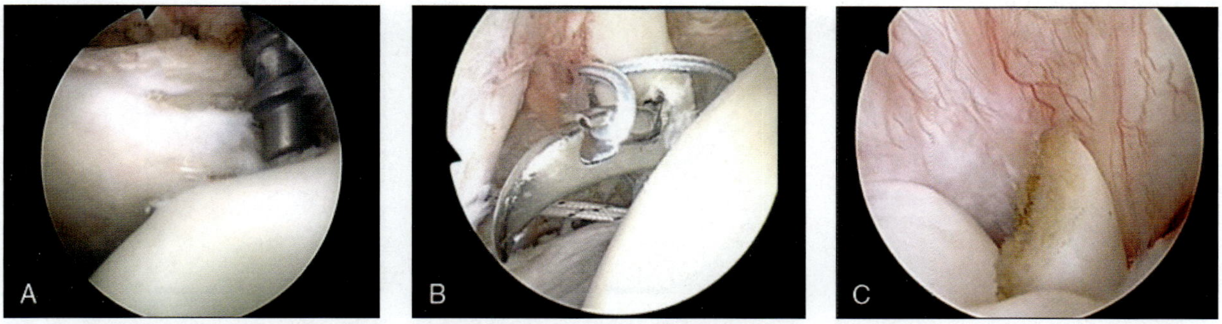

Arthroscopic views of all-inside tenodesis using a suture anchor. **A,** A double-loaded 5.5-mm bioabsorbable suture anchor is placed at the entrance of the bicipital groove next to the insertion of the subscapularis tendon. **B,** The long head of the biceps tendon is penetrated with a suture passer and suture limbs are shuttled through the tendon. **C,** Final view shows tendon stump fixation after detachment from the superior glenoid.

tenodesis have been described in the literature. Generally, the tendon stump can be reattached in one of three anatomic positions. Proximal reattachment refers to arthroscopic intra-articular LHB tenodesis; suprapectoral reattachment describes arthroscopic LHB tenodesis inferior to the entrance of the bicipital groove, above the superior edge of the pectoralis tendon;[14] and subpectoral LHB tenodesis involves fixation of the LHB tendon underneath the pectoralis tendon via an incision in the axilla, which was performed as an open procedure in almost all publications.

The patient is placed in the beach chair position and a standard posterior portal is established for initial evaluation of the glenohumeral joint and visualization of the LHB. A probe should be used to examine the intertubercular portion of the tendon by pulling the tendon into the joint. It is important to ensure that no lesions are found distal to the planned tenodesis and that no loose bodies are left within the sulcus. The tendon is cut at its proximal insertion and the proximal stump is débrided, taking care to avoid lacerating the labral structures.

Surgeons can also choose from various fixation methods and devices that range from suturing the tendon to the rotator cuff or the soft-tissue structures of the pulley sling to using suture anchors or intraosseous screw fixation. Suturing the tendon to adjacent soft-tissue structures such as the rotator cuff may be a simple, inexpensive procedure. However, the authors of this chapter believe that this technique may have an increased risk of failure because the resulting biomechanical stresses may function as a potential pain generator. Verma et al[15] described an arthroscopic technique of suturing the LHB tendon to the short head of the biceps tendon. This may result in good clinical outcome without interfering with other intra-articular structures. However, the described surgical technique is demanding and may be time-consuming, with an increased risk of extensive soft-tissue swelling, because the rotator interval needs to be opened.

Tenodesis is easily performed with a double-loaded 5.5-mm bioabsorbable suture anchor. A second suture anchor can be used to augment the tenodesis or for additional fixation of the cranial subscapularis or the anterior supraspinatus tendon (**Figure 1, A**). The tendon is pierced with a needle for placement of a shuttle suture. This suture can be used to transport the sutures for the anchor through the tendon. An arthroscopic penetrating device can be used instead of the needle to transport the sutures directly through the tendon (**Figure 1, B**). Some surgeons prefer to transport the suture in a sling-type fashion to improve the fixation strength and minimize slippage. The suture is fixed at the tendon with a knot.

The anchor should be placed at the entrance of the bicipital groove distal enough to prevent any impingement of the stump. If one of the two rotator cuff tendons needs to be reattached, it can be included in the repair by placing the anchor slightly more toward the adjoining tendon footprint. To improve biologic healing, the area is decorticated with an arthroscopic

FIGURE 2

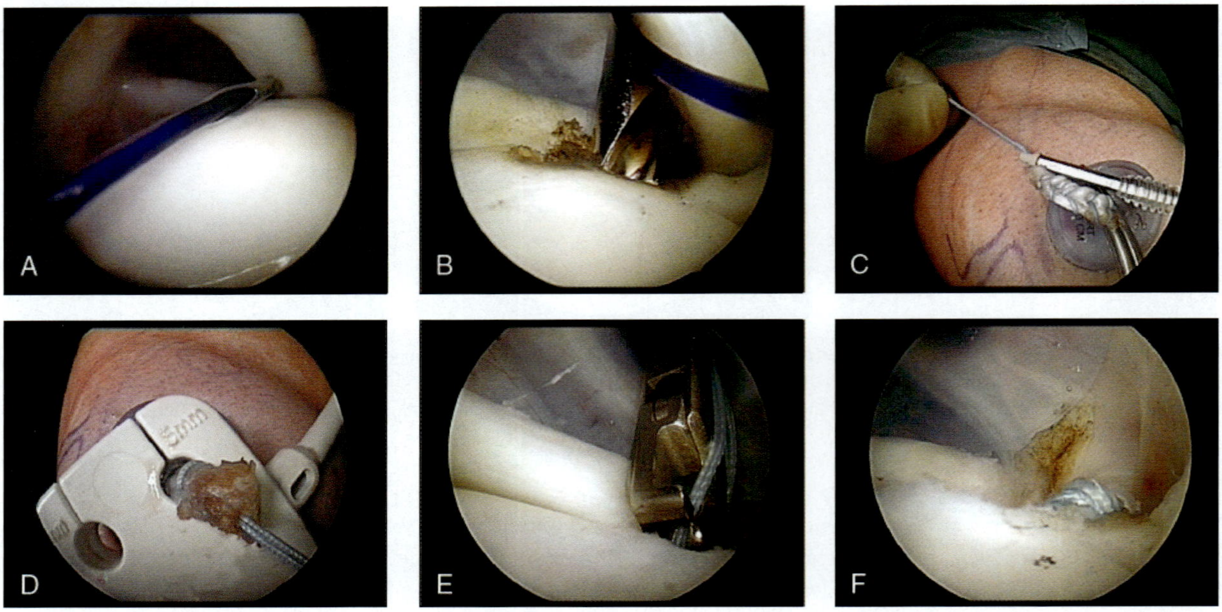

Arthroscopic views of tenodesis using screw fixation. **A,** A needle loaded with a shuttle suture is passed through the long head of the biceps tendon. **B,** The bone socket is drilled at the entrance of the intertubercular groove. **C,** Following detachment of the tendon from its origin, the tendon stump diameter is measured to calculate the bone socket size. **D,** Both suture limbs are loaded into the tip of the swivel lock tenodesis screw. **E,** The free limbs are cut after tendon stump fixation using the tenodesis screw. **F,** Final view of the fixed tendon stump.

shaver/burr to allow minimal bleeding. After the suture anchor is in place, the tendon can be fixed by tying knots using a knot pusher (**Figure 1, C**).

If the tendon needs to be fixed at a higher primary strength, intraosseous tenodesis may be performed using tenodesis screws.[16,17] This intraosseous fixation may increase primary stability and facilitate improved healing. The tendon length is marked at the planned tenodesis site and a holding suture is placed through the tendon (**Figure 2, A**). The tendon is cut proximal to its origin at the labrum and removed via the anterior portal. The proximal 20 mm of the tendon are removed to eliminate any tendon pathology from the tenodesis and to re-create an appropriate length. The diameter of the tendon stump is measured to ensure an optimal fit in the bone socket (**Figure 2, B**) and the suture limbs are loaded into the anchor (**Figure 2, C**).

The entrance of the intertubercular groove is localized and a 2-mm guidewire is inserted. The guidewire is then reamed over using a 7-mm cannulated reamer to a depth of 30 mm (**Figure 2, D**). The screw is inserted into the bone socket and the remaining suture limbs are cut over the top of the screw (**Figure 2, E**). The portal is then closed in the usual manner (**Figure 2, F**).

Rehabilitation

The postoperative rehabilitation is based mainly on any additional lesions found and any surgical procedures, which are often combined with LHB surgery, such as rotator cuff repair. Following arthroscopic tenotomy without additional surgery, the patient should rest the arm for the first 5 to 7 days. Range of motion does not have to be restricted, but active loading of the biceps should be avoided for the first 4 to 6 weeks following tenotomy.

Following tenodesis, patients should begin passive range-of-motion exercises but can progress quickly to active assisted exercises and active range of motion. Full range of motion at the elbow and grip strengthening are allowed immediately postoperatively. Strengthening exercises for elbow flexion or forward elevation of the arm should be restricted until 6 weeks postoperatively.

Clinical Outcome

Although no consensus currently exists regarding whether LHB tendon pathology should be treated with tenotomy or tenodesis, both procedures have shown good clinical results.[5] Gill et al[18] demonstrated significant reduction in pain, an improvement in function, and a complication rate of 13.3% after tenotomy. A recent systematic review by Slenker et al[5] showed favorable results for both tenotomy and tenodesis. The only relevant difference may be the increased cosmetic deformity reported in the patients who underwent biceps tenotomy. Osbahr et al[19] reported identical clinical results, but with a 30% incidence of cosmetic changes following tenotomy. Cramping and weakness with vigorous activities have also been reported following tenotomy.[11] No significant clinically relevant differences in strength for elbow flexion or forearm pronation and supination were reported.[9] Other authors have suggested tenotomy as effective for pain relief related to LHB tendon lesions. The authors of this chapter think that tenotomy is indicated largely in older patients or those with serious comorbidities.

Conclusion

Because the LHB is located near other critical structures of the shoulder such as the rotator cuff, surgical management often involves additional glenohumeral structures. Arthroscopic treatment, usually tenotomy or tenodesis, allows optimal glenohumeral visualization as well as additional simultaneous treatment, if needed.

References

1. Walch G, Nové-Josserand L, Boileau P, Levigne C: Subluxations and dislocations of the tendon of the long head of the biceps. *J Shoulder Elbow Surg* 1998;7(2): 100-108.
2. Werner A, Mueller T, Boehm D, Gohlke F: The stabilizing sling for the long head of the biceps tendon in the rotator cuff interval: A histoanatomic study. *Am J Sports Med* 2000;28(1):28-31.
3. Habermeyer P, Magosch P, Pritsch M, Scheibel MT, Lichtenberg S: Anterosuperior impingement of the shoulder as a result of pulley lesions: A prospective arthroscopic study. *J Shoulder Elbow Surg* 2004;13(1):5-12.
4. Elser F, Braun S, Dewing CB, Giphart JE, Millett PJ: Anatomy, function, injuries, and treatment of the long head of the biceps brachii tendon. *Arthroscopy* 2011;27(4):581-592.
5. Slenker NR, Lawson K, Ciccotti MG, Dodson CC, Cohen SB: Biceps tenotomy versus tenodesis: Clinical outcomes. *Arthroscopy* 2012;28(4):576-582.
6. Heckman DS, Creighton RA, Romeo AA: Management of failed biceps tenodesis or tenotomy: Causation and treatment. *Sports Med Arthrosc* 2010;18(3):173-180.
7. Ahrens PM, Boileau P: The long head of biceps and associated tendinopathy. *J Bone Joint Surg Br* 2007;89(8):1001-1009.
8. Boileau P, Baqué F, Valerio L, Ahrens P, Chuinard C, Trojani C: Isolated arthroscopic biceps tenotomy or tenodesis improves symptoms in patients with massive irreparable rotator cuff tears. *J Bone Joint Surg Am* 2007;89(4):747-757.
9. Shank JR, Singleton SB, Braun S, et al: A comparison of forearm supination and elbow flexion strength in patients with long head of the biceps tenotomy or tenodesis. *Arthroscopy* 2011;27(1):9-16.
10. Hsu AR, Ghodadra NS, Provencher MT, Lewis PB, Bach BR: Biceps tenotomy versus tenodesis: A review of clinical outcomes and biomechanical results. *J Shoulder Elbow Surg* 2011;20(2):326-332.
11. Barber A, Field LD, Ryu R: Biceps tendon and superior labrum injuries: Decision-making. *J Bone Joint Surg Am* 2007;89(8):1844-1855.
12. Frost A, Zafar MS, Maffulli N: Tenotomy versus tenodesis in the management of pathologic lesions of the tendon of the long head of the biceps brachii. *Am J Sports Med* 2009;37(4):828-833.
13. Hitchcock HH, Bechtol CO: Painful shoulder; observations on the role of the tendon of the long head of the biceps brachii in its causation. *J Bone Joint Surg Am* 1948;30A(2):263-273.
14. Lutton DM, Gruson KI, Harrison AK, Gladstone JN, Flatow EL: Where to tenodese the biceps: Proximal or distal? *Clin Orthop Relat Res* 2011;469(4):1050-1055.
15. Verma NN, Drakos M, O'Brien SJ: Arthroscopic transfer of the long head biceps to the conjoint tendon. *Arthroscopy* 2005;21(6):764.
16. Romeo AA, Mazzocca AD, Tauro JC: Arthroscopic biceps tenodesis. *Arthroscopy* 2004;20(2):206-213.

17. Kilicoglu O, Koyuncu O, Demirhan M, et al: Time-dependent changes in failure loads of 3 biceps tenodesis techniques: In vivo study in a sheep model. *Am J Sports Med* 2005;33(10):1536-1544.
18. Gill TJ, McIrvin E, Mair SD, Hawkins RJ: Results of biceps tenotomy for treatment of pathology of the long head of the biceps brachii. *J Shoulder Elbow Surg* 2001;10(3):247-249.
19. Osbahr DC, Diamond AB, Speer KP: The cosmetic appearance of the biceps muscle after long-head tenotomy versus tenodesis. *Arthroscopy* 2002;18(5):483-487.

CHAPTER *14*

Open Treatment of Biceps Tendon Injuries: Keyhole, Subpectoral Tenodesis, and Suture Anchor Techniques

Lauren E. Geaney, MD
Mandeep S. Virk, MBBS
Augustus D. Mazzocca, MS, MD

Introduction

The anatomy of the biceps tendon is unique. Proximally, it has two tendons, one intra-articular (the long head of the biceps [LHB]) and one extra-articular (the short head of the biceps), which combine to form the muscle and a single distal biceps tendon. The LHB is susceptible to pathology, including inflammatory tenosynovitis occurring in the bicipital groove, bicipital instability, and traumatic rupture.[1,2] Biceps tendinitis rarely occurs in isolation and most commonly presents in combination with other shoulder pathology. Although debate exists regarding the function of the LHB, this tendon is generally accepted to be a pain-generating anatomic structure in the shoulder. In cases of bicipital tearing, dislocation, and pain refractory to nonsurgical management, biceps tenodesis or tenotomy is indicated. Young, active patients may be candidates for biceps tenodesis. Options for tenodesis include open or arthroscopic techniques. This chapter describes three surgical techniques for open bicipital tenodesis: keyhole, subpectoral interference screw, and suture anchor.

Anatomy

The LHB originates at the supraglenoid tubercle and posterosuperior labrum; the short head originates at the apex of the coracoid process. The LHB is approximately 9 cm long and is intra-articular but extrasynovial at its proximal portion.[3,4] The tendon runs in the bicipital groove and is covered by the transverse humeral ligament, which was previously believed to be a significant contributor to the stability of the LHB in the bicipital groove.[2] However, anatomic studies have demonstrated that the rotator cuff interval, including the superior glenohumeral ligament, the coracohumeral ligament and fibers of the subscapularis tendon, and the insertion of the pectoralis major on the humerus, maintains the biceps position in the groove, as opposed to the transverse humeral ligament.[5,6]

Dr. Geaney or an immediate family member serves as a board member, owner, officer, or committee member of the Connecticut Orthopaedic Society. Dr. Mazzocca or an immediate family member serves as a paid consultant to or is an employee of Arthrex; and has received research or institutional support from Arthrex and Arthrosurface. Neither Dr. Virk nor any immediate family member has received anything of value from or has stock or stock options held in a commercial company or institution related directly or indirectly to the subject of this chapter.

The arterial supply of the LHB has always been of significant interest because of its implication in the pathogenesis of biceps tendon ruptures and tendinitis. The blood supply to the LHB derives from the branches of the brachial, thoracoacromial, and anterior circumflex humeral arteries.[7,8] Cheng et al[9] conducted a study of vascular contrast injections in cadavers and demonstrated that the proximal osseotendinous junction is supplied by the branches of the thoracoacromial artery; the distal musculotendinous junction, by the branches of the brachial artery; and the LHB tendon, by the branches of the anterior circumflex humeral artery via the mesotenon. A distinct hypovascular region was consistently found approximately 1.5 to 3.0 cm distal to the origin of LHB.

The function of the biceps is distinct proximally and distally. The distal tendon is the major supinator of the forearm and its secondary function is elbow flexion. In the shoulder, the role of the LHB tendon is still controversial. Some studies have demonstrated the importance of the LHB in providing stability to superior translation of the humeral head during abduction and contributing to overall stability of the glenohumeral joint.[10-12] Electromyographic studies in normal shoulders and shoulders with rotator cuff tears have demonstrated minimal activity in the LHB tendon in normal shoulders when elbow motion is restricted by a locked brace.[13]

Clinical Evaluation

The pathology of the LHB encompasses a variety of conditions including biceps inflammation, instability, or traumatic rupture, all of which may present differently. In general, patients with tenosynovitis or instability report progressive anterior shoulder pain. Patients with instability may describe an event followed by clicking and popping in the anterior shoulder.[1] Subluxation or dislocation usually occurs in association with a subscapularis tear, except in the rare case of extra-articular dislocation with the tendon lying superficial to the subscapularis.[14] Pain due to LHB pathology can be reproduced on physical examination by direct palpation over the bicipital groove. The LHB tendon can also be palpated by placing the index finger in the axilla under the pectoralis muscle–tendon unit (the preferred technique of ADM, senior author of this chapter). Resolution of pain and tenderness in the bicipital or subpectoral region after a lidocaine injection into the glenohumeral joint is definitive for the diagnosis of LHB tendon pathology. In cases of biceps rupture, physical examination reveals a bulbous mass proximal to the elbow, also called a Popeye deformity, with hollowness proximally. Extensive ecchymosis in the arm is a common finding. Instability may be reproduced with the shoulder fully abducted and externally rotated.

Physical examination tests for biceps pathology lack specificity. Palpation of the biceps tendon at its subpectoral position may elicit pain and is the anatomic location preferred by the authors of this chapter for the palpation of the LHB tendon instead of the bicipital groove proximally. The Speed test is considered positive when pain is reproduced with resisted forward flexion at 90° with the elbow in extension and supination. The Yergason test is considered positive when bicipital groove pain is reproduced with resisted supination with the elbow at 90°. It is important to understand that biceps pathology frequently presents with other shoulder conditions, so the physical examination also reveals findings consistent with these other injuries.

Diagnosis is primarily clinical, but imaging studies may help confirm the diagnosis or rule out associated pathology. Three radiographic views of the shoulder (AP, axillary, and supraspinatus outlet) should be obtained. MRI helps identify associated shoulder pathology, but may show fluid surrounding the LHB, alterations in tendon diameter, and signal intensity changes within the tendon. The role of MRI in diagnosing biceps tendinopathy is limited and has poor sensitivity.[15] Dynamic ultrasonography may help diagnose LHB instability as well as effusions within the biceps sheath but is operator dependent.[16,17]

Treatment

Nonsurgical treatment includes rest, NSAIDs, physical therapy, and corticosteroid injections into the glenohumeral joint or directly into the tendon sheath. Nonsurgical management also may be used for associated rotator cuff tears. Patients with traumatic LHB tears rarely require surgery. Pain is uncommon and patients can expect approximately 20% loss of supination strength and minimal loss of elbow flexion strength.[18]

Surgical intervention includes tenotomy or tenodesis. Tenotomy is generally indicated in older, low-demand patients. Following tenotomy, patients may report fatigue, cramps, or soreness with resisted elbow flexion and difficulty performing overhead work or sports.[19] Biceps tenodesis is advantageous when compared with tenotomy[20] regarding maintenance of the length-tension relationship of the biceps muscle, maintenance of elbow flexion and supination strength for maximum elbow function, and improved cosmesis.[21]

The indications for biceps tenodesis include tears involving more than 50% of the LHB tendon, medial subluxation of the LHB tendon, and subluxation in association with a subscapularis tear.[22,23] Other indications include severe proximal biceps tendinopathy resistant to nonsurgical treatment and occurring in association with some superior labrum anterior to posterior (SLAP) tears.[24] Multiple techniques exist for biceps tenodesis, including open[20,24,25] or arthroscopic,[22,23,26,27] performed proximal or distal to the bicipital groove. Techniques that involve fixation of the tendon proximal to the biceps groove may result in residual pain secondary to persistent tenosynovitis within the bicipital groove.[28]

Although arthroscopic approaches may be advantageous because they are less invasive, most techniques involve fixation of the tendon proximal to the bicipital groove.[26,29-31] Suprapectoral LHB tenodesis in the bicipital groove is associated with residual bicipital groove pain, and open subpectoral tenodesis has demonstrated a low reoperation rate. Because of this, the senior author of this chapter (ADM) prefers open procedures with fixation distal to the bicipital groove.

Techniques

Patients are placed in the beach chair or lateral position after induction of general anesthesia with or without a supplementary interscalene block. Before the procedure begins, a bilateral shoulder examination is performed and preoperative antibiotic prophylaxis is administered. The surgical arm is draped free and a padded Mayo stand is used to secure the arm. Irrespective of the preferred technique, a standard diagnostic glenohumeral arthroscopic examination is performed via the posterior portal. The LHB tendon should be evaluated with no fluid inflow (a dry scope) to avoid washing out the hypervascularity of the inflamed tenosynovium with high intra-articular pressure. A standard anterior portal is created and a probe inserted to pull the bicipital portion of the biceps tendon into the joint and evaluate its mobility and appearance. Once it is determined that a tenodesis will be performed, the biceps is tenotomized at the bicipitolabral junction with an arthroscopic basket or electrocautery. The stump is débrided with a shaver. The subpectoral approach is more reproducible and results in better cosmesis for the senior author (ADM). The author avoids the deltoid split and the deltopectoral approach because these may place the biceps tenodesis in an undesirable suprapectoral location.

Keyhole Tenodesis

For keyhole tenodesis,[28,32] the anterior shoulder is exposed using the deltopectoral approach. The LHB is palpated in the bicipital groove and the transverse humeral ligament is incised centrally to expose the LHB tendon (**Figure 1, A**). To maintain the length-tendon relationship, a marking stitch is placed in the tendon at the inferior margin of the transverse humeral ligament with the arm in neutral adduction and 90° of flexion.

The base of the groove is prepared by elevating the periosteum. A 4.5-mm bit is used to drill a unicortical hole in the floor of the groove and a burr is used to enlarge the hole to approximately 1 cm in diameter. A narrow key slot is then made with the burr distal to the circular bone window, usually approximately 5 mm in width (**Figure 1, B**). A curet may be needed to deepen the hole and remove cancellous bone.

The proximal tendon is prepared either by tying it into a knot or rolling it into a ball, holding it in place with a suture (**Figure 1, C**). The knot is pushed into the larger, proximal portion of the keyhole and pushed distally into the distal slot as the elbow is extended (**Figure 1, D**). Stable fixation of the tenotomized tendon in the keyhole can be confirmed by slowly extending and flexing the elbow.

If possible, the periosteum or transverse humeral ligament should be closed over the tenodesis. The wound is closed in the standard manner and the arm is placed in a sling. Potential complications associated with this procedure include fixation failure secondary to proximal humerus fracture through the keyhole, an intrasubstance tendon split, and dislodging of the tendon from the keyhole.

FIGURE 1

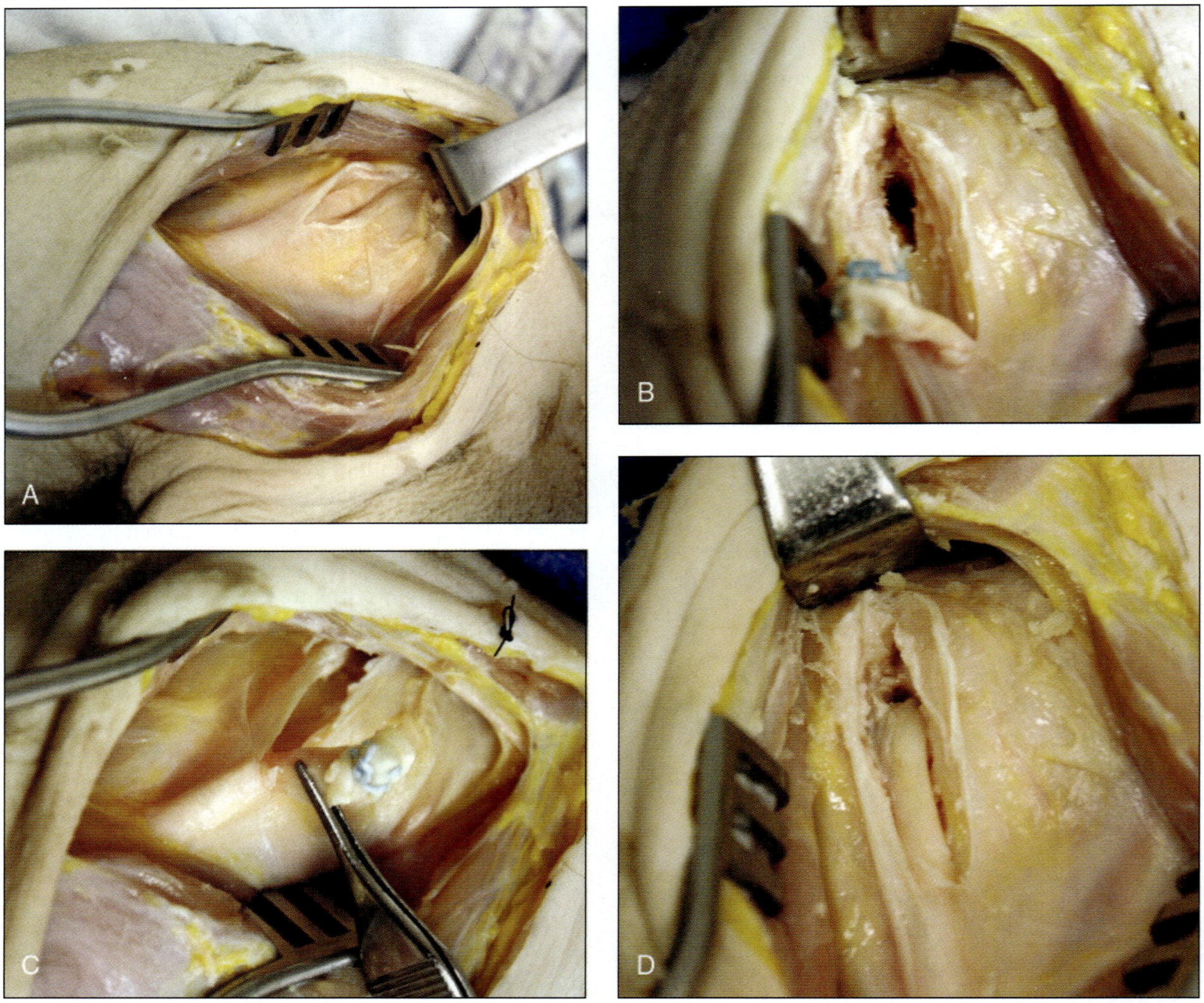

Photographs of the keyhole technique. **A,** Exposure is attained using the deltopectoral approach and the transverse humeral ligament is split. **B,** The keyhole is drilled with a 4.5-mm bit and enlarged to approximately 1 cm in diameter using a burr. The narrow key slot is made using the burr (usually approximately 5 mm wide). **C,** The proximal tendon is prepared by holding it in place with suture. **D,** The knot is inserted into the larger, proximal portion of the keyhole and pushed distally to deliver the tendon into the slot as the elbow is extended.

Subpectoral Interference Screw Technique

The goal of the subpectoral interference screw technique[20,24,33,34] is to perform tenodesis at the musculotendinous junction of the LHB to the bone at the level of the inferior border of the pectoralis major muscle, which provides an anatomic length-tension relationship for the remaining musculotendinous unit. The patient is placed in the beach chair position with the surgical arm in abduction and internal rotation. The inferior border of the pectoralis major tendon is palpated and a 4-cm longitudinal incision is started 1 cm superior to the inferior border of the pectoralis tendon (**Figure 2, A**). Prior to incision, the site is injected with subcutaneous local anesthetic with epinephrine for hemostasis and perioperative analgesia. The skin is incised and bleeding is controlled with electrocautery. A self-retainer is usually helpful with visualization at this point. The fascia overlying the conjoint tendon is visualized and incised proximal to distal. The pectoralis tendon is retracted proximally with an Army Navy retractor or a pointed Hohmann retractor. A blunt Chandler retractor is placed medially around the humerus to expose the LHB.

The LHB can now be palpated and delivered out of the incision using a right-angle clamp (**Figure 2, B**). The musculotendinous junction is identified, and a No. 2 nonabsorbable Krackow stitch (running lock stitch) is placed 15 mm proximal to the musculotendinous junction. The most proximal portion of the tendon is excised, leaving 20 to 25 mm of tendon remaining (**Figure 2, C**). A guidewire is placed through the anterior humerus 1 cm proximal to the pectoralis major tendon and overreamed with an 8-mm drill to a depth of 15 mm in the unicortical bone (**Figure 2, D**). One end of the Krackow suture is passed through an 8 × 12–mm interference screw (**Figure 2, E**). The authors of this chapter use an 8 × 12–mm polyether ether ketone screw, but titanium and biocomposite screws can also be used. The driver is placed in the bone tunnel and the screw is advanced until flush with the anterior cortex (**Figure 2, F**). The two ends of the suture are then tied together (**Figure 2, G**).

Complications are few and occur rarely. Fixation failure is reported in less than 1% of cases[1] and occurs because of screw pullout from the tunnel, tendon slippage at the bone-screw interface, or proximal humerus fracture through the bone tunnel.[35]

Suture Anchor Techniques

Suture anchor fixation has been used both arthroscopically and with the open subpectoral approach.[22,36-39] In the open approach, the biceps and bicipital groove are identified using the subpectoral approach described above. One option uses two double-loaded suture anchors placed in the bicipital groove, with the second anchor deployed approximately 5 mm distal to the first (**Figure 3, A**). No. 2 nonabsorbable sutures are sewn through the tendon in a mattress pattern (**Figure 3, B** and **C**). Alternately, the two anchors can be placed side-by-side and secured with modified Mason-Allen stitches. Another technique uses a single anchor and a Kessler suture pattern. Fixation failure occurs because of sutures cutting through the tendon substance or the mechanical failure of the suture anchor eyelet.

Postoperative Rehabilitation

Rehabilitation following tenodesis is determined largely by the associated pathology and surgical treatment. With isolated biceps tendinopathy and tenodesis, patients are placed in a sling for the first 4 weeks. From 4 to 12 weeks, the sling is discontinued and active elbow range of motion is begun. Simultaneously, rotator cuff, deltoid, and parascapular muscle strengthening is begun. Resistance strengthening exercises of the elbow are initiated at week 12 and should extend to month 6.

Outcomes

Biceps tenodesis can be performed using many different approaches and fixation methods. Multiple biomechanical studies have reported on the outcomes of these different techniques. Ozalay et al[39] and Kusma et al[40] used animal models to determine that the interference screw technique was stronger than the keyhole, suture anchor, or bone tunnel techniques in primary fixation strength. Similarly, Golish et al[36] showed that the interference screw had a statistically higher load-to-failure and stiffness than the corkscrew anchor in a cadaver model. Richards and Burkhart[38] also showed that the interference screw had greater resistance to pullout in a cadaver model. Mazzocca et al[37] found that the bone tunnel technique had the greatest displacement in a cadaver model when compared with interference screws and suture anchors. However, this was contrary to the results of Jayamoorthy et al,[41] who found that using the keyhole technique resulted in a significantly stronger repair than a metallic interference screw in a sheep model.

Although it appears that biomechanical models support the use of interference screws for superior strength, clinical outcome data are limited. Two systemic reviews have compared tenotomy with tenodesis.[21,42] All articles in the review except one were level IV evidence. The only consistent conclusion between the two reviews was the higher incidence of cosmetic deformity with tenotomy.

In the original description of the keyhole technique, Froimson and Oh[28] reported excellent results in 8 of 11 patients and good results in the remaining 3. All patients returned to work within 2 weeks. Mazzocca et al[33]

FIGURE 2

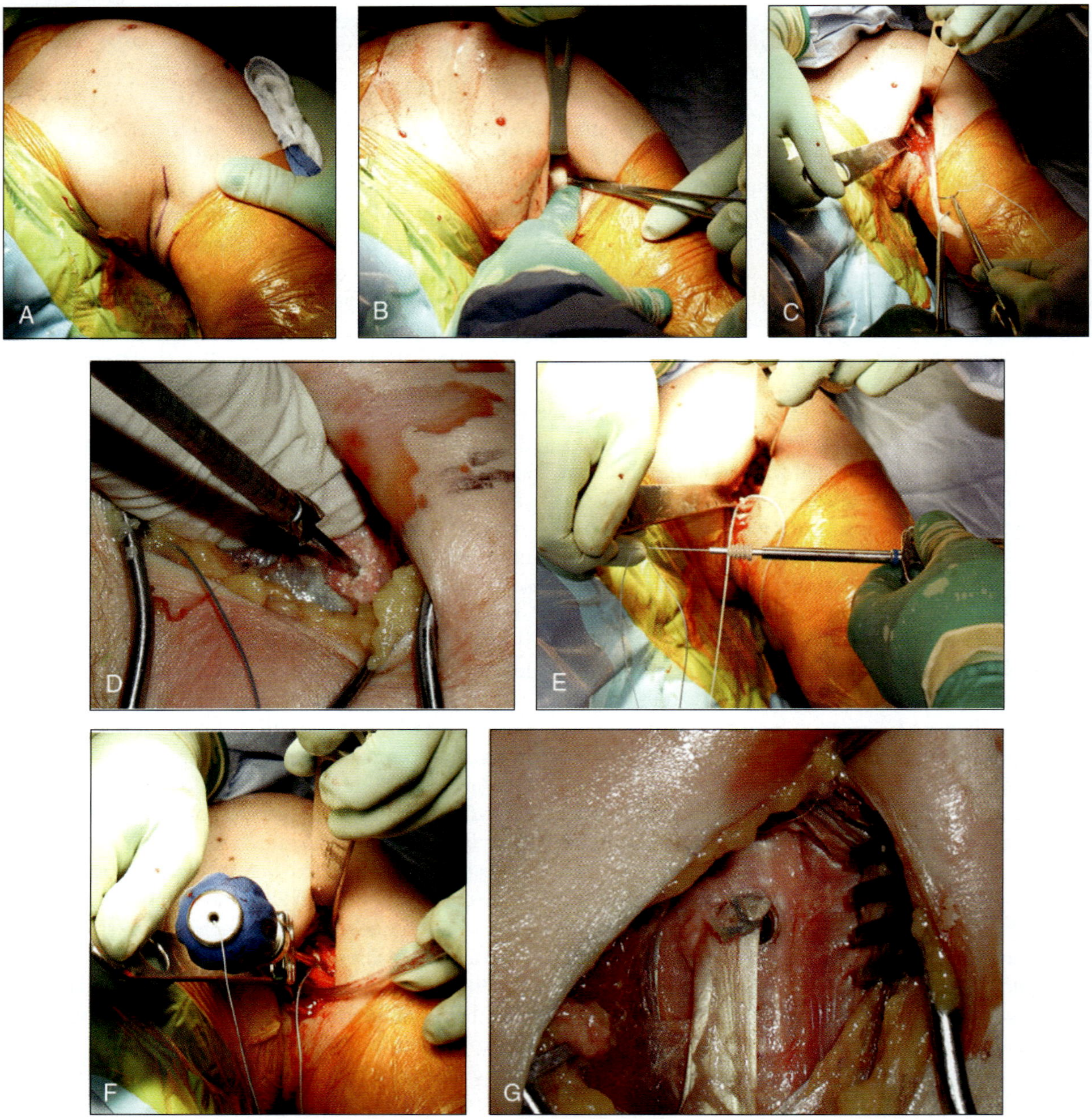

Photographs of the subpectoral tenodesis technique. **A,** The 4-cm incision is marked 1 cm superior to the inferior border of the pectoralis tendon. **B,** The pectoralis tendon is retracted proximally and the biceps tendon is identified with a right-angle clamp. **C,** The musculotendinous junction is identified and a Krackow stitch is placed. The most proximal portion of the tendon is excised, leaving 20 to 25 mm of tendon. **D,** A guidewire is placed through the anterior humerus 1 cm proximal to the pectoralis major tendon and is overreamed with an 8-mm drill. **E,** One end of the Krackow suture is passed through an 8 × 12–mm interference screw. **F,** The screwdriver is placed into the bone tunnel and the screw is advanced until flush with the anterior cortex. **G,** The two ends of the suture are tied together.

FIGURE 3

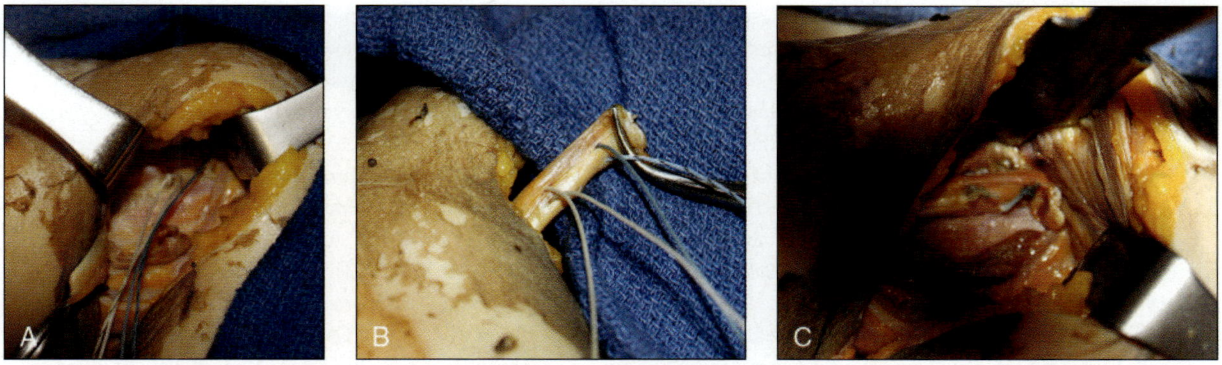

A, Suture anchors are placed in the bicipital groove. The second anchor is approximately 5 mm distal to the first. **B,** No. 2 nonabsorbable sutures from the suture anchor are sewn through the tendon in a mattress pattern. **C,** The sutures are tied to hold the biceps tendon in place.

followed 41 patients after subpectoral biceps tenodesis with an interference screw for a mean of 29 months. Only one failure was reported, and three patients (11%) reported pain. Nho et al[43] reported 7 complications in 353 patients following subpectoral tenodesis with interference screw after a mean follow-up of 2 years: 2 patients reported bicipital pain, 2 experienced failure of fixation, 1 had transient musculocutaneous nerve palsy, 1 had an infection, and 1 had reflex sympathetic dystrophy.

Conclusion

Biceps tenodesis is a good surgical option for patients with a biceps tear involving more than 50% of the tendon, medial subluxation of the biceps tendon, biceps subluxation in association with a subscapularis tear,[22,23] severe biceps tendinopathy resistant to nonsurgical treatment, and in association with some SLAP tears.[24] Clinical case series have shown reliable improvement in bicipital groove pain and good functional outcomes with open techniques that involve distal fixation of the tendon. Biomechanical studies have suggested that interference screws provide the strongest fixation. Prospective randomized studies with adequate follow-up are required to test the superiority of any fixation technique (open versus arthroscopic, proximal versus distal fixation, and screw fixation versus interference screw versus keyhole).

References

1. Nho SJ, Strauss EJ, Lenart BA, et al: Long head of the biceps tendinopathy: Diagnosis and management. *J Am Acad Orthop Surg* 2010;18(11):645-656.
2. Friedman DJ, Dunn JC, Higgins LD, Warner JJ: Proximal biceps tendon: Injuries and management. *Sports Med Arthrosc* 2008;16(3):162-169.
3. Sethi N, Wright R, Yamaguchi K: Disorders of the long head of the biceps tendon. *J Shoulder Elbow Surg* 1999;8(6):644-654.
4. Cooper DE, Arnoczky SP, O'Brien SJ, Warren RF, DiCarlo E, Allen AA: Anatomy, histology, and vascularity of the glenoid labrum: An anatomical study. *J Bone Joint Surg Am* 1992;74(1):46-52.
5. Gleason PD, Beall DP, Sanders TG, et al: The transverse humeral ligament: A separate anatomical structure or a continuation of the osseous attachment of the rotator cuff? *Am J Sports Med* 2006;34(1):72-77.
6. Walch G, Nove-Josserand L, Levigne C, Renaud E: Tears of the supraspinatus tendon associated with "hidden" lesions of the rotator interval. *J Shoulder Elbow Surg* 1994;3(6):353-360.
7. Cone RO, Danzig L, Resnick D, Goldman AB: The bicipital groove: Radiographic, anatomic, and pathologic study. *AJR Am J Roentgenol* 1983;141(4):781-788.
8. Hitchcock HH, Bechtol CO: Painful shoulder; observations on the role of the tendon of the long head of the biceps brachii in its causation. *J Bone Joint Surg Am* 1948;30-A(2):263-273.

9. Cheng NM, Pan WR, Vally F, Le Roux CM, Richardson MD: The arterial supply of the long head of biceps tendon: Anatomical study with implications for tendon rupture. *Clin Anat* 2010;23(6):683-692.
10. Warner JJ, McMahon PJ: The role of the long head of the biceps brachii in superior stability of the glenohumeral joint. *J Bone Joint Surg Am* 1995;77(3):366-372.
11. Kumar VP, Satku K, Balasubramaniam P: The role of the long head of biceps brachii in the stabilization of the head of the humerus. *Clin Orthop Relat Res* 1989;244:172-175.
12. Yamaguchi K, Riew KD, Galatz LM, Syme JA, Neviaser RJ: Biceps activity during shoulder motion: An electromyographic analysis. *Clin Orthop Relat Res* 1997;336:122-129.
13. Sakurai G, Ozaki J, Tomita Y, Nishimoto K, Tamai S: Electromyographic analysis of shoulder joint function of the biceps brachii muscle during isometric contraction. *Clin Orthop Relat Res* 1998;354:123-131.
14. Gambill ML, Mologne TS, Provencher MT: Dislocation of the long head of the biceps tendon with intact subscapularis and supraspinatus tendons. *J Shoulder Elbow Surg* 2006;15(6):e20-e22.
15. Mohtadi NG, Vellet AD, Clark ML, et al: A prospective, double-blind comparison of magnetic resonance imaging and arthroscopy in the evaluation of patients presenting with shoulder pain. *J Shoulder Elbow Surg* 2004;13(3):258-265.
16. Middleton WD, Reinus WR, Totty WG, Melson CL, Murphy WA: Ultrasonographic evaluation of the rotator cuff and biceps tendon. *J Bone Joint Surg Am* 1986;68(3):440-450.
17. Papatheodorou A, Ellinas P, Takis F, Tsanis A, Maris I, Batakis N: US of the shoulder: Rotator cuff and non-rotator cuff disorders. *Radiographics* 2006;26(1):e23.
18. Mariani EM, Cofield RH, Askew LJ, Li GP, Chao EY: Rupture of the tendon of the long head of the biceps brachii: Surgical versus nonsurgical treatment. *Clin Orthop Relat Res* 1988;228:233-239.
19. Kelly AM, Drakos MC, Fealy S, Taylor SA, O'Brien SJ: Arthroscopic release of the long head of the biceps tendon: Functional outcome and clinical results. *Am J Sports Med* 2005;33(2):208-213.
20. Mazzocca A, Noerdlinger MA, Romeo AA: Mini open and subpectoral biceps tenodesis. *Oper Tech Sports Med* 2003;11:24-31.
21. Slenker NR, Lawson K, Ciccotti MG, Dodson CC, Cohen SB: Biceps tenotomy versus tenodesis: Clinical outcomes. *Arthroscopy* 2012;28(4):576-582.
22. Gartsman GM, Hammerman SM: Arthroscopic biceps tenodesis: Operative technique. *Arthroscopy* 2000;16(5):550-552.
23. Kim SH, Yoo JC: Arthroscopic biceps tenodesis using interference screw: End-tunnel technique. *Arthroscopy* 2005;21(11):1405.
24. Provencher MT, LeClere LE, Romeo AA: Subpectoral biceps tenodesis. *Sports Med Arthrosc* 2008;16(3):170-176.
25. Edwards TB, Walch G: Biceps tenodesis: Indications and techniques. *Oper Tech Sports Med* 2002;10:99-104.
26. Boileau P, Krishnan SG, Coste JS, Walch G: Arthroscopic biceps tenodesis: A new technique using bioabsorbable interference screw fixation. *Arthroscopy* 2002;18(9):1002-1012.
27. Mazzocca A, Romeo AA: Arthroscopic Biceps tenodesis in the beach chair position. *Oper Tech Sports Med* 2003;11:6-14.
28. Froimson AI, O I: Keyhole tenodesis of biceps origin at the shoulder. *Clin Orthop Relat Res* 1975;112:245-249.
29. Guelich D, Lintner D: Arthroscopic intraosseous biceps tenodesis. *Oper Tech Sports Med* 2007;15:16-19.
30. Paulos L, Mendez KT, Berg T: A novel approach to arthroscopic biceps tenodesis. *Oper Tech Sports Med* 2007;15:27-34.
31. Klepps S, Hazrati Y, Flatow E: Arthroscopic biceps tenodesis. *Arthroscopy* 2002;18(9):1040-1045.
32. Lowe W, Craft JA, Milos S: Keyhole technique for tenodesis of the biceps tendon. *Oper Tech Sports Med* 2007;15:7-9.
33. Mazzocca AD, Cote MP, Arciero CL, Romeo AA, Arciero RA: Clinical outcomes after subpectoral biceps tenodesis with an interference screw. *Am J Sports Med* 2008;36(10):1922-1929.
34. Mazzocca AD, Rios CG, Romeo AA, Arciero RA: Subpectoral biceps tenodesis with interference screw fixation. *Arthroscopy* 2005;21(7):896.
35. Heckman DS, Creighton RA, Romeo AA: Management of failed biceps tenodesis or tenotomy: Causation and treatment. *Sports Med Arthrosc* 2010;18(3):173-180.
36. Golish SR, Caldwell PE III, Miller MD, et al: Interference screw versus suture anchor fixation for subpectoral tenodesis of the proximal biceps tendon: A cadaveric study. *Arthroscopy* 2008;24(10):1103-1108.

37. Mazzocca AD, Bicos J, Santangelo S, Romeo AA, Arciero RA: The biomechanical evaluation of four fixation techniques for proximal biceps tenodesis. *Arthroscopy* 2005;21(11):1296-1306.
38. Richards DP, Burkhart SS: A biomechanical analysis of two biceps tenodesis fixation techniques. *Arthroscopy* 2005;21(7):861-866.
39. Ozalay M, Akpinar S, Karaeminogullari O, et al: Mechanical strength of four different biceps tenodesis techniques. *Arthroscopy* 2005;21(8):992-998.
40. Kusma M, Dienst M, Eckert J, Steimer O, Kohn D: Tenodesis of the long head of biceps brachii: Cyclic testing of five methods of fixation in a porcine model. *J Shoulder Elbow Surg* 2008;17(6):967-973.
41. Jayamoorthy T, Field JR, Costi JJ, Martin DK, Stanley RM, Hearn TC: Biceps tenodesis: A biomechanical study of fixation methods. *J Shoulder Elbow Surg* 2004;13(2):160-164.
42. Hsu AR, Ghodadra NS, Provencher MT, Lewis PB, Bach BR: Biceps tenotomy versus tenodesis: A review of clinical outcomes and biomechanical results. *J Shoulder Elbow Surg* 2011;20(2):326-332.
43. Nho SJ, Reiff SN, Verma NN, Slabaugh MA, Mazzocca AD, Romeo AA: Complications associated with subpectoral biceps tenodesis: Low rates of incidence following surgery. *J Shoulder Elbow Surg* 2010;19(5):764-768.

CHAPTER 15

Special Patients: The Overhead Athlete

Christopher S. Ahmad, MD
Eric C. Makhni, MD
Neal S. ElAttrache, MD

Introduction

More than 60 years ago, Bennett[1] stated that professional baseball pitchers were uniquely susceptible to developing distinctive lesions in the shoulder. The overhead athlete places extreme force and repetitive demands on his or her shoulder at the extremes of range of motion (ROM), resulting in an increased risk of injury. In 1985, Andrews et al[2] identified the superior labrum as a common source of injury in overhead athletes; since then, significant emphasis has been placed on understanding the pathophysiology and pathomechanics of these injuries. Clinicians must not only alleviate symptoms of pain and discomfort in these athletes, they also must rehabilitate these high-demand patients to preinjury levels of performance and competition. Despite current increased awareness and diagnostic capacity, controversy exists regarding optimal treatment for this patient population. This chapter reviews current concepts, including functional anatomy of the biceps-labral complex, as well as the etiology, pathomechanics, diagnosis, and treatment of injuries to this structure in the overhead athlete.

Functional Anatomy of the Biceps-Labral Complex

Understanding the function of the biceps-labral complex requires understanding the individual components independently as well as how they interact during throwing. The superior labrum has several known anatomic variations that must not be confused with true pathology[3] (**Figure 1**). Anterosuperiorly, the superior labrum serves as the attachment site for the superior glenohumeral ligament (SGHL), the middle glenohumeral ligament (MGHL), and occasionally, fibers of the inferior glenohumeral ligament (IGHL).[4] The anterosuperior labrum may show normal thinning or be absent. The Buford complex is another natural variant that consists of an absent anterosuperior labrum with a cord-like MGHL that attaches to the base of the biceps tendon.[3,5] Unnecessary repair of these variants adversely restricts shoulder motion and causes significant morbidity.

Functionally, the labrum deepens the concavity of the shoulder joint, thereby resisting subluxation or dislocation of the humeral head through functional and ath-

Dr. Ahmad or an immediate family member serves as a paid consultant to or is an employee of Acumed and Arthrex; and has received research or institutional support from Arthrex, Major League Baseball, and Stryker. Dr. ElAttrache or an immediate family member has received royalties from Arthrex; has received research or institutional support from Omeros; and serves as a board member, owner, officer, or committee member of the American Orthopaedic Society for Sports Medicine. Neither Dr. Makhni nor any immediate family member has received anything of value from or has stock or stock options held in a commercial company or institution related directly or indirectly to the subject of this chapter.

FIGURE 1

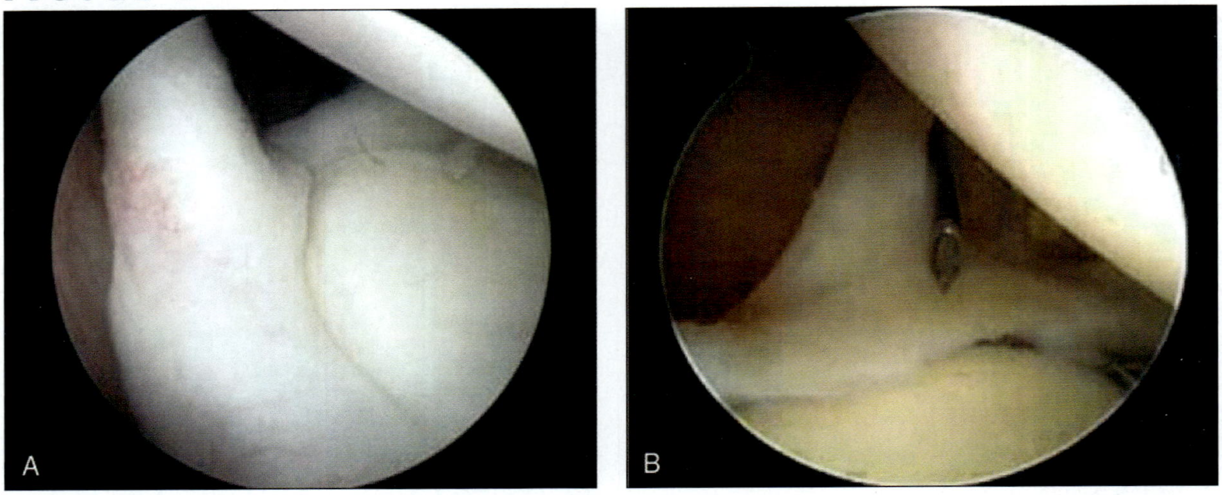

Arthroscopic views show the round morphology (**A**) and the meniscoid morphology (**B**) of the superior labrum.

letic ROM, especially in the superoinferior direction.[6] The labrum also absorbs forces in the joint,[7] acting as a "bumper" for the humeral head.[8] In overhead athletes, the role of the superior labrum is particularly important. Given the insertion of the SGHL and the MGHL at the superior labrum, concern exists that injury to this structure may result in increased glenohumeral laxity. Moreover, increased translation in patients with superior labral injury may facilitate edge loading of the glenoid, resulting in pain at extremes of motion and symptoms of instability.

Vangsness et al[9] demonstrated that the biceps anchor originates at both the supraglenoid tubercle and the superior labrum with roughly equal frequency. When originating at the labrum, it is typically found centrally or posteriorly. The intra-articular portion of the tendon is extrasynovial, and the amount of tendon that is intra-articular depends on the humeral position. In adduction and extension, this portion measures 35 mm, which is its maximum length.[10] As the tendon exits the joint and moves through the rotator interval, it is stabilized by the biceps pulley proximally and the bicipital groove distally. The pulley mechanism comprises the coracohumeral ligament and the SGHL; in the bicipital groove, the pulley is bordered superiorly by the transverse humeral ligament, which may actually be a confluence of terminal fibers of various structures rather than one discrete entity.[10]

In contrast to the labrum, the function of the long head of the biceps (LHB) tendon is less defined. Previous studies have indicated that the LHB tendon plays a role in humeral head depression and compression,[11,12] along with anterior[13-15] and posterior stabilization,[16] limitation of external rotation,[15] and stress shielding for the IGHL.[17] In a cadaver study by Youm et al,[17] successive loads were applied to the proximal biceps tendon, and the "path of glenohumeral articulation" was studied in each loading condition. The authors found that the LHB tendon had a tethering effect on glenohumeral rotation and all directions of translation, most markedly at the extremes of ROM. Moreover, dynamic loading of the biceps shifted the humeral head and center of rotation more toward the center of the glenoid through this arc of motion, which is consistent with findings from other studies.[18-20]

Given its role as a centering agent, the LHB tendon may play an integral role in overhead athletes, whose shoulders are routinely subjected to stress at the extremes of ROM. As the humerus moves from internal to external rotation, the biceps tendon similarly rotates from an anterosuperior position to a posterosuperior position as it maintains its position in the bicipital

FIGURE 2

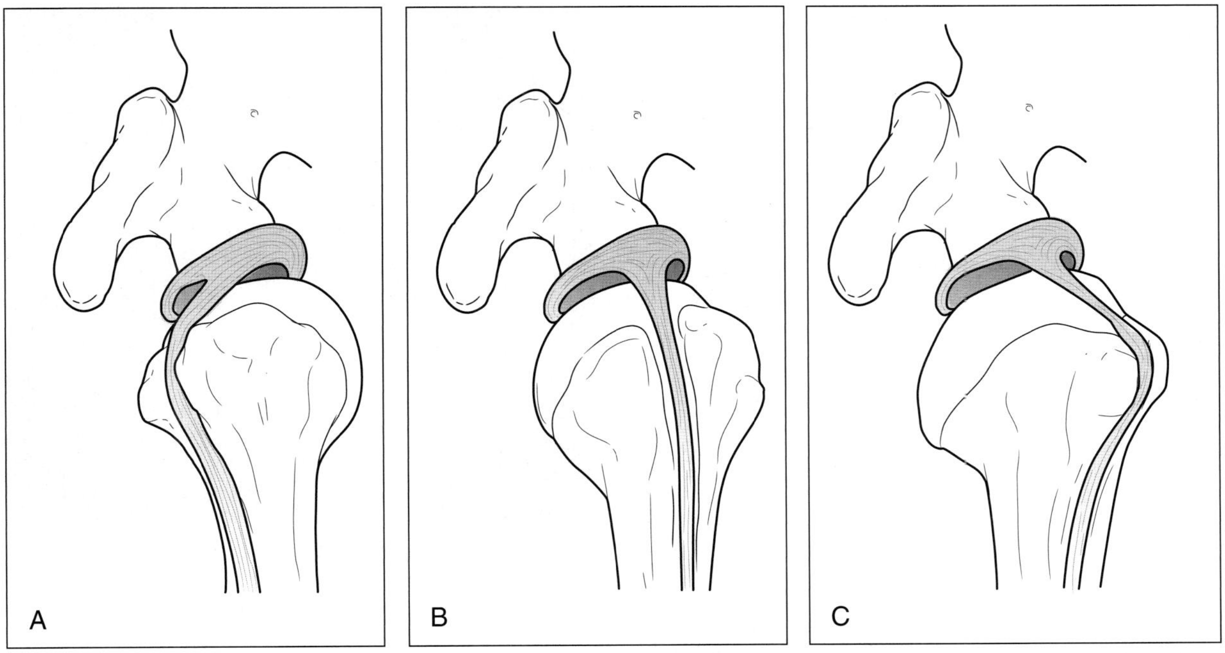

Illustration shows a superior view of the position of the long head of the biceps tendon in the glenohumeral joint with internal (**A**), neutral (**B**), and external rotation (**C**) of the humerus.

groove (**Figure 2**). At the extremes of external rotation and abduction, the intra-articular portion of the biceps is at its shortest length and highest tension, therefore achieving maximum compression of the humeral head.[17]

The role of the biceps during overhead motion has been further clarified using electromyographic (EMG) analysis. The biceps has been shown to be at maximum activation during the late cocking stage, when the humerus is in abduction and external rotation. EMG studies have also helped confirm the role of the biceps as a centering agent, as described by Youm et al.[17] Glousman et al[21] found increased EMG activity in the biceps of pitchers with anterior instability compared with those with normal shoulders. These findings were confirmed by Kim et al[22] in a study of patients with instability. However, other reports have discounted the role of the proximal biceps in shoulder motion, particularly for control of the elbow and forearm.[23] Yamaguchi et al[23] found no significant EMG activity in the LHB tendon throughout shoulder motion with the elbow immobilized in neutral rotation and 100° of flexion. These findings downplay the role of the LHB tendon as a shoulder stabilizer during throwing.

Youm et al[17] highlighted the importance of the function of the biceps tendon as a dynamic ligament at the extremes of ROM. However, this function depends on a stable superior labrum. Panossian et al[24] investigated this theory in simulated type II superior labrum anterior to posterior (SLAP) tears in cadaver specimens and found that lesions in both the superior labrum and the biceps anchor resulted in increased external rotation and glenohumeral translation. This excess rotation and translation was significantly decreased after repair using suture anchors. Pagnani et al[14] also demonstrated increased translation (anteroposterior and superoinferior) on loading in cadaver specimens with simulated lesions to the superior labrum and biceps anchor. Interestingly, the authors did not find increased translation with tears of the superior labrum that spared the biceps attachment, further signifying the role of the superior labrum and biceps anchor acting in concert to limit glenohumeral translation. Therefore, instances of injury or avulsion at the superior labrum increase the risk of compromise of both the secondary stabilizing effects of the LHB tendon (particularly in instances of posterosuperior injury) as well as the stabilizing effects of the attachments of the SGHL, MGHL, and IGHL (in instances of anterosuperior injury).

Etiology of SLAP Injuries in the Overhead Athlete

During the pitching motion, the shoulder experiences enormous stresses. Professional pitchers create up to 92 Nm of humeral torque during the throwing motion, which can exceed the failure limit of soft tissue in cadaver specimens.[25] Much of this repetitive stress during the late cocking phase is placed on the superior labrum, predisposing it to injury.[26] In a cadaver model, Shepard et al[27] demonstrated that posteriorly loaded biceps anchors—simulating the late cocking phase—resulted in type II SLAP lesions, and those shoulders with in-line loading—simulating deceleration—sustained no type II SLAP lesions. In addition, the biceps anchor was weaker when loaded in the late cocking position compared with loading in the deceleration position (262 versus 508 N). Kuhn et al[28] also demonstrated an increased likelihood of failure of the biceps-labral complex and development of type II SLAP lesions in shoulders loaded in the late cocking position compared with those loaded in the early deceleration position.

The most common labral injury in overhead athletes is the type II SLAP lesion, which involves the biceps anchor[29] (**Figure 3**). Concomitant partial-thickness articular-side rotator cuff tears are common in throwers,[30] and several theories have attempted to explain the overall constellation of pathology in throwers. Burkhart et al[31] proposed posterior capsule contraction as an inciting fundamental factor in shoulder pathology among overhead throwers. The authors theorized that the posterior capsule contracts as a result of chronically withstanding high tensile forces during deceleration and follow-through. This causes a posterosuperior shift in the humeral head center of rotation during external rotation and abduction, resulting in increased external rotation. This shift in positioning may be sustained by a tight posterior band of the IGHL, providing a posterosuperiorly directed force (**Figure 4**). This position of excessive external rotation may increase the shear forces at the labrum and biceps anchor, resulting in injury to the biceps-labral complex. Excessive shear may also occur at the posterosuperior rotator cuff, resulting in undersurface tears. Moreover, the loss of internal rotation (glenohumeral internal rotation deficit [GIRD]) results in decreased arm acceleration and velocity.

Figure 3

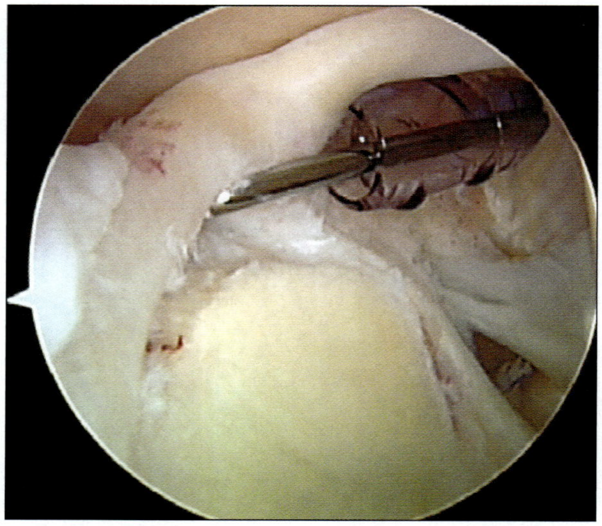

Arthroscopic view of a type II SLAP tear.

Burkhart and Morgan[32] also described the peel-back phenomenon in overhead throwers. With the arm in a position of abduction and external rotation (reproduced intraoperatively when the arm is removed from traction and into this position), a change occurs in the biceps tendon force vector to a more posterior and vertical position. This force is transmitted to the posterior labrum, causing it to peel back. This stress may cause injury to the biceps-labral complex, resulting in a type II SLAP tear. However, the role of peel-back toward initiation and progression of labral pathology remains theoretical, and newer theories suggest that the peel-back may be a physiologic response to the stresses of the throwing cycle in mobile labral segments and does not represent actual pathology.

Internal impingement was first described by Walch et al[33] in 1992. This phenomenon occurs when the shoulder is in 90° of abduction and 90° of external rotation.

FIGURE 4

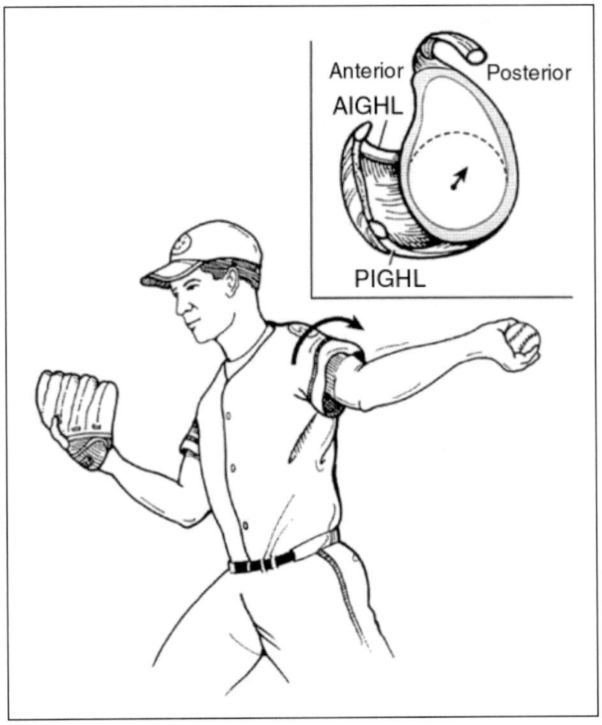

Illustration of the late cocking phase of throwing. Inset: the posterior band of the inferior glenohumeral ligament (PIGHL) is bowstrung beneath the humeral head, causing a posterosuperior shift in the glenohumeral rotation point (AIGHL = anterior inferior glenohumeral ligament). Also during late cocking, the biceps vector shifts posteriorly and twists at its base, maximizing peel-back forces. The pitcher depicted here shows classic derangements of pitching mechanics as a result of the tight posteroinferior capsule: external hyperrotation, horizontal hyperabduction (out of the scapular plane), dropped elbow, and premature trunk rotation. (Reproduced with permission from Burkhart SS, Morgan CD, Kibler WB: The disabled throwing shoulder: Spectrum of pathology. Part I: Pathoanatomy and biomechanics. *Arthroscopy* 2003;19[4]:404-420.)

FIGURE 5

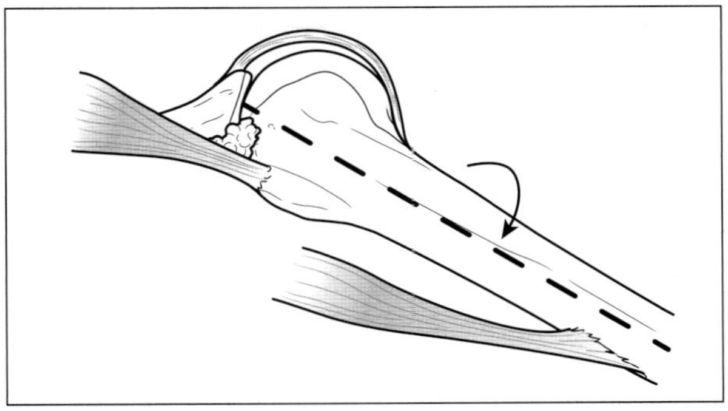

Illustration shows internal impingement that results when the humerus is placed in abduction and external rotation (curved arrow), causing the posterosuperior rotator cuff to come into contact with the posterosuperior glenoid labrum. Dashed line = axis of rotation.

This position creates contact between the posterosuperior rotator cuff and the posterosuperior labrum; the impingement of the rotator cuff between the labrum and the greater tuberosity may occur (**Figure 5**). This impingement may be tolerated in the static position, although repetitive, forceful impingement may result in partial-thickness rotator cuff tears and SLAP lesions.[34-37] Despite this evidence, however, the role of internal impingement in labral pathology in overhead athletes is less clear.[38] Some studies have documented the coexistence of undersurface rotator cuff lesions and labral tears in nonoverhead athletes.[39]

The biceps may also be damaged distal to the origin at the biceps-labral complex, and injury to the biceps is often concomitant with other shoulder pathology. Overhead athletes may be susceptible to the development of isolated tendinitis of the biceps resulting from repetitive forces and/or flaws in their throwing mechanics.

EVALUATION

The diagnosis of injury to the proximal biceps and superior labrum is made following a thorough history and physical examination, with appropriate imaging as needed. Overhead athletes with shoulder pathology may initially report vague symptoms related to their performance such as loss of control, loss of velocity, or even difficulty warming up and a feeling of tightness.[40,41] These athletes may also report pain and, at times, mechanical catching during certain provocative maneuvers in the pitching or overhead sequence. Posterosuperior pain during the late cocking phase may be due to instability or internal impingement in patients with type II SLAP lesions. Lesions that involve the anterosuperior labrum and its ligamentous attachments may also cause symptoms of instability, although frank dislocation is atypical, and unstable lesions may induce popping or locking. Patients with pain during follow-through may have rotator cuff tears or posterior capsular tightness.

Physical examination must include assessment of the entire kinetic chain involved in throwing, including the knee, hip, and low back, to determine strength, balance, and flexibility. Examination of the upper extermity should include visual inspection to discern any muscle atrophy or scapular winging. The acromioclavicular joint, the coracoid process, the LHB tendon, and the glenohumeral joint line should be palpated for tenderness. ROM assessment should include documentation of the basic arcs of forward elevation in the scapular plane, along with internal and external rotation with the arm held in 0° and 90° of abduction. In particular, differences in internal rotation between both shoulders should be noted. Scapular asymmetry should also be noted with the arm held at the side, in 45° of abduction (for example, with the hand on the hip), and in 90° of abduction. Isolated muscle strength testing should be assessed and compared between the dominant and nondominant sides.

Certain physical examination maneuvers may be used to identify injury specific to the biceps-labral complex. Tenderness to palpation of the LHB tendon may indicate tendon pathology or a SLAP lesion. A positive Speed test result (pain with the forearm in supination and the arm in 90° of forward elevation) may further indicate biceps tendon disease and can also indicate the possibility of a SLAP lesion.[41] A positive Yergason test result (pain with resisted forearm supination) may also indicate proximal biceps pathology. The active compression test, perhaps the most useful test for the identification of SLAP lesions, is performed by moving the patient's arm to 90° of forward elevation, 10° to 15° of adduction, and pronation with the thumb pointing down. The clinician applies a downward force on the forearm, and repeats with the arm in supination (and the thumb pointing up). The test result is considered positive if the patient reports worsened pain with pronation. This maneuver has been shown to have good sensitivity and specificity for diagnosing type II SLAP lesions.[42] The Jobe relocation test may reproduce symptoms of internal impingement. The patient is positioned supine on the examining table, and the arm is placed in 90° of abduction and 10° of forward elevation. The test is considered positive if the patient reports pain when the examiner exerts anterior force on the shoulder. Additionally, a positive apprehension relocation sign may indicate posterior SLAP injury in patients with internal impingement.[41] The examiner also should document findings of external impingement using the Neer and Hawkins tests.

Clinical suspicion of SLAP lesions following history and physical examination is usually confirmed with imaging. Standard shoulder radiographs, including true AP and axillary views, are obtained to identify possible bony defects. Magnetic resonance arthrography (**Figure 6**) is used most often to evaluate the labrum. Bencardino et al[43] found a 90% accuracy, a sensitivity of 89%, and a specificity of 91% for magnetic resonance arthrography in the diagnosis of SLAP tears. Concomitant rotator cuff tears may also be identified using MRI. MRI obtained with the arm in abduction and external rotation may be particularly helpful in the diagnosis of articular-side rotator cuff injury.[41]

Treatment of SLAP Lesions

Nonsurgical Treatment

When a SLAP injury is diagnosed in an overhead athlete, the initial treatment should be nonsurgical, designed to decrease pain and inflammation, improve motion and flexibility, and subsequently increase strength and facilitate a return to overhead activity.

Typically, rehabilitation begins with a period of rest in which the athlete avoids provocative maneuvers; NSAIDs may also help relieve pain. An intra-articular corticosteroid injection also may be considered for pain relief and reduction of inflammation. Patients with posterior capsular contraction must undergo a comprehensive stretching program to improve GIRD symptoms. Sleeper stretches are commonly used, and comprehensive stretching programs have been shown to significantly improve GIRD symptoms and posterior shoulder tightness.[44]

Once pain has been resolved and motion is improved, the patient may begin to focus on strengthening to eventually return to overhead activity. Physical therapy, along with a home exercise program, may help patients strengthen the rotator cuff muscles. Therapy is also directed toward scapular stabilization and strengthening. As strength is restored, a structured, gradual return to throwing may commence.

Nonsurgical treatment of SLAP lesions can be successful in overhead athletes. In a recent study of 39 pa-

FIGURE 6

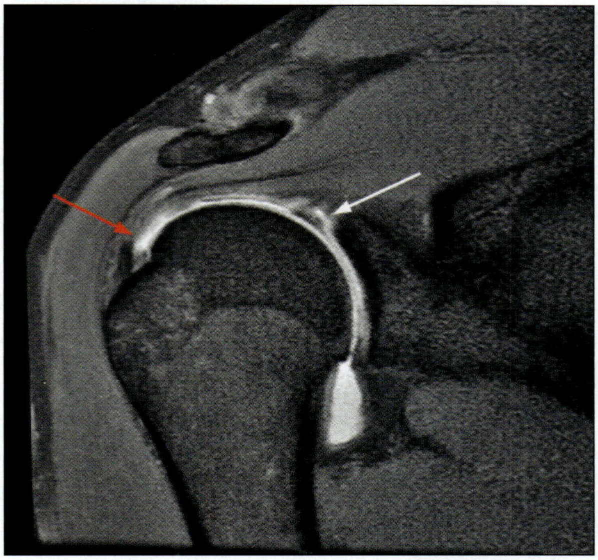

Coronal oblique magnetic resonance arthrogram shows a superior labral tear (white arrow) with dye tracking into the space between the glenoid and the labrum, and a partial-thickness rotator cuff tear (red arrow). (Courtesy of Columbia University, Department of Orthopaedics, New York, NY.)

tients undergoing nonsurgical treatment (which consisted of NSAIDs, scapular stabilization exercises, and posterior capsular stretching), Edwards et al[45] reported improvement in functional outcome and quality of life, as well as a decrease in pain in the 19 patients who did not undergo surgery. Even though the remaining 20 patients eventually underwent surgery, the authors showed that nonsurgical treatment can indeed be successful in a subpopulation of patients with SLAP tears.

Surgical Treatment of SLAP Lesions

Patients with recurrent or refractory symptoms whose comprehensive nonsurgical course of therapy has failed are candidates for surgical treatment. SLAP lesions are best classified during diagnostic arthroscopy. In general, type I SLAP tears are treated with débridement alone. Type II SLAP lesions are typically treated with arthroscopic repair of the labrum to the underlying glenoid. Type III SLAP tears often require excision of the bucket-handle component of the lesion, with repair of the lesion reserved for larger fragments with good tissue quality. Type IV SLAP tears are repaired if the fragment is large and has good-quality tissue, but biceps tenodesis or tenotomy may also be considered.

Type II SLAP Repair in the Overhead Athlete

The standard treatment of type II SLAP lesions is arthroscopic repair with suture anchors. In the overhead athlete, critical technical points may provide an advantageous outcome. The authors of this chapter prefer to place the patient in the lateral position because this provides optimal visualization and access to the entire labrum. It is essential to limit iatrogenic damage to the rotator cuff during surgery, particularly during portal placement, because throwers rely on the rotator cuff for maximal function and performance. A port of Wilmington portal for anchor placement and suture passing should be created medial to the rotator cuff cable to facilitate proper healing of the portal site. Alternately, anchor placement and suture passing may be performed percutaneously using a transtendinous approach that avoids creation of a traditional portal[46] (**Figure 7**).

Low-profile knots placed away from the articular surface and knotless repairs help avoid potential painful irritation related to the hardware.[47] Biomechanical studies have confirmed the adequacy of knotless devices compared with more traditional suture anchors.[48] A knotless repair with a vertical mattress suture configuration is shown in **Figure 8**.

Outcomes Following Labral Repair

The reported outcomes of arthroscopic repair for SLAP lesions for overhead athletes have been variable.[49-52] In a case series of 40 overhead athletes, Ide et al[53] reported a 95% return to sport and a 75% return to preinjury level of competition. Brockmeier et al[49] conducted a study of 34 athletes undergoing labral repair (28 of whom were overhead athletes) and reported a 74% return to preinjury level of competition. Friel et al[54] conducted a series of 22 overhead athletes and reported a 59% return to preinjury level of performance; 21 of these 22 patients indicated that they would undergo the same surgery again.

Concomitant rotator cuff pathology may play a role in preventing some overhead athletes, especially elite overhead throwers, from achieving preinjury level of perfor-

FIGURE 7

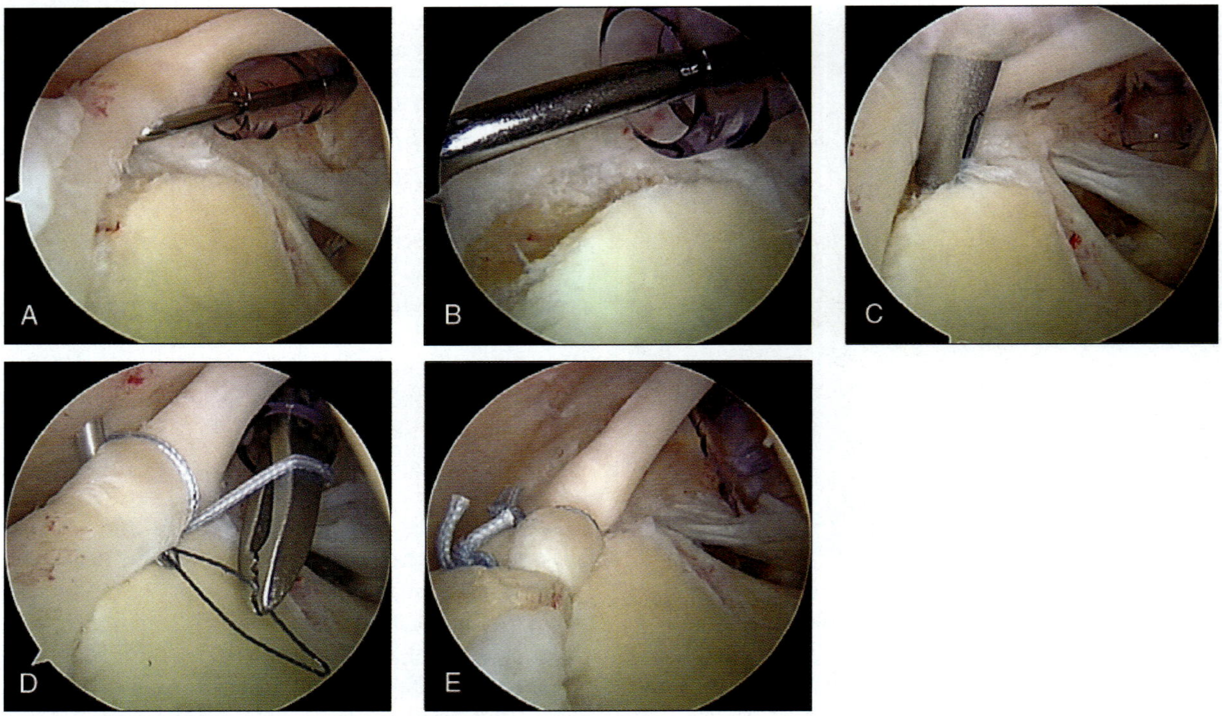

Arthroscopic views of a right shoulder obtained with the patient in the lateral decubitus position show the percutaneous SLAP repair technique used by the authors of this chapter. **A,** A motorized shaver is introduced via the anterior working portal and is used to prepare the superior neck of the glenoid beneath the detached labrum of a type II SLAP tear. **B,** The superior labrum is débrided and the bone is abraded to a cancellous surface. **C,** The anchor guide is positioned on the superior aspect of the glenoid. **D,** Percutaneous suture passage is demonstrated using a suture shuttling device. **E,** Completed repair shows anatomic restoration of the superior labrum. Note the secure fixation, with knots medial to the glenohumeral articulation. (Courtesy of Columbia University, Department of Orthopaedics, New York, NY.)

mance following surgery. Neri et al[55] reported on a series of 23 elite (collegiate or professional) athletes following labral repair for type II SLAP lesions, demonstrating a 57% return to preinjury level of performance. However, the authors also reported a significant correlation between concomitant partial-thickness rotator cuff tear and the inability to return to this level of activity in the 8 patients with this additional rotator cuff pathology.

Biceps Tenodesis for Type II SLAP Lesions

The causes of surgical failure of SLAP repairs in overhead athletes are not well understood. Boileau et al[56] postulated that rigid labral fixation prevents physiologic movement of the superior labrum and biceps anchor that normally occurs during overhead motion. The authors also stated that the patient may experience residual pain after securing the proximal biceps tendon and its rich network of sensory fibers. As a result, biceps tenodesis has recently been offered as an alternative treatment option for selected patients with type II SLAP lesions.[3,56] Boileau et al[56] reported on outcomes of 25 patients who underwent either arthroscopic labral repair or biceps tenodesis for type II SLAP lesions. Only 2 of 10 patients who underwent labral repair returned to his or her preinjury level of sport. In the tenodesis group, 13 of 15 patients returned to his or her preinjury level of performance. In addition, 3 patients in the repair group who required reoperation because of pain were treated with subsequent tenodesis; each of these patients successfully returned to his or her preinjury level of per-

FIGURE 8

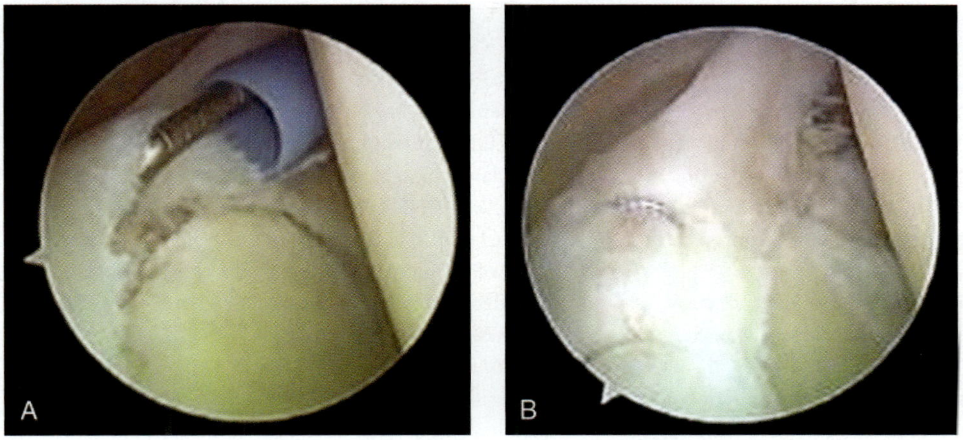

Arthroscopic views of a knotless repair of a type II SLAP lesion. **A,** A probe indicates an unstable type II SLAP tear. **B,** Vertical mattress knotless anchor repair results in a meniscoid-shaped superior labrum.

formance. However, the study had several limitations. The study was nonrandomized, and the decision to proceed with tenodesis versus repair was made intraoperatively. The treatment groups were different at baseline; patients in the tenodesis group were much older than those in the repair group (mean age, 52 and 37 years, respectively), and tenodesis was intentionally chosen for older, less active patients. Therefore, these results may not be applicable when considering young, overhead athletes, particularly elite athletes.

Given the number of biomechanical studies that promote the biceps tendon as a stabilizer during overhead motion, concern exists that tenodesis performed in the setting of type II SLAP lesions may result in residual instability. This theory was tested in a recent cadaver study.[57] The authors reported that simulation of type II SLAP lesions resulted in increased glenohumeral translation that was unchanged following tenodesis. The author concluded that the treatment of type II SLAP lesions using biceps tenodesis without labral repair should be approached with caution: the residual instability following such treatment may be acceptable in low-demand, recreational patients, but may be intolerable in younger, high-level overhead athletes who rely on optimal glenohumeral kinematics for maximal performance.

Conclusion

The authors of this chapter prefer to treat type II SLAP lesions using primary arthroscopic labral repair with suture anchor fixation. The authors prefer to avoid compromising the biceps tendon because of its potential functional role. However, biceps tenodesis may be considered as an option in patients whose prior SLAP repair has failed or in cases of lesions with complex biceps pathology. Further evidence of the role of tenodesis in the treatment of superior labral pathology, especially in elite, overhead athletes, is needed before tenodesis can be recommended as a primary treatment of type II SLAP lesions in this patient population.

The overhead athlete subjects his or her shoulder to significant repetitive stresses at the extremes of ROM, predisposing the structures in the shoulder to injury. The biceps-labral complex is especially susceptible, and injury most often occurs during the late cocking phase, with the shoulder in abduction and external rotation. The most common shoulder injury in this patient population is the type II SLAP lesion, affecting both the superior labrum and the proximal biceps. These lesions produce pain and instability and may be a significant obstacle in returning to competitive sports. When this type of injury does not respond to nonsurgical treatment, anatomic arthroscopic repair of the superior labrum to the underlying glenoid should be performed. However, evidence suggests that return to preinjury level of performance and competition is not always a predictable event in overhead athletes, especially in patients with concomitant partial-thickness rotator cuff tears. Although biceps tenodesis without labral repair has been offered as an alternative treatment option, it should be reserved for patients whose conventional repair has failed patients with complex pathology at the biceps root.

REFERENCES

1. Bennett GE: Shoulder and elbow lesions distinctive of baseball players. *Ann Surg* 1947;126(1):107-110.
2. Andrews JR, Carson WG Jr, McLeod WD: Glenoid labrum tears related to the long head of the biceps. *Am J Sports Med* 1985;13(5):337-341.
3. Burns JP, Bahk M, Snyder SJ: Superior labral tears: Repair versus biceps tenodesis. *J Shoulder Elbow Surg* 2011;20(Suppl 2,):S2-S8.
4. Tuoheti Y, Itoi E, Minagawa H, et al: Attachment types of the long head of the biceps tendon to the glenoid labrum and their relationships with the glenohumeral ligaments. *Arthroscopy* 2005;21(10):1242-1249.
5. Rao AG, Kim TK, Chronopoulos E, McFarland EG: Anatomical variants in the anterosuperior aspect of the glenoid labrum: A statistical analysis of seventy-three cases. *J Bone Joint Surg Am* 2003;85-A(4):653-659.
6. Liu SH, Boynton E: Posterior superior impingement of the rotator cuff on the glenoid rim as a cause of shoulder pain in the overhead athlete. *Arthroscopy* 1993;9(6):697-699.
7. Abrams GD, Safran MR: Diagnosis and management of superior labrum anterior posterior lesions in overhead athletes. *Br J Sports Med* 2010;44(5):311-318.
8. Howell SM, Galinat BJ: The glenoid-labral socket: A constrained articular surface. *Clin Orthop Relat Res* 1989;243:122-125.
9. Vangsness CT Jr, Jorgenson SS, Watson T, Johnson DL: The origin of the long head of the biceps from the scapula and glenoid labrum: An anatomical study of 100 shoulders. *J Bone Joint Surg Br* 1994;76(6):951-954.
10. Hsu SH, Miller SL, Curtis AS: Long head of biceps tendon pathology: Management alternatives. *Clin Sports Med* 2008;27(4):747-762.
11. Itoi E, Kuechle DK, Newman SR, Morrey BF, An KN: Stabilising function of the biceps in stable and unstable shoulders. *J Bone Joint Surg Br* 1993;75(4):546-550.
12. Kido T, Itoi E, Konno N, Sano A, Urayama M, Sato K: The depressor function of biceps on the head of the humerus in shoulders with tears of the rotator cuff. *J Bone Joint Surg Br* 2000;82(3):416-419.
13. Itoi E, Newman SR, Kuechle DK, Morrey BF, An KN: Dynamic anterior stabilisers of the shoulder with the arm in abduction. *J Bone Joint Surg Br* 1994;76(5): 834-836.
14. Pagnani MJ, Deng XH, Warren RF, Torzilli PA, Altchek DW: Effect of lesions of the superior portion of the glenoid labrum on glenohumeral translation. *J Bone Joint Surg Am* 1995;77(7):1003-1010.
15. Rodosky MW, Harner CD, Fu FH: The role of the long head of the biceps muscle and superior glenoid labrum in anterior stability of the shoulder. *Am J Sports Med* 1994;22(1):121-130.
16. Blasier RB, Soslowsky LJ, Malicky DM, Palmer ML: Posterior glenohumeral subluxation: Active and passive stabilization in a biomechanical model. *J Bone Joint Surg Am* 1997;79(3):433-440.
17. Youm T, ElAttrache NS, Tibone JE, McGarry MH, Lee TQ: The effect of the long head of the biceps on glenohumeral kinematics. *J Shoulder Elbow Surg* 2009;18(1):122-129.
18. Burkart A, Debski RE, Musahl V, McMahon PJ: Glenohumeral translations are only partially restored after repair of a simulated type II superior labral lesion. *Am J Sports Med* 2003;31(1):56-63.
19. McMahon PJ, Burkart A, Musahl V, Debski RE: Glenohumeral translations are increased after a type II superior labrum anterior-posterior lesion: A cadaveric study of severity of passive stabilizer injury. *J Shoulder Elbow Surg* 2004;13(1):39-44.
20. Pagnani MJ, Deng XH, Warren RF, Torzilli PA, O'Brien SJ: Role of the long head of the biceps brachii in glenohumeral stability: A biomechanical study in cadavera. *J Shoulder Elbow Surg* 1996;5(4):255-262.
21. Glousman R, Jobe F, Tibone J, Moynes D, Antonelli D, Perry J: Dynamic electromyographic analysis of the throwing shoulder with glenohumeral instability. *J Bone Joint Surg Am* 1988;70(2):220-226.
22. Kim SH, Ha KI, Kim HS, Kim SW: Electromyographic activity of the biceps brachii muscle in shoulders with anterior instability. *Arthroscopy* 2001;17(8):864-868.
23. Yamaguchi K, Riew KD, Galatz LM, Syme JA, Neviaser RJ: Biceps activity during shoulder motion: An electromyographic analysis. *Clin Orthop Relat Res* 1997;(336):122-129.
24. Panossian VR, Mihata T, Tibone JE, Fitzpatrick MJ, McGarry MH, Lee TQ: Biomechanical analysis of isolated

type II SLAP lesions and repair. *J Shoulder Elbow Surg* 2005;14(5):529-534.

25. Sabick MB, Torry MR, Kim YK, Hawkins RJ: Humeral torque in professional baseball pitchers. *Am J Sports Med* 2004;32(4):892-898.
26. Pradhan RL, Itoi E, Hatakeyama Y, Urayama M, Sato K: Superior labral strain during the throwing motion: A cadaveric study. *Am J Sports Med* 2001;29(4): 488-492.
27. Shepard MF, Dugas JR, Zeng N, Andrews JR: Differences in the ultimate strength of the biceps anchor and the generation of type II superior labral anterior posterior lesions in a cadaveric model. *Am J Sports Med* 2004;32(5):1197-1201.
28. Kuhn JE, Lindholm SR, Huston LJ, Soslowsky LJ, Blasier RB: Failure of the biceps superior labral complex: A cadaveric biomechanical investigation comparing the late cocking and early deceleration positions of throwing. *Arthroscopy* 2003;19(4):373-379.
29. Snyder SJ, Karzel RP, Del Pizzo W, Ferkel RD, Friedman MJ: SLAP lesions of the shoulder. *Arthroscopy* 1990;6(4):274-279.
30. Andrews JR, Broussard TS, Carson WG: Arthroscopy of the shoulder in the management of partial tears of the rotator cuff: A preliminary report. *Arthroscopy* 1985;1(2):117-122.
31. Burkhart SS, Morgan CD, Kibler WB: The disabled throwing shoulder: Spectrum of pathology Part I: Pathoanatomy and biomechanics. *Arthroscopy* 2003;19(4):404-420.
32. Burkhart SS, Morgan CD: The peel-back mechanism: Its role in producing and extending posterior type II SLAP lesions and its effect on SLAP repair rehabilitation. *Arthroscopy* 1998;14(6):637-640.
33. Walch G, Boileau P, Noel E, Donell ST: Impingement of the deep surface of the supraspinatus tendon on the posterosuperior glenoid rim: An arthroscopic study. *J Shoulder Elbow Surg* 1992;1(5):238-245.
34. Davidson PA, Elattrache NS, Jobe CM, Jobe FW: Rotator cuff and posterior-superior glenoid labrum injury associated with increased glenohumeral motion: A new site of impingement. *J Shoulder Elbow Surg* 1995;4(5):384-390.
35. Jobe CM: Posterior superior glenoid impingement: Expanded spectrum. *Arthroscopy* 1995;11(5):530-536.
36. Jobe CM: Superior glenoid impingement. *Orthop Clin North Am* 1997;28(2):137-143.
37. Jobe CM: Superior glenoid impingement: Current concepts. *Clin Orthop Relat Res* 1996;330:98-107.
38. Drakos MC, Rudzki JR, Allen AA, Potter HG, Altchek DW: Internal impingement of the shoulder in the overhead athlete. *J Bone Joint Surg Am* 2009;91(11): 2719-2728.
39. Budoff JE, Nirschl RP, Ilahi OA, Rodin DM: Internal impingement in the etiology of rotator cuff tendinosis revisited. *Arthroscopy* 2003;19(8):810-814.
40. ElAttrache NS, Gonzalez-Lomas G, Ahmad CS: *The Shoulder in Athletes*. Philadelphia, PA, Elsevier, 2009.
41. Greiwe RM, Ahmad CS: Management of the throwing shoulder: Cuff, labrum and internal impingement. *Orthop Clin North Am* 2010;41(3):309-323.
42. O'Brien SJ, Pagnani MJ, Fealy S, McGlynn SR, Wilson JB: The active compression test: A new and effective test for diagnosing labral tears and acromioclavicular joint abnormality. *Am J Sports Med* 1998;26(5):610-613.
43. Bencardino JT, Beltran J, Rosenberg ZS, et al: Superior labrum anterior-posterior lesions: Diagnosis with MR arthrography of the shoulder. *Radiology* 2000;214(1):267-271.
44. Tyler TF, Nicholas SJ, Lee SJ, Mullaney M, McHugh MP: Correction of posterior shoulder tightness is associated with symptom resolution in patients with internal impingement. *Am J Sports Med* 2010;38(1):114-119.
45. Edwards SL, Lee JA, Bell JE, et al: Nonoperative treatment of superior labrum anterior posterior tears: Improvements in pain, function, and quality of life. *Am J Sports Med* 2010;38(7):1456-1461.
46. Galano GJ, Ahmad CS, Bigliani L, Levine W: Percutaneous SLAP lesion repair technique is an effective alternative to portal of Wilmington. *Orthopedics* 2010;33(11):803.
47. Dines JS, Elattrache NS: Horizontal mattress with a knotless anchor to better recreate the normal superior labrum anatomy. *Arthroscopy* 2008;24(12):1422-1425.
48. Uggen C, Wei A, Glousman RE, et al: Biomechanical comparison of knotless anchor repair versus simple suture repair for type II SLAP lesions. *Arthroscopy* 2009;25(10):1085-1092.
49. Brockmeier SF, Voos JE, Williams RJ III, et al: Outcomes after arthroscopic repair of type-II SLAP lesions. *J Bone Joint Surg Am* 2009;91(7):1595-1603.

50. Gorantla K, Gill C, Wright RW: The outcome of type II SLAP repair: A systematic review. *Arthroscopy* 2010;26(4):537-545.

51. Kim SH, Ha KI, Kim SH, Choi HJ: Results of arthroscopic treatment of superior labral lesions. *J Bone Joint Surg Am* 2002;84(6):981-985.

52. Sayde WM, Cohen SB, Ciccotti MG, Dodson CC: Return to play after Type II superior labral anterior-posterior lesion repairs in athletes: A systematic review. *Clin Orthop Relat Res* 2012;470(6):1595-1600.

53. Ide J, Maeda S, Takagi K: Sports activity after arthroscopic superior labral repair using suture anchors in overhead-throwing athletes. *Am J Sports Med* 2005;33(4):507-514.

54. Friel NA, Karas V, Slabaugh MA, Cole BJ: Outcomes of type II superior labrum, anterior to posterior (SLAP) repair: Prospective evaluation at a minimum two-year follow-up. *J Shoulder Elbow Surg* 2010;19(6):859-867.

55. Neri BR, ElAttrache NS, Owsley KC, Mohr K, Yocum LA: Outcome of type II superior labral anterior posterior repairs in elite overhead athletes: Effect of concomitant partial-thickness rotator cuff tears. *Am J Sports Med* 2011;39(1):114-120.

56. Boileau P, Parratte S, Chuinard C, Roussanne Y, Shia D, Bicknell R: Arthroscopic treatment of isolated type II SLAP lesions: Biceps tenodesis as an alternative to reinsertion. *Am J Sports Med* 2009;37(5):929-936.

57. Strauss EJ, Salata MJ, Sershon RA, et al: Role of the superior labrum after biceps tenodesis in glenohumeral stability. *J Shoulder Elbow Surg* 2013;Sep30[Epub ahead of print].

CHAPTER 16

Special Patients: The Industrial Athlete

Wendell M.R. Heard, MD
Gregory P. Nicholson, MD

Introduction

The long head of the biceps (LHB) tendon has been the subject of extensive research. However, it does not have a well-defined function and the management of its disorders has not been clearly outlined for any group of patients. The industrial athlete is a subset of patients who require strength, agility, and stamina in a spectrum of industrial sectors. Workers such as painters, electricians, and plumbers who perform overhead tasks are susceptible to proximal LHB tendinopathy. These patients often endure high levels of physical stress and perform repetitive actions, making them susceptible to injury. This relates to the proximal LHB because the continuum of disease from inflammatory tendinitis to degenerative tendinosis is thought to result from repetitive traction, friction, and glenohumeral rotation at specific, anatomically narrow sites along the tendon's course.[1] LHB tendinopathy can be seen in isolation; however, it is more commonly seen in combination with other shoulder pathology such as impingement, rotator cuff disorders, superior labrum anterior to posterior (SLAP) lesions, bursitis and acromioclavicular joint disorders. Treatment starts with nonsurgical measures including physical therapy, NSAIDs, and possibly steroid or platelet-rich plasma (PRP) injections. If nonsurgical measures are unsuccessful, surgical options, mainly biceps tenotomy or tenodesis, may be explored.

History and Physical Examination

Patients often report chronic overuse-type symptoms secondary to repetitive activities, resulting in progressively worsening anterior shoulder pain and decreased function. It is important to perform a complete history and physical examination to ascertain the origin and timing of the pathology, especially in workers' compensation cases because of the potentially large financial implications. Particular tasks involved in the industrial athlete's daily work, the onset of symptoms, specific injuries, and functional limitations are fundamental to determining the correct diagnosis. Proximal LHB pain typically begins in the bicipital groove and radiates anteriorly to the biceps muscle belly, and rotator cuff pain tends to radiate toward the deltoid insertion. Overhead activities, particularly with flexion and horizontal adduction, can irritate the LHB tendon. The best way to verify the pathology and its origin is by evaluating the symptoms, determining the onset of symptoms, and using physical examination findings to establish whether the injury is consistent with this information.

At minimum, a complete cervical spine, shoulder, and upper extremity physical examination should be completed. Examination maneuvers specific to the proximal LHB tendon are included here, but LHB tendon pathology is often found in conjunction with other

Dr. Nicholson or an immediate family member has received royalties from Innomed and Zimmer; serves as a paid consultant to or is an employee of Zimmer and Tornier; has stock or stock options held in Zimmer; and has received research or institutional support from EBI, Tornier, and Zimmer. Neither Dr. Heard nor any immediate family member has received anything of value from or has stock or stock options held in a commercial company or institution related directly or indirectly to the subject of this chapter.

shoulder pathology, and a complete shoulder examination is therefore required. To perform the subpectoral LHB tendon test, the examiner palpates the proximal biceps tendon while the patient internally rotates the arm against resistance. If pain is greater on the affected side, and is alleviated with an intra-articular injection of lidocaine, pathology likely exists within the bicipital groove.[2] Several physical examination maneuvers have been described to evaluate LHB tendinitis, but no specific test has proved reliable for diagnosis. The Yergason test is considered to have a positive result when pain is experienced on palpation of the proximial biceps with resisted supination and the elbow in 90° of flexion. The Speed test is considered to have a positive result with pain in the bicipital groove on resisted forward flexion of the arm with the elbow in extension, the forearm in supination, and the humerus in 90° of forward flexion. These two tests are specific for but not sensitive in the diagnosis of biceps tendinitis, rupture, and SLAP lesions.[3]

FIGURE 1

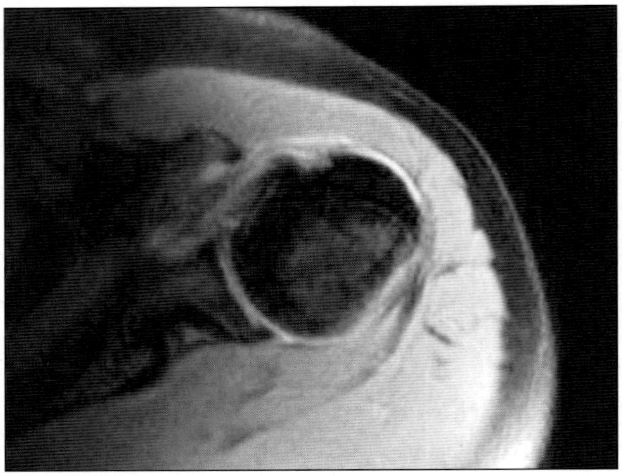

Axial MRI shows an empty bicipital groove with medial dislocation of the long head of the biceps tendon.

Imaging

Generally, no specific findings on plain radiographs can be seen that suggest a diagnosis of LHB tendinitis or rupture. MRI visualizes the biceps tendon, bicipital groove, osteophytes, and any fluid (**Figure 1**). However, correlation between arthroscopic findings and MRI has been poor to moderate when evaluating biceps pathology, inflammation, partial-thickness tear, and rupture.[4] Although ultrasonography is cost effective and accurate in the diagnosis of shoulder pathology, it is highly operator dependent. Ultrasonography is reliable for detection of biceps dislocation, subluxation, and rupture, but less accurate for the detection of partial-thickness tears of the biceps tendon.[5]

Nonsurgical Treatment

LHB tendinopathy in the industrial athlete should initially be treated nonsurgically with rest and activity modification combined with NSAIDs and physical therapy that should address any scapular dyskinesia, reduced range of motion, and rotator cuff weakness. The initial course of nonsurgical treatment should last 4 weeks. The industrial athlete can perform desktop duties if they do not provoke symptoms. Elbow flexion, forward shoulder elevation, and forearm supination should not be performed with more than 5 lb, and only if this weight does not exacerbate symptoms. No overhead lifting activities should be performed.

Corticosteroid injection into the subacromial space and the glenohumeral joint can help reduce inflammation associated with concomitant pathologies. Intra-articular glenohumeral injections affect the LHB tendon because it is an intra-articular structure. For isolated LHB tendon injuries, the tendon sheath within the bicipital groove also can be injected, taking care not to inject the tendon itself. Injections can help alleviate pain and facilitate rehabilitation, but more importantly, can also help eliminate potential pain generators and isolate others. Thus, the injection can be diagnostic to help determine if LHB pain is prevalent.

Laboratory studies have shown that tendon and cartilage cells show increased cell viability after exposure to allogenic PRP and ketorolac tromethamine. PRP was also shown to reverse the negative effect that methylprednisolone had on cells. Although not clinically proved, these injections may provide a useful alternative to the steroid injections that are currently used.[6]

Surgical Treatment

Surgical treatment should be considered when nonsurgical management of LHB tendon pathology fails. During arthroscopy (**Figure 2**), an LHB tendon noted to have a tear greater than 30% of the tendon, one that shows subluxation, or is associated with a degenerative type II SLAP lesion, is treated definitively with surgery. The two most commonly performed procedures are biceps tenotomy and biceps tenodesis, but the surgical management of LHB tendon pathology is controversial.

Biceps tenotomy is a relatively simple operation that provides predictable pain relief and requires minimal postoperative restrictions and rehabilitation. Complications include the occurrence of a cosmetic Popeye deformity in 3% to 70% of tenotomy cases.[7-9] Probably of greater concern to the industrial athlete is fatigue cramping of the biceps muscle belly. Kelly et al[7] evaluated 40 patients who underwent arthroscopic tenotomy to treat biceps tendinitis. The authors found that 15 patients (38%) had fatigue discomfort in the biceps after resisted elbow flexion activities at 2-year follow-up; 7 of the patients were younger than 40 years and 8 were between 40 and 60 years. No patient older than 60 years experienced fatigue discomfort. Overall, the mean American Shoulder and Elbow Surgeon (ASES) score was 77.6; 35% of patients had a poor result (ASES score <70.0).[7] The authors concluded that arthroscopic release of the LHB tendon is an option for patients with chronic, refractory biceps tendinitis; however, it was not advocated for younger patients and those who work as laborers.[7]

Gill et al[9] also examined tenotomy for the treatment of LHB tendon pathology in 30 patients. At a mean follow-up of 19 months, 97% of patients required no pain medication, 90% returned to their previous level of sport with minimal or no pain, 97% returned to his or her previous occupation, and the mean ASES score was 81.8. However, strength testing was not performed, the type of work the patients returned to was not specified, and no recommendations specific to laborers were made.

Biceps tenodesis, either arthroscopic or open, is performed to preserve the length-tension relationship of the biceps muscle, which may prevent muscle atrophy and fatigue cramping and maintain the normal contour of the biceps muscle. Tenodesis can be performed either proximally with the tendon maintained in the bicipital groove, or distally with the tendon removed from the groove. Removing the LHB tendon from the bicipital groove is thought to decrease postoperative pain

FIGURE 2

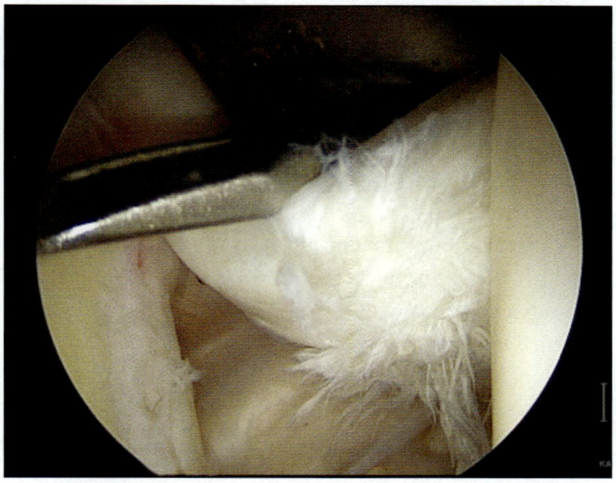

Arthroscopic view of a right shoulder, from the posterior portal, shows a frayed long head of the biceps tendon. The tendon is pulled into the glenohumeral joint to reveal the pathology.

secondary to residual tenosynovitis within the biceps sheath.[10,11] No studies have been conducted comparing tenodesis locations and outcomes or pain.

Despite several studies that have evaluated the outcomes of LHB tenotomy and various tenodesis techniques, no consensus exists on which surgical treatment is the best. Slenker et al[12] performed a systematic review that evaluated the results of 699 biceps tenotomies and 433 tenodesis procedures for the management of LHB tendon lesions. Good or excellent results were seen in 77% of tenotomy and 74% of tenodesis procedures, and the Popeye deformity was seen in 43% and 8% of patients, respectively. Only a few of the studies in the review reported on bicipital pain and/or cramping: among these, 19% of tenodesis patients and 24% of tenotomy patients reported these complications. The review included patients with a large variety of initial pathologies and age groups, but the authors concluded that little difference in outcomes exists between tenotomy and tenodesis when used for the treatment of LHB tendon lesions. The only consistent difference was the increased presence of a Popeye deformity in the tenotomy group.[12] Whether this cosmetic deformity is important to the industrial athlete is unclear, but it is unlikely to be clinically relevant.

Shank et al[13] compared forearm supination and elbow flexion strength in 17 patients who underwent isolated arthroscopic LHB tenotomy and 19 patients who underwent isolated arthroscopic LHB tenodesis. The authors noted no statistical difference in either forearm supination or elbow flexion strength among patients in the tenotomy, tenodesis, and control groups. The authors stated that tenodesis may be a reasonable consideration in patients who need to maintain supination strength. Peak strength was evaluated, but exercise-to-fatigue testing, which is important for the industrial athlete, was not evaluated.

Koh et al[14] evaluated 43 patients who underwent LHB tenodesis (mean follow-up, 28 months) and 41 patients who underwent LHB tenotomy (mean follow-up, 27 months). Two patients in the tenodesis group and 4 in the tenotomy group reported arm pain with resisted elbow flexion; this difference was not considered significant. Clinical scores showed no statistical differences between the two groups.

Postoperative Considerations

Postoperative protocols for biceps tenodesis often require sling use for 3 to 4 weeks, and possibly longer, depending on concomitant procedures. Elbow range of motion and grip strength exercises may begin immediately postoperatively. Active elbow flexion and supination exercises are often prohibited until 6 weeks. Light biceps strengthening can begin after 6 weeks. Patients are usually able to return to full activity at 3 to 4 months, which is the time an industrial athlete can expect to return to work. Jobs with tasks that involve resisted elbow flexion may require additional time to regain strength and endurance. Maximum medical improvement following biceps tenotomy is usually achieved at 6 months. If a type II SLAP tear is fixed in conjunction with a biceps tenodesis procedure, the rehabilitation for the SLAP tear can proceed as normal, but active elbow flexion should be avoided for 6 weeks to protect the tenodesis.

After isolated biceps tenotomy, minimal restrictions are required and often minimal physical therapy is needed. Patients are allowed to add activities as tolerated. Patients who have undergone tenotomy can potentially return to work sooner than those who have undergone tenodesis, and maximum medical improvement is usually achieved at 2 to 3 months. Postoperative care and the timing of return to work are certainly considerations when deciding to perform tenodesis or tenotomy.

Conclusion

Biceps tenotomy and tenodesis have both shown favorable clinical results for proximal LHB tendon lesions. In the industrial athlete, it is important to consider the postoperative ability of the biceps to function effectively and painlessly, optimizing the patient's ability to return to work. Although still debated, the consensus is that biceps tenotomy is indicated in patients older than 55 to 60 years, and biceps tenodesis is indicated in patients younger than 50 years or those of any age who work in industrial sectors.[7,14]

References

1. Refior HJ, Sowa D: Long tendon of the biceps brachii: Sites of predilection for degenerative lesions. *J Shoulder Elbow Surg* 1995;4(6):436-440.
2. Mazzocca AD, Rios CG, Romeo AA, Arciero RA: Subpectoral biceps tenodesis with interference screw fixation. *Arthroscopy* 2005;21(7):896.
3. Holtby R, Razmjou H: Accuracy of the Speed's and Yergason's tests in detecting biceps pathology and SLAP lesions: Comparison with arthroscopic findings. *Arthroscopy* 2004;20(3):231-236.
4. Mohtadi NG, Vellet AD, Clark ML, et al: A prospective, double-blind comparison of magnetic resonance imaging and arthroscopy in the evaluation of patients presenting with shoulder pain. *J Shoulder Elbow Surg* 2004;13(3):258-265.
5. Teefey SA, Hasan SA, Middleton WD, Patel M, Wright RW, Yamaguchi K: Ultrasonography of the rotator cuff: A comparison of ultrasonographic and arthroscopic findings in one hundred consecutive cases. *J Bone Joint Surg Am* 2000;82(4):498-504.
6. Beitzel K, McCarthy MB, Cote MP, et al: The effect of ketorolac tromethamine, methylprednisolone, and platelet-rich plasma on human chondrocyte and tenocyte viability. *Arthroscopy* 2013;29(7):1164-1174.
7. Kelly AM, Drakos MC, Fealy S, Taylor SA, O'Brien SJ: Arthroscopic release of the long head of the biceps tendon: Functional outcome and clinical results. *Am J Sports Med* 2005;33(2):208-213.

8. Frost A, Zafar MS, Maffulli N: Tenotomy versus tenodesis in the management of pathologic lesions of the tendon of the long head of the biceps brachii. *Am J Sports Med* 2009;37(4):828-833.
9. Gill TJ, McIrvin E, Mair SD, Hawkins RJ: Results of biceps tenotomy for treatment of pathology of the long head of the biceps brachii. *J Shoulder Elbow Surg* 2001;10(3):247-249.
10. Friedman DJ, Dunn JC, Higgins LD, Warner JJ: Proximal biceps tendon: Injuries and management. *Sports Med Arthrosc* 2008;16(3):162-169.
11. Mazzocca AD, Bicos J, Santangelo S, Romeo AA, Arciero RA: The biomechanical evaluation of four fixation techniques for proximal biceps tenodesis. *Arthroscopy* 2005;21(11):1296-1306.
12. Slenker NR, Lawson K, Ciccotti MG, Dodson CC, Cohen SB: Biceps tenotomy versus tenodesis: Clinical outcomes. *Arthroscopy* 2012;23(4):576-582.
13. Shank JR, Singleton SB, Braun S, et al: A comparison of forearm supination and elbow flexion strength in patients with long head of the biceps tenotomy or tenodesis. *Arthroscopy* 2011;27(1):9-16.
14. Koh KH, Ahn JH, Kim SM, Yoo JC: Treatment of biceps tendon lesions in the setting of rotator cuff tears: Prospective cohort study of tenotomy versus tenodesis. *Am J Sports Med* 2010;38(8):1584-1590.

CHAPTER 17

Special Considerations: The Proximal Biceps Tendon, Superior Labrum Anterior to Posterior Tears, Rotator Cuff Tears, and Shoulder Stiffness

Arash Dini, MD
Michael J. O'Brien, MD
Felix H. Savoie III, MD

Introduction

The proximal biceps tendon has been an area of intense interest and research in recent years. Walch et al[1] showed improvement in pain in massive rotator cuff tears with biceps tenotomy. Also, an increased interest in superior labrum anterior to posterior (SLAP) tears and the incidence of stiffness in failed SLAP repairs have focused attention on the role of the biceps tendon in the shoulder. This chapter examines the biceps and its association with SLAP tears, rotator cuff tears, and stiffness.

SLAP Lesions and Instability

Current arthroscopic techniques have made possible the diagnosis and treatment of intra-articular lesions of the shoulder that cause instability. The glenoid labrum increases the bony contact area and congruity in the glenohumeral joint; its firm fixation to both the scapula and the glenohumeral ligaments have been described as a tension brake that enhances stability.[2] The incidence of SLAP lesions is higher in shoulders with recurrent instability compared with shoulders that sustained a first-time dislocation. The incidence of Bankart lesions has been reported as high: 72% to 100% in various case reviews of patients with anterior instability, but SLAP lesions are encountered less often.[3] A recent review reported an incidence of SLAP lesions of 24% in patients with recurrent dislocations compared with 12% in patients with primary dislocations.[4]

Dr. O'Brien or an immediate family member has received nonincome support (such as equipment or services), commercially derived honoraria, or other non–research-related funding (such as paid travel) from DePuy, a Johnson & Johnson company, Mitek, and Smith & Nephew. Dr. Savoie or an immediate family member is a member of a speakers' bureau or has made paid presentations on behalf of Mitek and Smith & Nephew; serves as a paid consultant to or is an employee of Exactech; serves as an unpaid consultant to Cayenne Medical; has received research or institutional support from Amp Orthopedics; and serves as a board member, owner, officer, or committee member of the Arthroscopy Association of North America. Neither Dr. Dini nor any immediate family member has received anything of value from or has stock or stock options held in a commercial company or institution related directly or indirectly to the subject of this chapter.

Regarding labral pathology and instability, type II SLAP tears are most often associated with instability in younger patients.[5] The influence of SLAP and proximal biceps tendon lesions on shoulder instability is a subject of controversy. Dynamic cadaver models have shown that in a position of abduction and external rotation, the long head of the biceps tendon resists the generated torsional forces, and therefore contributes to shoulder stability in the overhead position.[6] Following detachment of the superior glenoid labrum, this position of abduction and external rotation placed significant strain on the inferior glenohumeral ligament. Electromyographic analysis in vivo has also suggested that the long head of the biceps is a humeral head stabilizer against superiorly and anteriorly directed forces.[7] Other authors have shown elimination of the arthroscopic drive-through sign following successful repair of the biceps anchor at the time of arthroscopy.[8] Although type IV SLAP lesions (bucket-handle tear with extension into the long head of the biceps tendon) are rarely described, surgical repair has been advocated over débridement to preserve as much of the proximal bicep tendon as possible because of its potential role as a dynamic stabilizer.[9]

Throwing athletes experience a unique progression of proximal biceps tendon pathology, ultimately resulting in an inability to throw. Burkhart et al[10] described the pathologic cascade in the throwing shoulder as vital to understanding the dead arm, which had previously been a career-ending condition. The acquired increase in abduction and external rotation observed in throwers is accompanied by a compensatory decrease in internal rotation resulting from contracture of the posteroinferior capsule. Additionally, contraction of the posterior inferior glenohumeral ligament produces both a glenohumeral internal rotation deficit (GIRD) and a comparatively decreased total arc of motion. Combined with a pattern of scapular dyskinesia, this results in internal impingement of the infraspinatus on the posterosuperior labrum. This can be visualized arthroscopically: in the setting of a SLAP lesion with significant posterior extension, as the arm is moved into a position of abduction and external rotation, the peel-back lesion of the superior labrum is visualized as it displaces medially over the glenoid.

The outcomes of SLAP repairs vary and depend on the preinjury activity level of the patient. Overall patient satisfaction has been reported as high, with decreased pain and improved range of motion in retrospective and prospective reviews. Gorantla et al[11] conducted a meta-review and reported a 64% return to preinjury level of performance in various overhead athletes. Studies that have specifically isolated elite overhead athletes have not demonstrated similar high rates of satisfaction because in this population, subsequent return to preinjury level of play is the critical outcome metric and determinant of patient satisfaction. Ide et al[12] showed a 63% return-to-play rate in baseball players compared with other overhead athletes.

Combined SLAP and Rotator Cuff Tears

The management of SLAP lesions in the setting of a rotator cuff tear is controversial. The incidence of associated intra-articular lesions with concomitant full-thickness rotator cuff tears has been reported as high as 74%.[13] Specifically, all SLAP lesion subtypes have been reported to occur in conjunction with full-thickness rotator cuff tears in up to 40% of cases, with a 31% incidence of concomitant rotator cuff tears in the setting of type II SLAP lesions.[14,15] Several reviews have reported postoperative stiffness as an outcome of treating these injuries concomitantly, most notably in middle-age patients.[16] Biceps tenotomy or tenodesis have been recommended to help avoid postoperative stiffness. Although simple débridement of the SLAP lesion has been shown to have poor results in younger patients, SLAP repair in older patients has been advocated against by several authors.[17-19] The results suggest improved pain and functional outcome with débridement when compared with repair.

Accurate diagnosis can be aided by specific examination (**Figure 1**) and imaging modalities (**Figure 2**). In addition to several provocative examination maneuvers described for the diagnosis of SLAP tears, the authors of this chapter combine these maneuvers with simple palpation of the biceps in the rotator interval and beneath the pectoralis insertion. The authors think that tenderness to palpation in one of these two areas is more predictive of the biceps as the cause of pain, rather than a SLAP tear. If the patient's history and physical examination results demonstrate a need for additional imaging, MRI has been shown to aid clinical decision

FIGURE 1

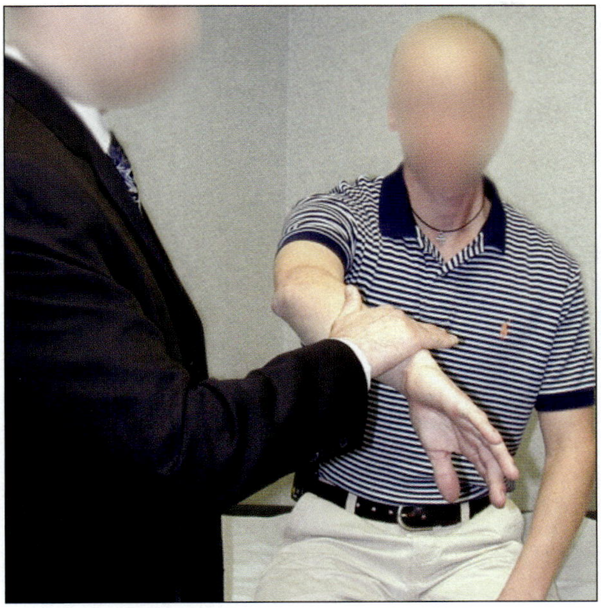

The O'Brien test. The patient's arm is placed in 10° to 15° of adduction and 90° of forward flexion. With the patient's thumb pointing toward the floor (full forearm pronation), the patient resists the examiner's downward pressure on the wrist of the outstretched arm. (Reproduced with permission from Rapley JH, Barber FA: Superior labrum anteroposterior [SLAP] tears, in Angelo RL, Esch JC, Ryu RKN, eds: *AANA Advanced Arthroscopy: The Shoulder.* Saunders Elsevier, Philadelphia, PA, 2010, pp 177-187.)

making. The improved accuracy of MRI interpretation by a fellowship-trained musculoskeletal radiologist has been validated.[20-22] Magnetic resonance arthrography with gadolinium has been shown to improve specificity when compared directly with conventional MRI and has been validated at arthroscopy, which suggests increased potential for arthrography to improve diagnostic accuracy. Additionally, in throwers, imaging with the arm in abduction and external rotation has been extremely useful in documenting the peel-back lesion and internal impingement.[23] When used with magnetic resonance arthrography, this position has shown positive and negative predictive values in a large series of patients comparing preoperative magnetic resonance arthrography with intraoperative arthroscopic findings. Excellent intraobserver reliability was also demonstrated.[24]

CT arthrography has been studied recently because of its decreased cost and increased accessibility compared with MRI or magnetic resonance arthrography. Waldt et al[25] compared multislice CT arthrography with magnetic resonance arthrography in cadaveric specimens and demonstrated similar diagnostic potential for superior labral anatomic variants and pathology. These results have been replicated in vivo;[26] Kim et al[27] showed a sensitivity of 95% and a specificity of 73% within similar diagnostic ranges reported for magnetic resonance arthrography. Additional studies evaluating CT arthrography are needed before it is widely used.

Several studies have compared treatment options for combined rotator cuff and SLAP tears. Franceschi et al[16] conducted a prospective review comparing biceps tenotomy with SLAP repair in patients older than 50 years with associated rotator cuff tears and type II SLAP lesions. Range of motion, function, and patient satisfaction were significantly greater in patients in the biceps tenotomy group. However, dissatisfaction with cosmetic outcome resulting from the distal migration of the tendon (the Popeye sign) and the decreased shoulder strength were noted in patients in the tentomy group. Biceps tenodesis has been shown to be a successful alternative when performed in isolation, but no study has compared the outcomes of biceps tenodesis with those of SLAP repair performed in the setting of a rotator cuff tear.

Contrary to the previous thinking that concomitant repair of rotator cuff tears and SLAP lesions resulted in shoulder stiffness, several more recent studies have shown no adverse outcomes with a combined procedure. An aggressive postoperative rehabilitation program has been suggested as a possible cause for these differing outcomes.[28] Most recently, Forsythe et al[29,30] showed no difference in outcomes of a large series of patients who underwent a single arthroscopic procedure for rotator cuff repair and SLAP repair compared with patients who underwent rotator cuff repair alone in the absence of a SLAP lesion. Patients with visible fraying of the biceps tendon underwent bicep tenodesis rather than SLAP repair. If the tendon was in good condition with an unstable biceps labral complex, repair was performed. Previously, better functional outcomes were shown for patients who underwent biceps tenodesis compared with type II SLAP repair when this injury was isolated from other intra-articular patholo-

FIGURE 2

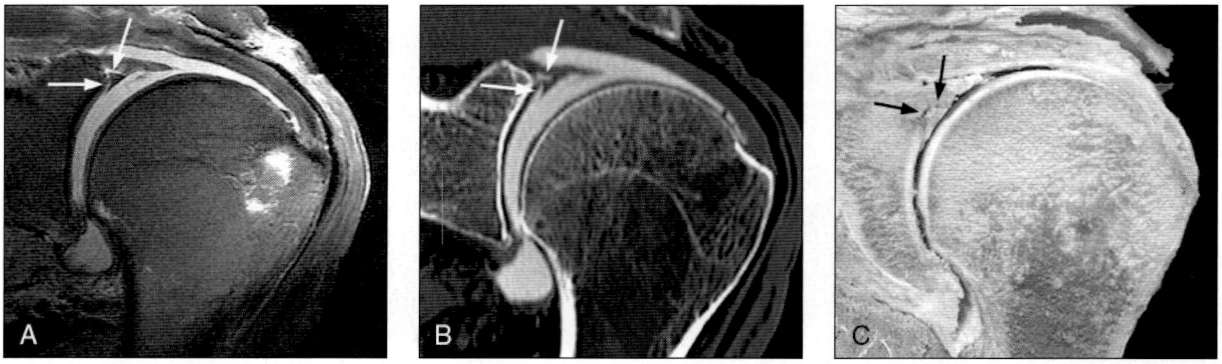

Images of a type III superior labrum anterior to posterior (SLAP) tear. **A,** Coronal oblique fat-saturated T1-weighted magnetic resonance arthrogram shows two interfaces (arrows) delineated by contrast medium: one between the preserved biceps anchor and the superior labrum and one between the glenoid rim and the superior labrum, which show a type III SLAP tear. **B,** Corresponding coronal oblique reformation after CT arthrography identically demonstrates a triangular segment of the superior labrum delineated by two contrast medium interfaces (arrows). **C,** Photograph of the shoulder specimen sectioned parallel to the biceps anchor demonstrates a bucket handle superior labral tear without displacement of the labral fragment into the joint space (arrows). (Reproduced with permission from Waldt S, Metz S, Burkart A, et al: Variants of the superior labrum and labro-bicipital complex: A comparative study of shoulder specimens using MR arthrography, multi-slice CT arthrography and anatomic dissection. *Eur Radiol* 2006;16[2]:451-458.)

gies such as rotator cuff tears or associated instability.[31] Research comparing the outcomes of rotator cuff repair with concomitant biceps tenodesis versus SLAP repair could help guide future treatment of combined rotator cuff and SLAP tears for the best outcome. The current treatment algorithm used by the authors of this chapter for most rotator cuff tears favors débridement without repair of the superior labrum. In this situation, the biceps can often remain in its original position.

In the throwing athlete, internal impingement also can cause combined rotator cuff and SLAP lesions, which must be recognized and treated differently than other combined lesions. Combined GIRD and SLAP lesions can substantially decrease the likelihood of a return to a high level of performance. Simultaneous arthroscopic repair of combined infraspinatus and SLAP lesions was reviewed in 20 overhead athletes younger than 25 years. Of these, only 8 (40%) were able to return to preinjury level of play; 3 athletes, all of whom were pitchers, were completely unable to return to play.[32]

Nonsurgical Treatment

Nonsurgical treatment of SLAP lesions has been reported infrequently in recent literature, likely because of the widely accepted (but never validated) notion of high patient dissatisfaction and poor functional improvement without surgery. NSAIDs are often prescribed at initial presentation, with or without intra-articular steroid injection. Physical therapy should include scapular stabilization exercises. A tight posterior capsule can be treated with stretching: the sleeper stretch has been described for this purpose, is tolerated well, and requires minimal patient education.[33,34] Edwards et al[35] reviewed a series of patients treated nonsurgically with NSAIDs, with or without intra-articular steroid injections, in addition to core and rotator cuff strengthening, and showed rates of return to play comparable with those who had undergone surgery, with somewhat inferior results for overhead athletes.

Surgical Treatment

Surgery may be indicated for the patient with a true type II SLAP lesion resulting from trauma or a specific activity. Repairing the superior labrum using stitch patterns that keep sutures away from the stump of the biceps is a reasonable solution in these cases, but achieving the correct preoperative and intraoperative diagnosis is more important than the nuances of surgical technique.

FIGURE 3

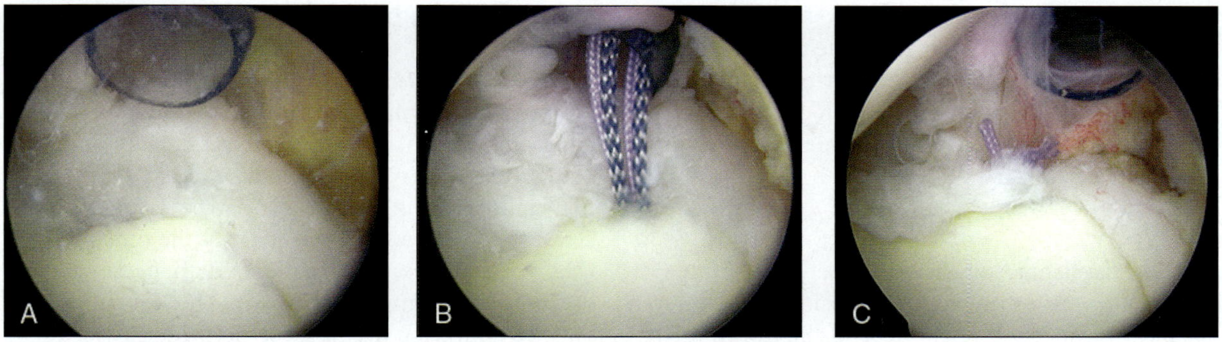

Arthroscopic views of a superior labrum anterior to posterior tear after biceps tenotomy. **A,** Chondromalacia of the glenoid and frayed edges of the labrum are visible. **B,** Anchor placement. **C,** The suture is tied and cut with reapproximation of the superior labrum to the glenoid.

Diagnostic arthroscopy demonstrates the labral avulsion in a type II SLAP tear. In a truly unstable superior labral tear, chondromalacia of the glenoid near the torn area, a frayed labral undersurface, and a corresponding area of injury on the superior glenoid devoid of articular cartilage are immediately visible. A smooth cartilaginous surface indicates a normal variant and not a superior labral tear. Repair should proceed in the same manner as with any labral repair: débridement of loose tissue, abrasion of the underlying glenoid, and anchor placement and suture passage. The anterosuperior anchor is placed via a superior rotator interval portal and the posterior anchor is placed via a port of Wilmington portal, which penetrates the muscle belly of the upper infraspinatus. A portal should never be created through the tendons of the rotator cuff.[36,37] In most cases, shuttling the sutures through the labrum using spinal needles and monofilament suture is fairly easy, although one can certainly use commercially available shuttles. Sutures cannot be passed through the biceps tendon. The authors of this chapter favor mattress sutures over simple sutures as a better re-creation of normal anatomy. In the anterosuperior quadrant, it is important to re-create the normal attachments of the superior glenohumeral ligament (SGHL) and middle glenohumeral ligament (MGHL). Posteriorly, stabilizing the labrum and eliminating the pathologic peel-back in abduction and external rotation is usually sufficient (**Figure 3**).

Combined Lesions

The real issue with combined lesions is determining the etiology of the lesions. In cases in which the labral tear occurred first, usually via acute or repetitive trauma, both lesions need to be repaired, as with the superior labrum anterior cuff (SLAC) lesion discussion above. In most cases, the rotator cuff is the primary lesion and the type I SLAP tear is a variant that results from abnormal superior tracking resulting from the deficient rotator cuff. In these cases, the labral tear associated with the full-thickness rotator cuff tear can be managed with simple débridement and biceps tenotomy or tenodesis, and the surgical emphasis is on rotator cuff repair using standard arthroscopic technique followed by biceps tenodesis when indicated.

SLAC Lesions

Savoie et al[38] described a SLAC lesion, a particular type of combined SLAP and rotator cuff tear in which the SGHL and MGHL are avulsed from the superior glenoid. The resultant instability of this SLAC lesion causes the supraspinatus to impinge against the acromion, resulting in a partial or sometimes full-thickness tear at its anterior edge. The anterior supraspinatus tear may result in biceps subluxation with subsequent symptoms.

In cases of combined tears, the anterosuperior labrum is repaired first, using a small suture anchor. The authors of this chapter recommend a mattress suture with one limb through the SGHL and one through the

MGHL to eliminate instability. Next, either a partial articular-side tendon avulsion repair is performed via a superior rotator interval portal or the tear is completed and a standard rotator cuff repair is performed. If the damage to the biceps is minimal with no instability, the biceps may be preserved. However, in most cases, tenodesis will be necessary.

Results

Good to excellent results have been reported, from 65% to 97%, for repair of type II SLAP lesions.[39-42] However, the outcome of SLAP repair depends highly on the patient's preinjury level of activity, and significant differences in patient satisfaction have been noted between overhead athletes and nonathletes. Further, when concurrent intra-articular pathologies are identified and treated at the time of surgery in addition to the SLAP repair, results begin to decline from uniformly excellent outcomes. Friel et al[39] evaluated 46 patients with type II SLAP tears repaired arthroscopically using suture anchor fixation and showed significant improvement in postoperative range of motion. Several patients underwent concurrent Bankart repair, subacromial decompression, distal clavicle excision, and intra-articular débridement. Overall, 79% of patients reported excellent results subjectively and 89% would undergo the same procedure again. Of 13 overhead collegiate athletes, only 54% (7 patients) returned to his or her previous level of sport. Of these 7, 6 baseball players returned to preoperative level of play, and only 1 of 4 tennis players returned to a high level of play. Low rates of return to sport have been consistently reported following SLAP repair.[40,41]

Neri et al[43] examined a group of collegiate and professional throwers who underwent arthroscopic SLAP repair using the Kerlan-Jobe Orthopaedic Clinic Shoulder and Elbow score, which is a targeted measure of outcomes tailored for high-performance overhead tasks. The study demonstrated a 57% return to high-performance overhead competition, which was consistent with previous investigations.[44] Concomitant partial articular-side tendon avulsion lesions that underwent débridement were identified as an independent risk factor for a greater likelihood of inability to return to play.[43] Although excellent results can be expected for the general population, high-demand patients and overhead athletes should be counseled regarding his or her likelihood of return to overhead activity.[40,41]

Complications

Postoperative complications can include pain at rest, pain with range of motion, decreased range of motion, and mechanical symptoms. Outcome studies suggest that complications increase and patient satisfaction decreases with increasing patient age at the time of SLAP tear. Specifically, among patients with declared poor outcomes following SLAP repair, 71% remained dissatisfied following a course of nonsurgical treatment before discussion of revision surgery.[45] Workers' compensation claims, involvement of the dominant arm, and history of trauma were shown to have poorer outcomes. Revision surgery may include biceps tenodesis, loose body removal, removal of loose suture material, manipulation, capsular release, and revision of the repair. Unlike the young patient with an isolated SLAP injury, an older patient likely undergoes treatment for concomitant intra-articular pathology at the time of surgery. This creates confounding circumstances when trying to determine the cause of the poor result.

Biceps and Shoulder Stiffness

Revision SLAP repair is rarely indicated. The usual findings at revision arthroscopy following SLAP repair are partial tears of the long head tendon of the biceps and inflammation within the rotator interval. These findings strongly suggest that the original SLAP repair was not necessary.

Surgical treatment of the stiff shoulder following SLAP repair should include débridement and removal of all sutures, rotator interval release, and, usually, biceps tenotomy or tenodesis. Older patients who may undergo SLAP repair should be counseled frankly regarding all possible outcomes. Incorrect diagnosis of a SLAP tear and resultant repair has been shown to result in poor outcomes. Weber et al[46] conducted a recent review of the American Board of Orthopaedic Surgery Part II database of cases submitted by Board candidates and showed an alarming number of SLAP repairs being performed nationwide. SLAP repairs comprised 9.4% of all shoulder cases submitted. The mean patient age was 36.4 years for men and 40.0 years for women; SLAP repairs were performed in patients much older than 80 years in both sexes. This study highlights the misplaced enthusiasm for SLAP repair. Many patients older than 40 years benefit from biceps tenodesis. SLAP repair performed in patients older than 40 years may be associated with an increased incidence of stiffness and overall postoperative morbidity.[47] Treatment must always be guided by the diagnosis, even if the diagnosis is established at arthroscopy. Gobezie et al[48] showed significant interobserver and intraobserver variability when differentiating between normal shoulders and various SLAP lesions among experienced shoulder surgeons, which emphasizes the difficulty in establishing the diagnosis of a SLAP tear. Further refinement in the education of surgeons regarding normal aging, normal anatomic variants, and true intra-articular pathology may help decrease the rates of misdiagnosis and failed repair.

Conclusion

Lesions of the superior labrum and proximal biceps tendon can be reliably treated, but correct diagnosis and treatment are essential to maximize the likelihood of a satisfactory result. Although treatment options such as SLAP repair or biceps tenodesis are often straightforward in both younger and older patients, further study is needed to determine the optimal treatment of middle-age patients. Currently, surgeons must rely on their own interpretation of the physical examination findings, the patient's physical demands and expectations, and the arthroscopic findings before choosing the appropriate treatment.

References

1. Walch G, Edwards TB, Boulahia A, Nové-Josserand L, Neyton L, Szabo I: Arthroscopic tenotomy of the long head of the biceps in the treatment of rotator cuff tears: Clinical and radiographic results of 307 cases. *J Shoulder Elbow Surg* 2005;14(3):238-246.
2. Huber WP, Putz RV: Periarticular fiber system of the shoulder joint. *Arthroscopy* 1997;13(6):680-691.
3. Sugaya H, Moriishi J, Kanisawa I, Tsuchiya A: Arthroscopic osseous Bankart repair for chronic recurrent traumatic anterior glenohumeral instability: Surgical technique. *J Bone Joint Surg Am* 2006;88(Suppl 1 Pt 2):159-169.
4. Gutierrez V, Monckeberg JE, Pinedo M, Radice F: Arthroscopically determined degree of injury after shoulder dislocation relates to recurrence rate. *Clin Orthop Relat Res* 2012;470(4):961-964.
5. Kim TK, Queale WS, Cosgarea AJ, McFarland EG: Clinical features of the different types of SLAP lesions: An analysis of one hundred and thirty-nine cases. *J Bone Joint Surg Am* 2003;85-A(1):66-71.
6. Rodosky MW, Harner CD, Fu FH: The role of the long head of the biceps muscle and superior glenoid labrum in anterior stability of the shoulder. *Am J Sports Med* 1994;22(1):121-130.
7. Sakurai G, Ozaki J, Tomita Y, Nishimoto K, Tamai S: Electromyographic analysis of shoulder joint function of the biceps brachii muscle during isometric contraction. *Clin Orthop Relat Res* 1998;354:123-131.
8. Pagnani MJ, Speer KP, Altchek DW, Warren RF, Dines DM: Arthroscopic fixation of superior labral lesions using a biodegradable implant: A preliminary report. *Arthroscopy* 1995;11(2):194-198.
9. Burkhart SS, Fox DL: Case report: Arthroscopic repair of a type IV SLAP lesion—the red-on-white lesion as a component of anterior instability. *Arthroscopy* 1993;9(5):488-497.
10. Burkhart SS, Morgan CD, Kibler WB: The disabled throwing shoulder: Spectrum of pathology: Part I. Pathoanatomy and biomechanics. *Arthroscopy* 2003;19(4):404-420.
11. Gorantla K, Gill C, Wright RW: The outcome of type II SLAP repair: A systematic review. *Arthroscopy* 2010;26(4):537-545.
12. Ide J, Maeda S, Takagi K: Sports activity after arthroscopic superior labral repair using suture anchors in overhead-throwing athletes. *Am J Sports Med* 2005;33(4):507-514.
13. Miller C, Savoie FH: Glenohumeral abnormalities associated with full-thickness tears of the rotator cuff. *Orthop Rev* 1994;23(2):159-162.
14. Morgan CD, Burkhart SS, Palmeri M, Gillespie M: Type II SLAP lesions: Three subtypes and their relationships to superior instability and rotator cuff tears. *Arthroscopy* 1998;14(6):553-565.
15. Snyder SJ, Banas MP, Karzel RP: An analysis of 140 injuries to the superior glenoid labrum. *J Shoulder Elbow Surg* 1995;4(4):243-248.

16. Franceschi F, Longo UG, Ruzzini L, Rizzello G, Maffulli N, Denaro V: No advantages in repairing a type II superior labrum anterior and posterior (SLAP) lesion when associated with rotator cuff repair in patients over age 50: A randomized controlled trial. *Am J Sports Med* 2008;36(2):247-253.
17. Altchek DW, Warren RF, Wickiewicz TL, Ortiz G: Arthroscopic labral debridement: A three-year follow-up study. *Am J Sports Med* 1992;20(6):702-706.
18. Cordasco FA, Steinmann S, Flatow EL, Bigliani LU: Arthroscopic treatment of glenoid labral tears. *Am J Sports Med* 1993;21(3):425-431.
19. Abbot AE, Li X, Busconi BD: Arthroscopic treatment of concomitant superior labral anterior posterior (SLAP) lesions and rotator cuff tears in patients over the age of 45 years. *Am J Sports Med* 2009;37(7):1358-1362.
20. Reuss BL, Schwartzberg R, Zlatkin MB, Cooperman A, Dixon JR: Magnetic resonance imaging accuracy for the diagnosis of superior labrum anterior-posterior lesions in the community setting: Eighty-three arthroscopically confirmed cases. *J Shoulder Elbow Surg* 2006;15(5):580-585.
21. Jee WH, McCauley TR, Katz LD, Matheny JM, Ruwe PA, Daigneault JP: Superior labral anterior posterior (SLAP) lesions of the glenoid labrum: Reliability and accuracy of MR arthrography for diagnosis. *Radiology* 2001;218(1):127-132.
22. Amin MF, Youssef AO: The diagnostic value of magnetic resonance arthrography of the shoulder in detection and grading of SLAP lesions: Comparison with arthroscopic findings. *Eur J Radiol* 2012;81(9):2343-2347.
23. Chhadia AM, Goldberg BA, Hutchinson MR: Abnormal translation in SLAP lesions on magnetic resonance imaging abducted externally rotated view. *Arthroscopy* 2010;26(1):19-25.
24. Borrero CG, Casagranda BU, Towers JD, Bradley JP: Magnetic resonance appearance of posterosuperior labral peel back during humeral abduction and external rotation. *Skeletal Radiol* 2010;39(1):19-26.
25. Waldt S, Metz S, Burkart A, et al: Variants of the superior labrum and labro-bicipital complex: A comparative study of shoulder specimens using MR arthrography, multi-slice CT arthrography and anatomical dissection. *Eur Radiol* 2006;16(2):451-458.
26. Bencardino JT, Beltran J, Rosenberg ZS, et al: Superior labrum anterior-posterior lesions: Diagnosis with MR arthrography of the shoulder. *Radiology* 2000;214(1):267-271.
27. Kim YJ, Choi JA, Oh JH, Hwang SI, Hong SH, Kang HS: Superior labral anteroposterior tears: Accuracy and interobserver reliability of multidetector CT arthrography for diagnosis. *Radiology* 2011;260(1):207-215.
28. Samani JE, Marston SB, Buss DD: Arthroscopic stabilization of type II SLAP lesions using an absorbable tack. *Arthroscopy* 2001;17(1):19-24.
29. Forsythe B, Martin SD: Concomitant arthroscopic SLAP and rotator cuff repair: Surgical technique. *J Bone Joint Surg Am* 2011;93(Suppl 1):1-9.
30. Forsythe B, Guss D, Anthony SG, Martin SD: Concomitant arthroscopic SLAP and rotator cuff repair. *J Bone Joint Surg Am* 2010;92(6):1362-1369.
31. Boileau P, Parratte S, Chuinard C, Roussanne Y, Shia D, Bicknell R: Arthroscopic treatment of isolated type II SLAP lesions: Biceps tenodesis as an alternative to reinsertion. *Am J Sports Med* 2009;37(5):929-936.
32. Van Kleunen JP, Tucker SA, Field LD, Savoie FH III: Return to high-level throwing after combination infraspinatus repair, SLAP repair, and release of glenohumeral internal rotation deficit. *Am J Sports Med* 2012;40(11):2536-2541.
33. Burkhart SS, Morgan CD, Kibler WB: The disabled throwing shoulder: Spectrum of pathology: Part II. Evaluation and treatment of SLAP lesions in throwers. *Arthroscopy* 2003;19(5):531-539.
34. Burkhart SS, Morgan CD, Kibler WB: Shoulder injuries in overhead athletes: The "dead arm" revisited. *Clin Sports Med* 2000;19(1):125-158.
35. Edwards SL, Lee JA, Bell JE, et al: Nonoperative treatment of superior labrum anterior posterior tears: Improvements in pain, function, and quality of life. *Am J Sports Med* 2010;38(7):1456-1461.
36. Lo IK, Lind CC, Burkhart SS: Glenohumeral arthroscopy portals established using an outside-in technique: Neurovascular anatomy at risk. *Arthroscopy* 2004;20(6):596-602.
37. Meyer M, Graveleau N, Hardy P, Landreau P: Anatomic risks of shoulder arthroscopy portals: Anatomic cadaveric study of 12 portals. *Arthroscopy* 2007;23(5):529-536.
38. Savoie FH III, Field LD, Atchinson S: Anterior superior instability with rotator cuff tearing: SLAC lesion. *Orthop Clin North Am* 2001;32(3):457-461, ix.

39. Friel NA, Karas V, Slabaugh MA, Cole BJ: Outcomes of type II superior labrum, anterior to posterior (SLAP) repair: Prospective evaluation at a minimum two-year follow-up. *J Shoulder Elbow Surg* 2010;19(6):859-867.
40. Sayde WM, Cohen SB, Ciccotti MG, Dodson CC: Return to play after Type II superior labral anterior-posterior lesion repairs in athletes: A systematic review. *Clin Orthop Relat Res* 2012;470(6):1595-1600.
41. Neuman BJ, Boisvert CB, Reiter B, Lawson K, Ciccotti MG, Cohen SB: Results of arthroscopic repair of type II superior labral anterior posterior lesions in overhead athletes: Assessment of return to preinjury playing level and satisfaction. *Am J Sports Med* 2011;39(9):1883-1888.
42. Rhee YG, Lee DH, Lim CT: Unstable isolated SLAP lesion: Clinical presentation and outcome of arthroscopic fixation. *Arthroscopy* 2005;21(9):1099-1104.
43. Neri BR, ElAttrache NS, Owsley KC, Mohr K, Yocum LA: Outcome of type II superior labral anterior posterior repairs in elite overhead athletes: Effect of concomitant partial-thickness rotator cuff tears. *Am J Sports Med* 2011;39(1):114-120.
44. Alberta FG, ElAttrache NS, Bissell S, et al: The development and validation of a functional assessment tool for the upper extremity in the overhead athlete. *Am J Sports Med* 2010;38(5):903-911.
45. Katz LM, Hsu S, Miller SL, et al: Poor outcomes after SLAP repair: Descriptive analysis and prognosis. *Arthroscopy* 2009;25(8):849-855.
46. Weber SC, Martin DF, Seiler JG III, Harrast JJ: Superior labrum anterior and posterior lesions of the shoulder: Incidence rates, complications, and outcomes as reported by American Board of Orthopedic Surgery. Part II candidates. *Am J Sports Med* 2012;40(7):1538-1543.
47. Weber SC, Kauffman JI: Arthroscopic biceps tenodesis: Experience with Castagna technique. Long-term follow-up. *Arthroscopy* 2008;24(6, Suppl)e9-e10.
48. Gobezie R, Zurakowski D, Lavery K, Millett PJ, Cole BJ, Warner JJ: Analysis of interobserver and intraobserver variability in the diagnosis and treatment of SLAP tears using the Snyder classification. *Am J Sports Med* 2008;36(7):1373-1379.

CHAPTER 18

Complications of Superior Labrum Anterior to Posterior and Biceps Tendon Repairs

Hans C. Bengtson, MD
Matthew L. Busam, MD
Samer S. Hasan, MD, PhD

Background

Adverse events and complications related to the surgical treatment of disorders of the biceps root and the long head of the biceps tendon are relatively uncommon and usually manageable. Many, but not all, can be avoided with basic strategies covered elsewhere in this monograph, such as proper diagnosis and indications for surgery, as well as thorough and precise treatment. This chapter reviews common complications encountered during and after the surgical treatment of biceps pathology, including superior labrum anterior to posterior (SLAP) repairs, biceps tenodesis, and biceps tenotomy.

Complications Following SLAP Repair

Complications following a SLAP repair can result from an incorrect diagnosis or indication for repair, pitfalls related to surgical technique and rehabilitation, and spurious intraoperative and postoperative events. Guidelines for the surgical treatment of various SLAP tears have been proposed,[1,2] but what constitutes pathologic detachment of the labrum is still undefined because intraobserver and interobserver variability remains high.[3] Multiple fixation methods have been described for SLAP repair, including transosseous sutures, staples, screws, bioabsorbable tacks, and suture anchors; however, this evolution in repair technique has revealed various associated complications.

Relaxed Indications for SLAP Repair

The incidence of SLAP repairs has been increasing during the past decade,[4,5] suggesting that the indications for SLAP repair may have relaxed considerably. In a recent review of the American Board of Orthopaedic Surgery (ABOS) Part II surgical case database, Weber et al[4] found that SLAP repairs comprised 9.4% of all shoulder arthroscopic procedures and were performed in patients as old as 88 years. In contrast, Snyder et

Dr. Busam or an immediate family member has received nonincome support (such as equipment or services), commercially derived honoraria, or other non–research-related funding (such as paid travel) from Arthrex, DePuy, a Johnson & Johnson company, DJ Orthopaedics, and OREF. Dr. Hasan or an immediate family member serves as a paid consultant to or is an employee of DJ Orthopaedics; has received research or institutional support from DJ Orthopaedics and Arthrex and serves as a board member, owner, officer, or committee member of the American Academy of Orthopaedic Surgeons Publications Committee. Neither Dr. Bengtson nor any immediate family member has received anything of value from or has stock or stock options held in a commercial company or institution related directly or indirectly to the subject of this chapter.

al[6] conducted a review of 2,375 shoulder arthroscopic procedures performed over 9 years at a single institution and reported an overall SLAP lesion incidence of 5.9%. Type II lesions encompassed approximately one half (55%), for a total type II SLAP lesion incidence of 3.25%.

Determining intraoperatively which SLAP lesion requires surgical treatment can be a challenge, especially when the lesion occurs concomitantly with a rotator cuff tear or in an older patient. Alpert et al[7] examined the effect of age on the outcome of isolated type II SLAP repairs using suture anchors. No significant difference was observed in patients older or younger than 40 years regarding various patient outcome scores or satisfaction levels, or willingness to undergo the same procedure again. Denard et al[8] showed a high rate of success for the repair of SLAP lesions in all age groups, but a trend toward poorer results with worker's compensation patients and those older than 40 years.

Abbot and Busconi[9] investigated 38 patients older than 45 years who underwent arthroscopic rotator cuff repair with concomitant type II SLAP repair (18 patients) or débridement (20 patients). The authors found that patients in the débridement group experienced significantly better overall UCLA shoulder rating scores ($P < 0.001$), function ($P < 0.005$), pain relief ($P < 0.001$), and range of motion in both internal and external rotation ($P < 0.001$) at 1 and 2 years postoperatively compared with patients in the repair group.

Franceschi et al[10] reached a similar conclusion from a randomized controlled trial of 63 patients. The authors noted that in patients older than 50 years with a type II SLAP lesion and a concurrent rotator cuff tear, repairing the SLAP lesion was not advantageous. In fact, the authors reported a significant difference in total postoperative UCLA shoulder rating scores and range of motion when comparing rotator cuff repair with tenotomy versus rotator cuff repair with a SLAP repair ($P < 0.05$).

In contrast, Strickland et al[11] reported on 11 patients (mean age, 47 years) who underwent concurrent arthroscopic rotator cuff repair and type II SLAP repair and concluded that in carefully selected active adults without workers' compensation claims, concurrent SLAP and rotator cuff repair can result in improved outcomes. However, the authors cautioned that an accelerated rehabilitation protocol was essential for success. Another study found that an unhealed SLAP lesion after concomitant rotator cuff and SLAP repair did not preclude a successful outcome after the rotator cuff repair.[12]

The review of the ABOS Part II surgical case database also reported an overall complication rate of 4.7% and described the complications as "neither uncommon nor insignificant."[4] Although these data included adverse events such as pneumonia, pulmonary embolism, and anesthetic complications, the data also encompassed many of the surgically specific complications in this chapter, showing that such events are, unfortunately, still encountered.

Postoperative Stiffness

Postoperative stiffness has been reported as the most common cause of failure of SLAP repairs.[13,14] Brockmeier et al[15] prospectively evaluated 47 patients who underwent SLAP repair using bioabsorbable suture anchors with minimum follow-up of 2 years. Five of 47 patients experienced complications (10.6%); 4 complications were refractory stiffness (8.5%), 1 of which required arthroscopic lysis of adhesions for severe postoperative adhesive capsulitis that did not respond to nonsurgical treatment. Provencher et al[16] studied 179 young military patients who underwent type II SLAP repairs and reported a 31% failure rate and a 27% revision rate, which showed that patients whose repairs failed had range of motion and outcome scores that were unchanged from the preoperative assessment.

Weber[17] reviewed 24 shoulders in 22 patients who experienced persistent pain following SLAP repair. Of the 10 patients who had preoperative stiffness, 7 had noteworthy chondral injuries thought to be related to implant failure or migration. Additionally, 8 of the 14 patients with chondral injuries seen during repeat arthroscopy had stiffness during physical examination.

Katz et al[14] reviewed 34 patients who were dissatisfied following SLAP repair and reported that although all patients had pain, 75% also reported stiffness. Of the 34 patients, 10 (29%) improved with nonsurgical management, including physical therapy. Of the 21 patients who progressed to surgical revision, 1 required manipulation under anesthesia and 4 required capsular release (**Figure 1**).

FIGURE 1

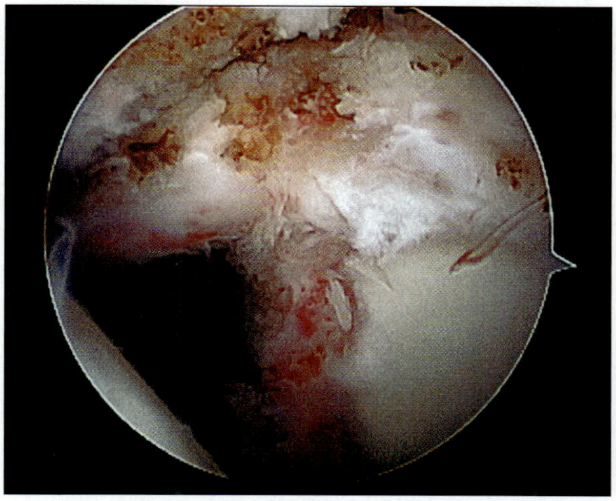

Arthroscopic view shows scarring of the biceps-labral complex and generalized capsulitis following arthroscopic superior labrum anterior to posterior injury repair.

FIGURE 2

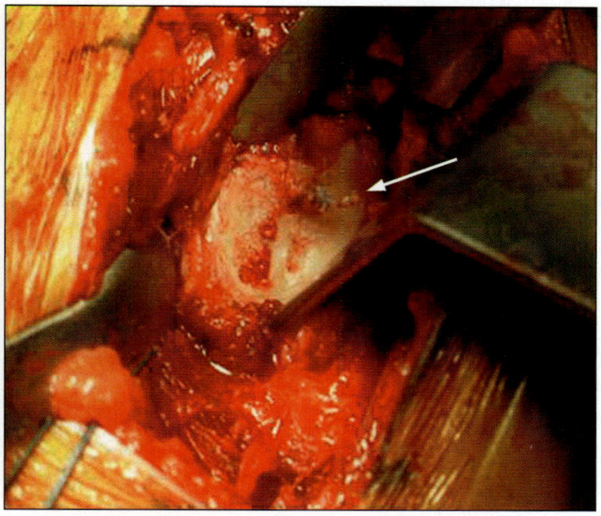

Photograph shows suture anchor erosion into the glenoid center and associated advanced chondrolysis (arrow) following arthroscopic superior labrum anterior to posterior injury repair. (Reprinted with permission from Hasan SS, Fleckenstein CM: Glenohumeral chondrolysis: Part 1. Clinical presentation and predictors of disease progression. *Arthroscopy* 2013;29[7]:1135-1140.)

Implant-Related Complications

Although not regularly encountered, when implant-related complications occur during SLAP repair, the results can be debilitating and, at times, destructive. The clinical presentation often mimics that of shoulder stiffness following SLAP repair, as patients describe postoperative pain that occurs weeks to months after the index procedure, often accompanied by decreasing range of motion.[18,19] Foreign-body reactions from exposed bioabsorbable devices such as tacks can produce painful, diffuse synovitis that can hamper recovery and mimic infection. The histologic appearance of this synovitis is characterized by the infiltration of histiocytes and multinucleated giant cells. Treatment may require repeat arthroscopy with débridement and synovectomy.[19]

In addition, bioabsorbable suture anchors that are recessed into the bone may also cause a foreign-body reaction as the anchor degrades. This foreign-body reaction has also been implicated in the etiology of glenoid osteolysis and subsequent implant loosening.[19] Treatment may require removal of the loose anchors and revision fixation of the labral tear.[18] Another implant-related complication is the formation of a suture granuloma that causes intra-articular posterosuperior impingement.[20] Moreover, arthroscopic knots made with stiff, permanent sutures that face the humeral head may cause cartilage abrasion[17] and mechanical irritation or squeaking.[21]

Of even greater concern are the full-thickness chondral injuries that can result from gross implant debris, including fragmented or whole anchors, within the glenohumeral joint.[19,22,23] Anchors that loosen and piston or become prominent or loose within the glenohumeral joint have also been implicated in glenohumeral chondrolysis,[24] a devastating condition characterized by rapid, diffuse cartilage loss and joint destruction. Finally, iatrogenic glenoid chondral injuries and even chondrolysis may result from errant glenoid drilling and anchor placement (**Figure 2**).

Nerve Injury

Neuropathies that result from SLAP lesions or their treatment are rare and most commonly isolated to the suprascapular nerve and caused by a spinoglenoid notch cyst.[25,26] However, iatrogenic nerve injury sus-

FIGURE 3

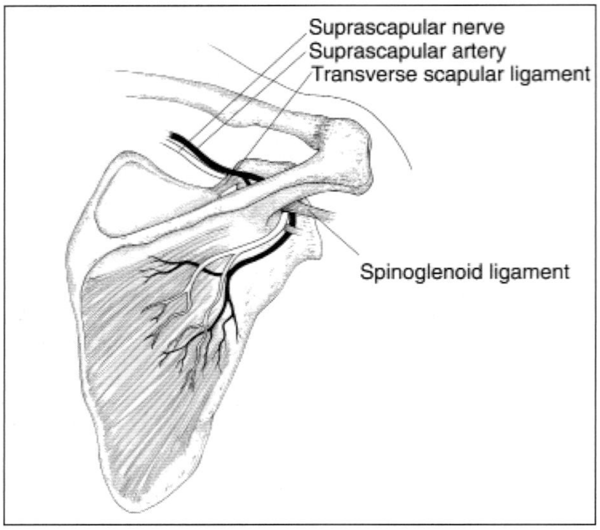

Line drawing depicts the course of the suprascapular nerve and its proximity to the superior glenoid rim. (Reproduced from Piasecki DP, Romeo AA, Bach BR Jr, Nicholson GP: Suprascapular neuropathy. *J Am Acad Orthop Surg* 2009;17[11]:665-676.)

tained during SLAP repair can occur and may result in substantial morbidity. Yoo et al[27] reported on a single case of suprascapular nerve injury located distal to the spinoglenoid notch, which caused isolated infraspinatus atrophy. The authors suspected that the cause was a 5.0-mm metal anchor that was improperly inserted during SLAP repair. The suprascapular nerve courses a mean (± SD) of 1.8 ± 0.2 cm medial to the glenoid surface at the spinoglenoid notch level[28] (**Figure 3**). Great care should be taken during suture anchor preparation and insertion to ensure secure fixation in the bone and avoid entering the spinoglenoid notch.

Rotator Cuff Injury

Intraoperative efforts to obtain the ideal suture anchor location and angle of anchor insertion can also contribute to complications following SLAP repair. Insertion of the suture anchor through the rotator interval minimizes rotator cuff injury, but it may not always provide the appropriate anchor trajectory and repair biomechanics. In a series of 31 patients, O'Brien et al[29] found that although 16 patients were able to return to their preinjury level of play, 3 (10%) were dissatisfied with the results of the surgery, and no patient had symptoms that suggested rotator cuff pathology. The authors contend that a transrotator cuff approach offers a more optimal device placement in the superior labrum without compromising rotator cuff function.

In contrast, Cohen et al[30] reviewed 41 patients with isolated type II SLAP lesions repaired arthroscopically with tack fixation at a mean follow-up of 3.7 years and found that the mean American Shoulder and Elbow Surgeons (ASES) outcomes scores were statistically inferior in patients who underwent rotator cuff piercing versus those who did not ($P < 0.05$). Additionally, almost all patients reporting night pain had undergone a cuff-piercing approach. The authors concluded that transrotator cuff portals may contribute to inferior surgical outcomes following SLAP repair.

These conflicting reports can be reconciled by noting that the potentially deleterious effect of a large rent through the tendons of the rotator cuff, such as that required to accommodate a plastic cannula, may be quite different from the effects of percutaneous insertion of a narrow drill guide and suture anchor through the rotator cuff muscles. Percutaneous suture anchor insertion using a portal at the port of Wilmington[31] with the arm internally oriented to deliver the infraspinatus muscle into the anchor trajectory may help avoid piercing the tendon.

Infection

Although postoperative infection is always a concern for surgeons, the overall rate of intra-articular infection after shoulder arthroscopy is low, reported as 1.6 per 1,000 cases in one study.[32] Weber et al[4] reviewed the ABOS Part II database and reported 14 infections among 4,975 SLAP repairs (0.28%). Multiple authors[33,34] have shown that chlorhexidine-based skin preparations reduce the overall bacterial count before shoulder surgery, a potentially important action toward infection prophylaxis, including lowering the bacterial load of *Propionibacterium acnes*, a common shoulder pathogen.

Complications Following Biceps Tenodesis

Tenodesis of the long head of the biceps tendon is commonly performed to alleviate pain caused by tearing, instability, or inflammation of the tendon, as well as certain SLAP tears. Multiple fixation techniques have been used for biceps tenodesis, but the complications for these different procedures are similar. Biceps tenodesis is thought to preserve the length-tension relationship of the biceps muscle by establishing a new origin at the appropriate length to prevent muscle atrophy. Biceps tenodesis helps maintain elbow flexion and supination strength to optimize elbow function and improve cosmesis by reproducing the biceps appearance.

For active patients (younger individuals, manual laborers, and athletes) with refractory biceps tendinosis, tenodesis to either the soft tissue or the humerus is the preferred surgical treatment.[35-38] Although the benefits of the location of fixation have been debated without clearly established guidelines, some authors contend that distal fixation beyond the bicipital groove avoids the potential residual tenosynovitis, and the associated pain, within the biceps sheath.[35,39,40]

Biceps tenodesis is also used for the treatment of symptomatic SLAP tears. Boileau et al[41] reported on 25 consecutive patients with isolated type II SLAP tears who were treated arthroscopically with either SLAP repair using suture anchors or with extra-articular biceps tenodesis with a bioabsorbable interference screw. Each Constant subscore was statistically similar between the SLAP repair and biceps tenodesis groups (pain, 11.7 versus 14.1; mobility, 39.1 versus 39.5; strength, 19.1 versus 17.5; $P > 0.05$) except for the activity subscore, which was higher in the tenodesis group (16.3 versus 19.5; $P < 0.001$). Although the authors noted that the sample size was small, the study was nonrandomized, and the groups were significantly different regarding age (the patients in the tenodesis group were older), the authors concluded that arthroscopic biceps tenodesis with an interference screw is an effective alternative to suture anchor repair of an isolated type II SLAP repair.

Nho et al[42] conducted the largest series published to date on complications in 353 patients who underwent open subpectoral biceps tenodesis. Of these, 2 patients (0.57%) had persistent pain, 2 experienced failure of fixation that resulted in a Popeye deformity (1 at 4 months, 1 at 6 months), a deep postoperative wound infection requiring surgical débridement and intravenous antibiotics developed in 1 (0.28%), 1 had postoperative musculocutaneous neuropathy, and complex regional pain syndrome requiring invasive pain management intervention developed in 1.

FIGURE 4

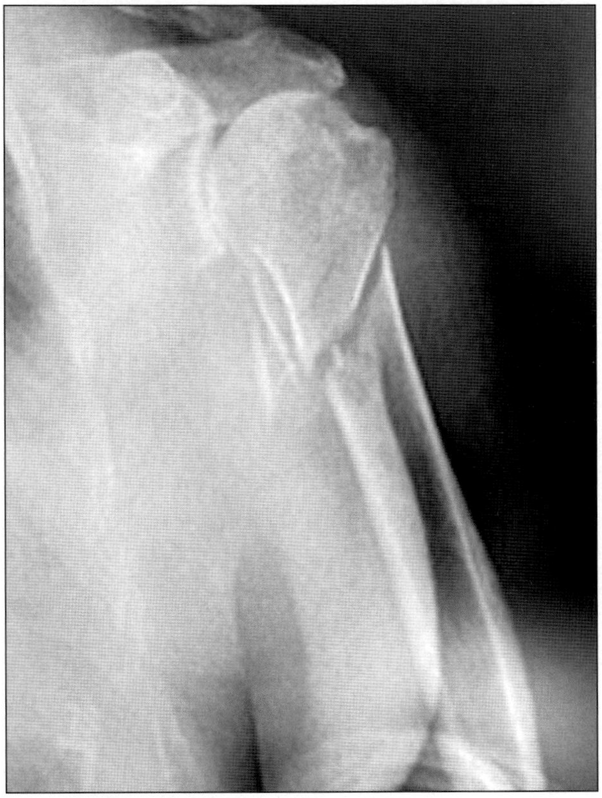

AP radiograph shows a proximal humerus fracture extending through the site of a subpectoral biceps tenodesis with an interference screw. (Courtesy of Dr. Greg Dairyko, Elmhurst, IL.)

Proximal Humerus Fracture

Interference screw fixation for proximal biceps tenodesis creates a rather large unicortical window that can act as a stress riser. Proximal humerus fracture following biceps tenodesis is a rare but potentially devastating complication following biceps tenodesis (**Figure 4**). Sears et al[43] reported on two patients who underwent open subpectoral biceps tenodesis with bioabsorbable interference screw fixation. One patient sustained a fracture when picking up a bag and a second patient sustained a fracture when falling down a small hill 6 months postoperatively. Both patients eventually underwent treatment with open reduction and humeral plate fixation.

Other authors[44-46] have reported proximal humerus fractures after arthroscopic biceps tenodesis in adults of various ages that occurred between 6 and 18 weeks postoperatively following low-energy injury. The theoretical concern with this specific technique relates to the additional humeral drill holes created for suture passage. Tension stresses can potentially result in a fracture propagating through the stress riser in the proximal humeral diaphysis.[40]

Nerve Injury

As with complications following SLAP repair, neuropathy after tenodesis of the long head of the biceps is rare and has been reported infrequently in the literature. Nho et al[42] noted musculocutaneous neuropathy that was diagnosed by forearm numbness and weakness with elbow flexion and forearm supination in 1 of 353 patients. The nerve was subsequently explored at 6 weeks and found to be intact; further intervention was not needed and complete recovery was seen at 6 months. Similarly, Ma et al[47] reported on a single patient in whom musculocutaneous neuropathy developed because of a nerve trapped behind the tenodesis site. During revision tenodesis and neurolysis, no neuroma was seen and the nerve was found to be in continuity but narrowed at the site of maximum stretch around the biceps. Immediate return of biceps function and resolution of the numbness and pain were noted; full recovery was seen at 1 year postoperatively.

A recent anatomic cadaver study[48] evaluated structures at risk during subpectoral biceps tenodesis and found that of all the structures evaluated, the musculocutaneous nerve was at the highest risk: it was closest to both the medial retractor (mean, 2.9 mm) and the tenodesis site (mean, 10.1 mm). In 18% of specimens, the nerve was in direct contact with the medial retractor during internal rotation of the arm. Furthermore, the deep brachial artery and the radial nerve were also noted to course near the medial retractor (mean distance, 5.7 and 7.4 mm, respectively); hence, the authors cautioned that if medial retraction is warranted, gentle retraction with a nonlevering retractor to reduce iatrogenic injury risk should be considered.

Loss of Fixation

Multiple fixation techniques with various devices have been used to secure the long head of the biceps during tenodesis, and the associated biomechanical strengths have been assessed in a laboratory model, showing that the interference screw techniques have the highest ultimate load to failure and the least amount of displacement on cyclic loading compared with other methods of fixation.[35,49] Despite the initial fixation strength provided by an interference screw, failure of biceps tenodesis (**Figure 5**) can occur, but the incidence appears to be very low.[42]

Arthroscopic Versus Open Biceps Tenodesis

Arthroscopic biceps tenodesis is an alternative to open biceps tenodesis, and can be performed using interference screws or suture anchors. Proponents of arthroscopic biceps tenodesis cite potential benefits such as improved cosmesis and a longer residual tendon that enables revision fixation. Detractors express concerns over axillary incisions required for open procedures and the associated potential for infection. However, proximal biceps tenodesis also has risks and concerns. The fixation strength of interference screws in cancellous bone is inferior to that in cortical bone. In addition, optimal tensioning of the biceps tendon may be less predictable, especially with most all-soft-tissue or suture anchor techniques.

Chronic Bicipital Groove Pain

One recognized complication of biceps tenodesis performed high within the bicipital groove is the potential for residual pain in the bicipital groove.[50,51] This pain may result from residual tenosynovitis and tendon abrasion within the groove (**Figure 6**). Sanders et al[51] reported a higher revision rate with arthroscopic tenodesis (45%) and open proximal tenodesis when the biceps sheath remained in place (16.7%) compared with open proximal tenodesis (0%) with the sheath released or open distal tenodesis (7.7%). The authors advocated arthroscopic débridement of the groove at the time of tenodesis. Multiple authors have recently reported promising early results following arthroscopic tenodesis at the lower portion of the groove, termed suprapectoral tenodesis.[52,53]

Millett et al[37] specifically investigated the differences in outcome and postoperative pain in 88 patients who

FIGURE 5

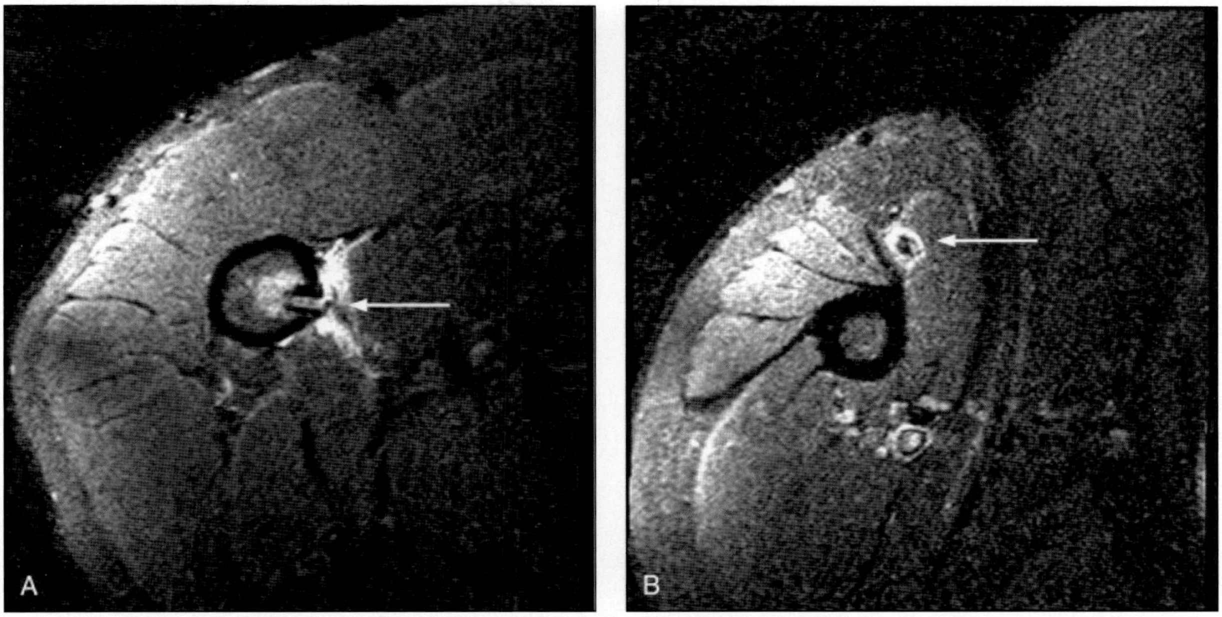

Coronal MRIs demonstrate failure of fixation after open subpectoral biceps tenodesis. **A,** Interference screw (arrow). **B,** Biceps tendon stump (arrow).

underwent subpectoral biceps tenodesis with either an interference screw or suture anchor fixation. No significant differences were seen between the two groups regarding visual analog scale, ASES, or modified Constant scores; persistent spasm; or persistent pain in the bicipital groove (3% for interference screw and 7% for suture anchor fixation). Nho et al[42] reported that persistent bicipital pain was seen in only 0.57% of patients following subpectoral biceps tenodesis.

Complications Following Biceps Tenotomy

Tenotomy of the long head of the biceps tendon is considered a reasonable alternative to tenodesis with predictable pain relief, relative ease of surgical treatment, and minimal postoperative rehabilitation.[40,54] Complications related to biceps tenotomy can be classified as surgical or postoperative.

Intraoperative complications are quite rare and relate primarily to iatrogenic injury to adjacent structures during transection of the biceps tendon. Using thermal

FIGURE 6

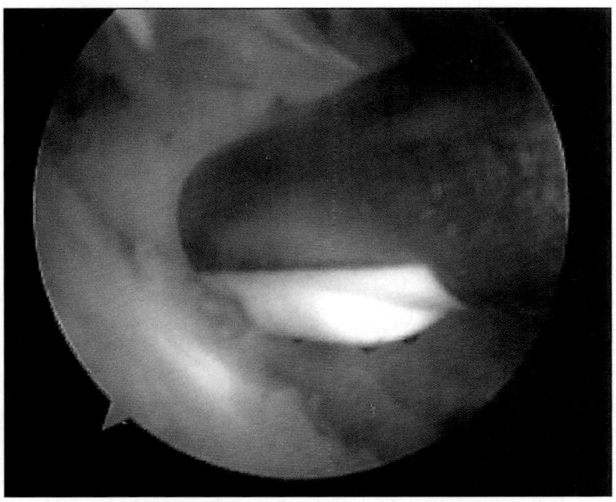

Arthroscopic view shows release of the biceps sheath and biceps tendon scarring following proximal biceps tenodesis. The scar was released, the intertubercular portion of the tendon was resected, and tenodesis of the distal tendon stump was performed in a subpectoral position.

probes to divide the tendon may injure adjacent cartilage and result in chondral lesions. Other authors have suggested that if the biceps tendon has an hourglass shape and cannot retract into the bicipital groove, simple transection of the biceps at its origin may not alleviate the pain generator and may result in an entrapped tendon.[55] In this situation, the intra-articular portion of the tendon should be removed completely.

Postoperative complications and adverse effects related to biceps tenotomy include cosmetic deformity (often referred to as a Popeye deformity), decrease in elbow flexion, and fatigue discomfort.[54-60] Cosmetic deformity has been reported after biceps tenotomy for 3% to 70% of cases.[54,57,58] Several authors have noted that this deformity occurs more commonly in men.[54,58,60] Lim et al[61] investigated the relationship between cosmetic deformity and other patient factors (age, sex, dominant arm involvement, and body mass index) and found that male sex was the only significant factor ($P < 0.001$). Walch et al[60] reviewed 307 biceps tenotomies and postulated that muscle atrophy and loss of muscle tone are possible reasons that cosmetic deformity does not occur in older patients. Frost et al[57] recommended that thin patients who are concerned about appearance should not undergo tenotomy.

Kelly et al[54] reported on 40 biceps tenotomy cases and noted a significant decrease in elbow flexion strength, more commonly in younger patients, and arm pain, similar to muscle cramping, that occurred in 37.5% of patients. Other authors have described arm pain in 21%[56] and 40%[59] of patients.

Conclusion

Disorders of the long head of the biceps tendon are a common source of shoulder pain and can be treated successfully using SLAP repair, biceps tenodesis, and biceps tenotomy. Because the indications for SLAP repair continue to be refined, some of the associated complications will likely cease to be an issue. Biceps tenodesis, biceps tenotomy, and SLAP repair can provide a durable and excellent clinical outcome. Each procedure has specific advantages and must be selected carefully for each patient and for each clinical indication. Conversely, each procedure has the risk of associated complications that must be understood by the surgeon so as to avoid them.

References

1. Mileski RA, Snyder SJ: Superior labral lesions in the shoulder: Pathoanatomy and surgical management. *J Am Acad Orthop Surg* 1998;6(2):121-131.
2. Nam EK, Snyder SJ: The diagnosis and treatment of superior labrum, anterior and posterior (SLAP) lesions. *Am J Sports Med* 2003;31(5):798-810.
3. Gobezie R, Zurakowski D, Lavery K, Millett PJ, Cole BJ, Warner JJ: Analysis of interobserver and intraobserver variability in the diagnosis and treatment of SLAP tears using the Snyder classification. *Am J Sports Med* 2008;36(7):1373-1379.
4. Weber SC, Martin DF, Seiler JG III, Harrast JJ: Superior labrum anterior and posterior lesions of the shoulder: Incidence rates, complications, and outcomes as reported by American Board of Orthopedic Surgery. Part II candidates. *Am J Sports Med* 2012;40(7): 1538-1543.
5. Zhang AL, Kreulen C, Ngo SS, Hame SL, Wang JC, Gamradt SC: Demographic trends in arthroscopic SLAP repair in the United States. *Am J Sports Med* 2012;40(5):1144-1147.
6. Snyder SJ, Banas MP, Karzel RP: An analysis of 140 injuries to the superior glenoid labrum. *J Shoulder Elbow Surg* 1995;4(4):243-248.
7. Alpert JM, Wuerz TH, O'Donnell TF, Carroll KM, Brucker NN, Gill TJ: The effect of age on the outcomes of arthroscopic repair of type II superior labral anterior and posterior lesions. *Am J Sports Med* 2010;38(11):2299-2303.
8. Denard PJ, Lädermann A, Burkhart SS: Long-term outcome after arthroscopic repair of type II SLAP lesions: Results according to age and workers' compensation status. *Arthroscopy* 2012;28(4):451-457.
9. Abbot AE, Li X, Busconi BD: Arthroscopic treatment of concomitant superior labral anterior posterior (SLAP) lesions and rotator cuff tears in patients over the age of 45 years. *Am J Sports Med* 2009;37(7):1358-1362.
10. Franceschi F, Longo UG, Ruzzini L, Rizzello G, Maffulli N, Denaro V: No advantages in repairing a type II superior labrum anterior and posterior (SLAP) lesion when associated with rotator cuff repair in patients over age 50: A randomized controlled trial. *Am J Sports Med* 2008;36(2):247-253.
11. Strickland JP, Fleckenstein CM, Ducker A, Hasan SS: Early results of concurrent arthroscopic repair of rotator

cuff and type II superior labral anterior posterior tears. *Sports Health* 2010;2(6):503-508.

12. Oh JH, Kim SH, Kwak SH, Oh CH, Gong HS: Results of concomitant rotator cuff and SLAP repair are not affected by unhealed SLAP lesion. *J Shoulder Elbow Surg* 2011;20(1):138-145.
13. Burkhart SS, Morgan CD: The peel-back mechanism: Its role in producing and extending posterior type II SLAP lesions and its effect on SLAP repair rehabilitation. *Arthroscopy* 1998;14(6):637-640.
14. Katz LM, Hsu S, Miller SL, et al: Poor outcomes after SLAP repair: Descriptive analysis and prognosis. *Arthroscopy* 2009;25(8):849-855.
15. Brockmeier SF, Voos JE, Williams RJ III, et al: Outcomes after arthroscopic repair of type-II SLAP lesions. *J Bone Joint Surg Am* 2009;91(7):1595-1603.
16. Provencher MT, McCormick F, Dewing CB, Solomon DJ: Paper #208: Revision rates and outcomes of superior labrum anterior posterior 2 repairs. A prospective analysis of 225 patients. *AAOS 2012 Annual Meeting Proceedings*. CD-ROM. Rosemont, IL, 2012.
17. Weber SC: Surgical management of the failed SLAP repair. *Sports Med Arthrosc* 2010;18(3):162-166.
18. Burkart A, Imhoff AB, Roscher E: Foreign-body reaction to the bioabsorbable Suretac device. *Arthroscopy* 2000;16(1):91-95.
19. Freehill MQ, Harms DJ, Huber SM, Atlihan D, Buss DD: Poly-L-lactic acid tack synovitis after arthroscopic stabilization of the shoulder. *Am J Sports Med* 2003;31(5):643-647.
20. Ifesanya A, Scheibel M: Posterosuperior suture granuloma impingement after arthroscopic SLAP repair using suture anchors: A case report. *Knee Surg Sports Traumatol Arthrosc* 2008;16(7):703-706.
21. Barber FA: Biodegradable shoulder anchors have unique modes of failure. *Arthroscopy* 2007;23(3): 316-320.
22. Rhee YG, Lee DH, Lim CT: Unstable isolated SLAP lesion: Clinical presentation and outcome of arthroscopic fixation. *Arthroscopy* 2005;21(9):1099.
23. Sassmannshausen G, Sukay M, Mair SD: Broken or dislodged poly-L-lactic acid bioabsorbable tacks in patients after SLAP lesion surgery. *Arthroscopy* 2006;22(6): 615-619.
24. Athwal GS, Shridharani SM, O'Driscoll SW: Osteolysis and arthropathy of the shoulder after use of bioabsorbable knotless suture anchors: A report of four cases. *J Bone Joint Surg Am* 2006;88(8):1840-1845.
25. Thompson RC Jr, Schneider W, Kennedy T: Entrapment neuropathy of the inferior branch of the suprascapular nerve by ganglia. *Clin Orthop Relat Res* 1982;(166): 185-187.
26. Westerheide KJ, Dopirak RM, Karzel RP, Snyder SJ: Suprascapular nerve palsy secondary to spinoglenoid cysts: Results of arthroscopic treatment. *Arthroscopy* 2006;22(7):721-727.
27. Yoo JC, Lee YS, Ahn JH, Park JH, Kang HJ, Koh KH: Isolated suprascapular nerve injury below the spinoglenoid notch after SLAP repair. *J Shoulder Elbow Surg* 2009;18(4):e27-e29.
28. Shishido H, Kikuchi S: Injury of the suprascapular nerve in shoulder surgery: An anatomic study. *J Shoulder Elbow Surg* 2001;10(4):372-376.
29. O'Brien SJ, Allen AA, Coleman SH, Drakos MC: The trans-rotator cuff approach to SLAP lesions: Technical aspects for repair and a clinical follow-up of 31 patients at a minimum of 2 years. *Arthroscopy* 2002;18(4):372-377.
30. Cohen DB, Coleman S, Drakos MC, et al: Outcomes of isolated type II SLAP lesions treated with arthroscopic fixation using a bioabsorbable tack. *Arthroscopy* 2006;22(2):136-142.
31. Morgan CD, Burkhart SS, Palmeri M, Gillespie M: Type II SLAP lesions: Three subtypes and their relationships to superior instability and rotator cuff tears. *Arthroscopy* 1998;14(6):553-565.
32. Randelli P, Castagna A, Cabitza F, Cabitza P, Arrigoni P, Denti M: Infectious and thromboembolic complications of arthroscopic shoulder surgery. *J Shoulder Elbow Surg* 2010;19(1):97-101.
33. Saltzman MD, Nuber GW, Gryzlo SM, Marecek GS, Koh JL: Efficacy of surgical preparation solutions in shoulder surgery. *J Bone Joint Surg Am* 2009;91(8): 1949-1953.
34. Murray MR, Saltzman MD, Gryzlo SM, Terry MA, Woodward CC, Nuber GW: Efficacy of preoperative home use of 2% chlorhexidine gluconate cloth before shoulder surgery. *J Shoulder Elbow Surg* 2011;20(6): 928-933.
35. Mazzocca AD, Bicos J, Santangelo S, Romeo AA, Arciero RA: The biomechanical evaluation of four fixation techniques for proximal biceps tenodesis. *Arthroscopy* 2005;21(11):1296-1306.

36. Mazzocca AD, Rios CG, Romeo AA, Arciero RA: Subpectoral biceps tenodesis with interference screw fixation. *Arthroscopy* 2005;21(7):896.
37. Millett PJ, Sanders B, Gobezie R, Braun S, Warner JJ: Interference screw vs. suture anchor fixation for open subpectoral biceps tenodesis: Does it matter? *BMC Musculoskelet Disord* 2008;9:121.
38. Verma NN, Drakos M, O'Brien SJ: Arthroscopic transfer of the long head biceps to the conjoint tendon. *Arthroscopy* 2005;21(6):764.
39. Friedman DJ, Dunn JC, Higgins LD, Warner JJ: Proximal biceps tendon: Injuries and management. *Sports Med Arthrosc* 2008;16(3):162-169.
40. Provencher MT, LeClere LE, Romeo AA: Subpectoral biceps tenodesis. *Sports Med Arthrosc* 2008;16(3):170-176.
41. Boileau P, Parratte S, Chuinard C, Roussanne Y, Shia D, Bicknell R: Arthroscopic treatment of isolated type II SLAP lesions: Biceps tenodesis as an alternative to reinsertion. *Am J Sports Med* 2009;37(5):929-936.
42. Nho SJ, Reiff SN, Verma NN, Slabaugh MA, Mazzocca AD, Romeo AA: Complications associated with subpectoral biceps tenodesis: Low rates of incidence following surgery. *J Shoulder Elbow Surg* 2010;19(5):764-768.
43. Sears BW, Spencer EE, Getz CL: Humeral fracture following subpectoral biceps tenodesis in 2 active, healthy patients. *J Shoulder Elbow Surg* 2011;20(6):e7-e11.
44. Friedel R, Markgraf E, Schmidt I, Dönicke T: Proximal humerus shaft fracture as a complication after keyhole-plasty. A case report. *Unfallchirurgie* 1995;21(4):198-201.
45. Gyulai M: Humeral fracture after keyhole tenodesis. *Magy Traumatol Orthop Helyreallito Seb* 1990;33(3):234-236.
46. Reiff SN, Nho SJ, Romeo AA: Proximal humerus fracture after keyhole biceps tenodesis. *Am J Orthop (Belle Mead NJ)* 2010;39(7):E61-E63.
47. Ma H, Van Heest A, Glisson C, Patel S: Musculocutaneous nerve entrapment: An unusual complication after biceps tenodesis. *Am J Sports Med* 2009;37(12):2467-2469.
48. Dickens JF, Kilcoyne KG, Tintle SM, Giuliani J, Schaefer RA, Rue JP: Subpectoral biceps tenodesis: An anatomic study and evaluation of at-risk structures. *Am J Sports Med* 2012;40(10):2337-2341.
49. Kusma M, Dienst M, Eckert J, Steimer O, Kohn D: Tenodesis of the long head of biceps brachii: Cyclic testing of five methods of fixation in a porcine model. *J Shoulder Elbow Surg* 2008;17(6):967-973.
50. Becker DA, Cofield RH: Tenodesis of the long head of the biceps brachii for chronic bicipital tendinitis: Long-term results. *J Bone Joint Surg Am* 1989;71(3):376-381.
51. Sanders B, Lavery KP, Pennington S, Warner JJ: Clinical success of biceps tenodesis with and without release of the transverse humeral ligament. *J Shoulder Elbow Surg* 2012;21(1):66-71.
52. Lo IK, Burkhart SS: Arthroscopic biceps tenodesis using a bioabsorbable interference screw. *Arthroscopy* 2004;20(1):85-95.
53. Lutton DM, Gruson KI, Harrison AK, Gladstone JN, Flatow EL: Where to tenodese the biceps: Proximal or distal? *Clin Orthop Relat Res* 2011;469(4):1050-1055.
54. Kelly AM, Drakos MC, Fealy S, Taylor SA, O'Brien SJ: Arthroscopic release of the long head of the biceps tendon: Functional outcome and clinical results. *Am J Sports Med* 2005;33(2):208-213.
55. Boileau P, Ahrens PM, Hatzidakis AM: Entrapment of the long head of the biceps tendon: The hourglass biceps—a cause of pain and locking of the shoulder. *J Shoulder Elbow Surg* 2004;13(3):249-257.
56. Boileau P, Baqué F, Valerio L, Ahrens P, Chuinard C, Trojani C: Isolated arthroscopic biceps tenotomy or tenodesis improves symptoms in patients with massive irreparable rotator cuff tears. *J Bone Joint Surg Am* 2007;89(4):747-757.
57. Frost A, Zafar MS, Maffulli N: Tenotomy versus tenodesis in the management of pathologic lesions of the tendon of the long head of the biceps brachii. *Am J Sports Med* 2009;37(4):828-833.
58. Gill TJ, McIrvin E, Mair SD, Hawkins RJ: Results of biceps tenotomy for treatment of pathology of the long head of the biceps brachii. *J Shoulder Elbow Surg* 2001;10(3):247-249.
59. Osbahr DC, Diamond AB, Speer KP: The cosmetic appearance of the biceps muscle after long-head tenotomy versus tenodesis. *Arthroscopy* 2002;18(5):483-487.
60. Walch G, Edwards TB, Boulahia A, Nové-Josserand L, Neyton L, Szabo I: Arthroscopic tenotomy of the long head of the biceps in the treatment of rotator cuff tears: Clinical and radiographic results of 307 cases. *J Shoulder Elbow Surg* 2005;14(3):238-246.
61. Lim TK, Moon ES, Koh KH, Yoo JC: Patient-related factors and complications after arthroscopic tenotomy of the long head of the biceps tendon. *Am J Sports Med* 2011;39(4):783-789.

CHAPTER 19

Rehabilitation for Tendinopathy of the Long Head of the Biceps Tendon

Mark P. Cote, PT, DPT, MSCTR
Michael F. Joseph, PhD, PT
Augustus D. Mazzocca, MS, MD

Introduction

The long head of the biceps (LHB) tendon is a common source of anterior shoulder pain.[1,2] Disorders of the LHB tendon include tendinitis, tendinosis, and rupture and have been reported to occur in isolation as well as with other shoulder conditions.[3-6] Rotator cuff tears, hyperlaxity, injury to the superior labrum (superior labrum anterior to posterior [SLAP] tears), and acromioclavicular joint disorders often result in secondary lesions of the LHB tendon.[5,7,8] Inflammatory conditions such as adhesive capsulitis and glenohumeral arthritis have also been associated with LHB tendon disorders.[9]

Treatment for disorders of the LHB tendon encompasses both nonsurgical management and surgical intervention and depends largely on the presence and nature of the concomitant pathology. The challenge for the clinician during rehabilitation of the patient is the comprehensive identification of the etiologic factors that contribute to LHB tendinopathy. Because many factors potentially contribute to LHB symptomatology, the ability to individualize intervention based on a comprehensive evaluation is required for optimal patient care.

Rehabilitation, both as part of nonsurgical management as well as postoperative care, plays an important role in the management of LHB tendon lesions. When formulating a rehabilitation program, the surgeon needs to consider guidelines for therapeutic intervention and progression based on anatomy, biomechanics, and healing timeframes, as well as the individual's overall health.

Terminology

Several terms have been used to describe the pathophysiology of LHB tendon disorders.[10-17] Tendinitis refers to inflammation within the tendon itself, whereas tendinosis describes chronic degeneration in the absence of an active inflammatory process.[17] Tenosynovitis of the LHB tendon consists of inflammation and thickening of the tendon sheath, which originates from the synovial lining of the glenohumeral joint and covers the intra-articular portion of the tendon. Research regarding the pathophysiology of the tendon has demonstrated both inflammatory as well as degenerative findings of the LHB tendon.[11] The term tendinopathy represents the process of tendon disease, often related to overuse, and

Dr. Mazzocca or an immediate family member serves as a paid consultant to or is an employee of Arthrex, Inc.; and has received research or institutional support from Arthrex and Arthrosurface. Neither of the following authors nor any immediate family member has received anything of value from or has stock or stock options held in a commercial company or institution related directly or indirectly to the subject of this chapter: Dr. Cote and Dr. Joseph.

FIGURE 1

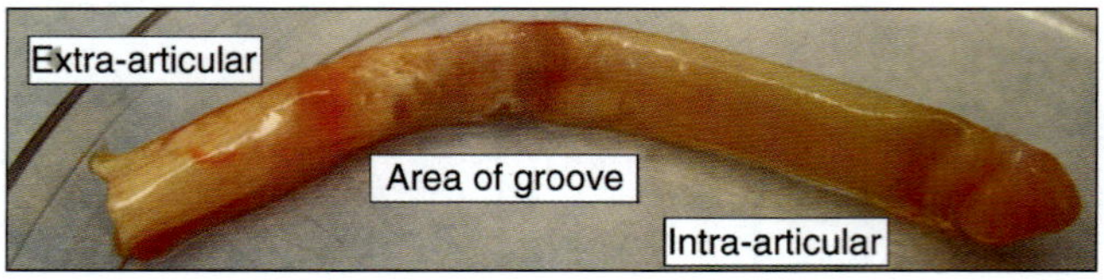

Photograph of the long head of the biceps tendon following tenotomy. The intra-articular part of the tendon is clearly tendinopathic, showing macroscopic signs of paratenon thickening proximally, as well as degeneration and structural damage where the tendon slides within the intertubercular groove.

is the preferred nomenclature for tendon pathology in the absence of histolopathologic examination.[17]

Classification

The management of biceps tendinopathy varies according to the suspected disorder and associated pathology. Various classification schemes to describe different etiologies and pathologic processes have been reported for the categorization of LHB tendon lesions. In general, disorders of the LHB tendon are classified as (1) inflammatory or degenerative in nature (tendinitis, tendinosis), (2) a result of instability (tendon damage occurring as a result of excessive motion of the LHB), or (3) traumatic (tear or rupture related to a trauma).[18] This classification has been further subgrouped to distinguish lesions by anatomic location, pathologic process, and the status of the biceps tendon.[19] Irrespective of classification, multiple conditions are often present, and from the perspective of rehabilitation, evaluation and intervention must target underlying modifiable factors that result in appropriate mechanical load of the tendon.

Pathophysiology of Biceps Tendinopathy

Mechanical load is essential in maintaining tendon health and homeostasis. The overloaded tendon is predisposed to structural damage that results in tendinopathy. Tendon overload may result from intrinsic failure of the tendon to counter external loading, as well as extrinsic mechanical damage due to subacromial impingement or bicipital groove instability.

Irrespective of mechanism, damage to tendon collagen fibers from aberrant loading results in local tenocyte and tendon progenitor cell dysfunction.[20,21] Tenocytes are the cells that maintain tendon homeostasis and repair, and rely on mechanical signals relayed via the extracellular matrix (ECM) for remodeling and survival.[22] Tendon morphologic changes such as the accumulation of proteoglycan, disorganized matrix, increased collagen III production, and decreased loading capability result from the disruption of the ECM/cell interface. Often, these events occur asymptomatically. Kannus and Józsa[23] examined spontaneous tendon ruptures and found that in almost all instances (97%), tendon degeneration preceded rupture. In samples from control patients, evidence of degeneration was seen in 34% of all tendons, and only 51% of the biceps tendons in patients in the control group were histologically normal.

To promote tendon health and healing, the clinician must identify modifiable factors that, when treated, result in appropriate tendon load. The anatomy of the intra-articular portion of the LHB and the mechanics of the shoulder girdle make this identification inherently challenging. The intra-articular and intertubercular portions of the tendon are often subjected to injurious forces, whereas the extra-articular portion of the tendon can appear quite healthy (**Figure 1**).[24] The intra-articular portion of the tendon attaches to the supraglenoid tubercle and superior labrum. The attachment of the LHB superiorly is predisposed to compression and distraction forces often associated with SLAP lesions.[25] Because the LHB slides within its groove during arm motion, the tendon is predisposed to adverse friction forces, along with inflammation of the paratenon, which may thicken and entrap the tendon. The LHB tendon also rotates up to 40° as it exits the joint, which creates adverse torsional forces.[8]

In addition to issues related directly to the anatomy of the LHB tendon, asymmetric and deleterious loading of the tendon occurs, along with damage to various dynamic and static restraints of the glenohumeral joint. The LHB contributes to anterior stability of the glenohumeral joint[26] and this function is amplified in the presence of rotator cuff tears[27,28] and anterior instability.[29] Because scapular dyskinesia can contribute to all of the conditions listed, it frequently coexists with abnormal loading of the LHB tendon.

Nonsurgical Management

To date, no studies have evaluated the efficacy of nonsurgical treatment of LHB tendinopathy. Nonsurgical management is often reported as the first course of treatment in review articles or surgical technique papers, which typically feature brief commentary on nonsurgical management.[30,31] Common treatment recommendations include activity modification, NSAIDs, and rehabilitation to treat underlying biomechanical issues. Rehabilitation represents an opportunity to identify modifiable contributing factors that are amenable to therapy-based interventions. Common findings during evaluation of anterior shoulder pain and LHB tendinopathy include subacromial impingement, rotator cuff dysfunction, posterior capsular tightness, SLAP lesions, anterior patholaxity, and scapular dyskinesis.

Primary LHB Tendinopathy

Primary LHB tendinopathy occurs without any associated injury to or disease in the shoulder. Primary LHB tendinopathy is thought to comprise only 5% of all cases of LHB tendinopathy and is primarily caused by inflammation of the LHB tendon within the intertubercular groove.[3] Groove walls that are shallow or oblique may expose the biceps tendon to excessive strain, resulting in pathologic changes.[10] Pfahler et al[32] examined the intertubercular groove of 67 consecutive patients with ultrasonography and radiography. Radiologic signs of groove degeneration, including shallow or oblique groove walls, correlated with a 43.6% incidence of biceps tendinopathy measured using ultrasonography.

By definition, primary LHB tendinopathy implies healthy surrounding structures of the shoulder. Although an active disease process or injury may not be present or apparent in adjacent structures, soft-tissue restrictions, strength deficits, or alterations in normal kinematics may exist that promote biceps pathology. Findings common among patients in this group include pectoralis minor tightness and scapular dyskinesis.

Secondary LHB Tendinopathy

More commonly, LHB tendinopathy is secondary to other shoulder conditions. Chronic degenerative changes in the LHB tendon have been largely associated with rotator cuff pathology and the diagnosis of subacromial impingement.[3-5,13] Murthi et al[13] examined the condition of the LHB tendon at the time of surgery in 200 shoulders undergoing arthroscopic subacromical decompression and found that 70% had a concomitant rotator cuff tear. Chen et al[4] reported similar findings among a group of patients undergoing rotator cuff repair. Of 122 rotator cuff repairs, visual evidence of LHB tendon pathology was observed in 76% of all cases.

Given the high incidence of associated pathology, it is not unusual for patients with LHB tendinopathy to present with symptoms of subacromial impingement. In this regard, it seems reasonable to conclude that successful management of LHB tendinopathy largely depends on effective treatment of the impingement. Several studies have demonstrated reduction in pain and improvements in function with exercise-based therapy for patients with subacromial impingement.[33-35] De Mey et al[33] investigated the effect of a 6-week exercise program consisting of the following four strengthening exercises: side-lying forward flexion, side-lying external rotation, prone horizontal abduction with external rotation, and prone extension in neutral position. Improvements in pain and function based on the Shoulder Pain and Disability Index (SPADI) scores and the reduction in relative trapezius muscle activation were demonstrated in the 40 participants who completed the program, suggesting exercise alone is an efficacious treatment for patients with impingement syndrome. Strengthening exercise programs for patients with secondary LHB tendinopathy associated with subacromial impingement should include these exercises.

As previously mentioned, scapular dyskinesia can contribute to a multitude of shoulder diagnoses. Several methods exist for the quantification of scapular dyskinesis. Kibler et al[36] described a system for the classification of scapular dysfunction based on three types of abnormal motion. To improve reliability, this system has been simplified as the scapular dyskinesis test, which classifies scapular dyskinesis as either present or absent.[37,38] The authors of this chapter have found this test useful for the identification of patients with scapular dyskinesis (online training for this test is located at http://www.arcadia.edu/academic/default.aspx?id=15080).

FIGURE 2

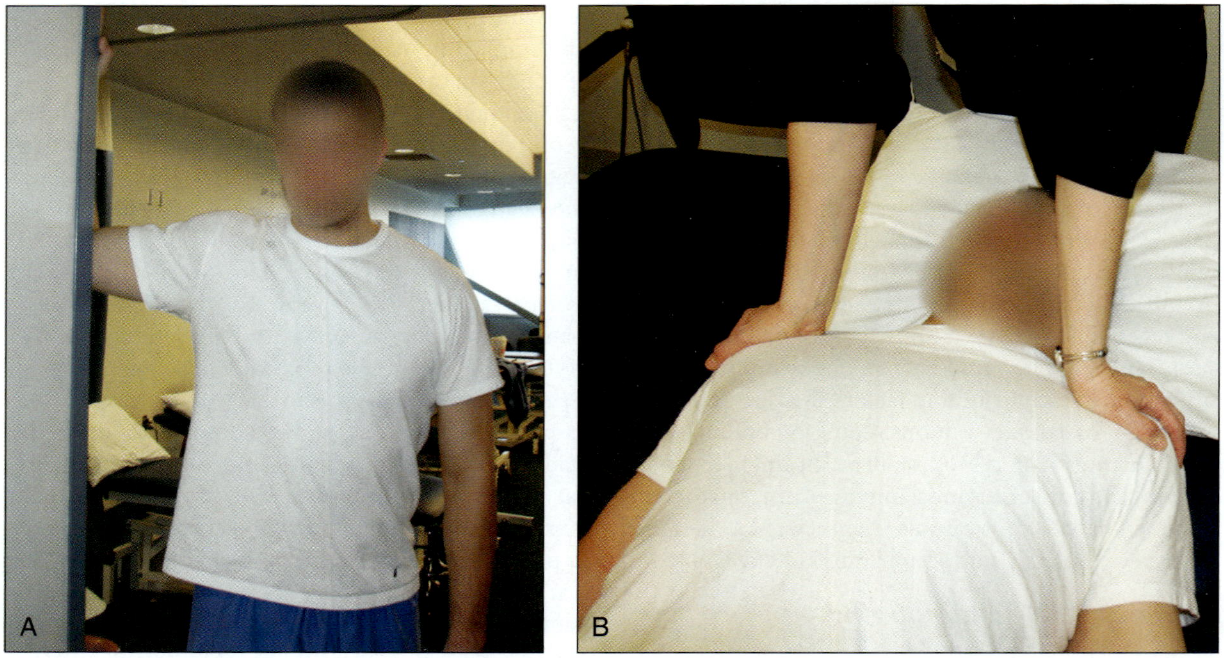

Photographs of stretches for the treatment of pectoralis minor tightness. **A,** The unilateral corner stretch. With the forearm positioned vertically on the doorjamb, the patient rotates his trunk in the opposite direction until a stretch is felt in the anterior chest wall. **B,** The supine manual stretch. The patient's shoulder is placed in abduction and external rotation, with a towel roll placed longitudinally down the spine. The clinician applies force through the coracoid process with the hypothenar eminence to stretch the anterior chest wall.

The causes of scapular dyskinesia include tightness of the pectoralis minor, posterior shoulder tightness, and weakness and aberrant activation patterns of the periscapular musculature. Quantification of pectoralis minor restrictions can be difficult because few methods of measurement exist. Borstad[39] described a clinical method using a tape measure to quantify the linear distance between the origin and the insertion of the pectoralis minor with the patient in the supine position. Although its routine clinical use has been debated, this method has been shown to have good concurrent validity and can help the clinician identify and monitor pectoralis minor tightness.

Several stretches have been described to relieve pectoralis minor tightness. Borstad and Ludwig[40] compared three stretches for the pectoralis minor and found the unilateral corner stretch to be the most effective, followed by the supine manual stretch (**Figure 2**). The authors of this chapter found these stretches to be very useful in eliminating pectoralis minor tightness. In prescribing these exercises, it is important to be mindful of the glenohumeral joint. The unilateral corner stretch places the glenohumeral joint in the terminal degrees of external rotation and horizontal abduction. Prior to stretching, patients should be screened for hyperlaxity to avoid excessive strain of the glenohumeral joint.

Posterior shoulder tightness has been associated with excessive scapular protraction and therefore may contribute to the manifestation of subacromial impingement and secondary LHB tendinopathy.[41] Several methods have been developed to measure posterior shoulder restrictions.[42-46] Obtaining measurements of glenohumeral internal rotation at 90° of abduction and at the side are two common methods that allow the clinician to evaluate the presence of posterior shoulder tightness. Clinically, both measurements should be used to facilitate a more comprehensive assessment of posterior shoulder tightness.

FIGURE 3

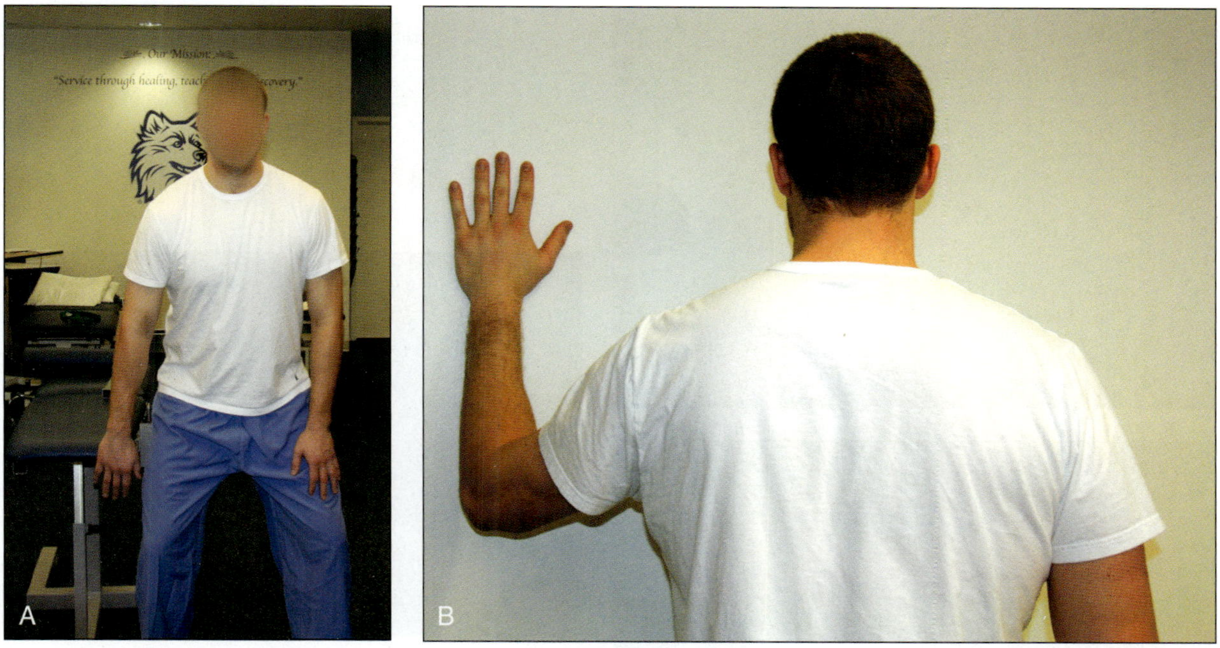

Photographs show closed chain scapular exercises. **A,** The isometric low row exercise. With the hand positioned on the edge of a table or plinth, the patient pushes back for 10 seconds while keeping the elbow extended. This exercise incorporates trunk extension, scapular retraction, and arm extension. **B,** The scapular clock exercise (to facilitate scapular motion and control). The patient performs scapular depression and retraction by moving his scapula to the 6 o'clock and 7:30 clock positions.

Several stretches have been described for posterior shoulder tightness.[47-49] The most common stretches are the horizontal adduction cross-body stretch and the sleeper stretch. In a randomized control trial, McClure et al[49] found the horizontal adduction cross-body stretch produced significant improvements over control patients, whereas the sleeper stretch did not. It is important to recognize that posterior shoulder tightness is common in many patients with shoulder pain and dysfunction. In patients with LHB tendinopathy, the horizontal adduction cross-body stretch may not be tolerated because this position may impinge the LHB on the coracoid and surrounding tissues of the chest wall. In these instances, internal rotation stretching performed in abduction and with the arm at the side in conjunction with posterior glenohumeral joint mobilization may help in improving posterior shoulder mobility.

To treat weakness and aberrant activation of periscapular musculature, the authors of this chapter prefer to begin with closed kinetic chain scapular activities that are easily tolerated and progress to open kinetic chain exercises that are functional for the individual patient's daily activities. Closed chain scapular exercises similar to those described by Burkhart et al[47] are recommended as introductory activities to help isolate scapular movements. These movements include the isometric low row exercise, which incorporates trunk extension, scapular retraction, and arm extension (**Figure 3, A**), and the scapular clock exercise, in which scapular depression and retraction are facilitated by instructing the patient to move the scapula toward a position that mimics the hours on a clock face (**Figure 3, B**).

Exercise is progressed with the addition of isotonic strengthening focusing on the scapular and rotator cuff musculature (**Figure 4**). Attention is given to exercises that recruit the middle and lower trapizeus muscles. Early integration of kinetic chain exercises is also recommended to enhance the recovery of shoulder

FIGURE 4

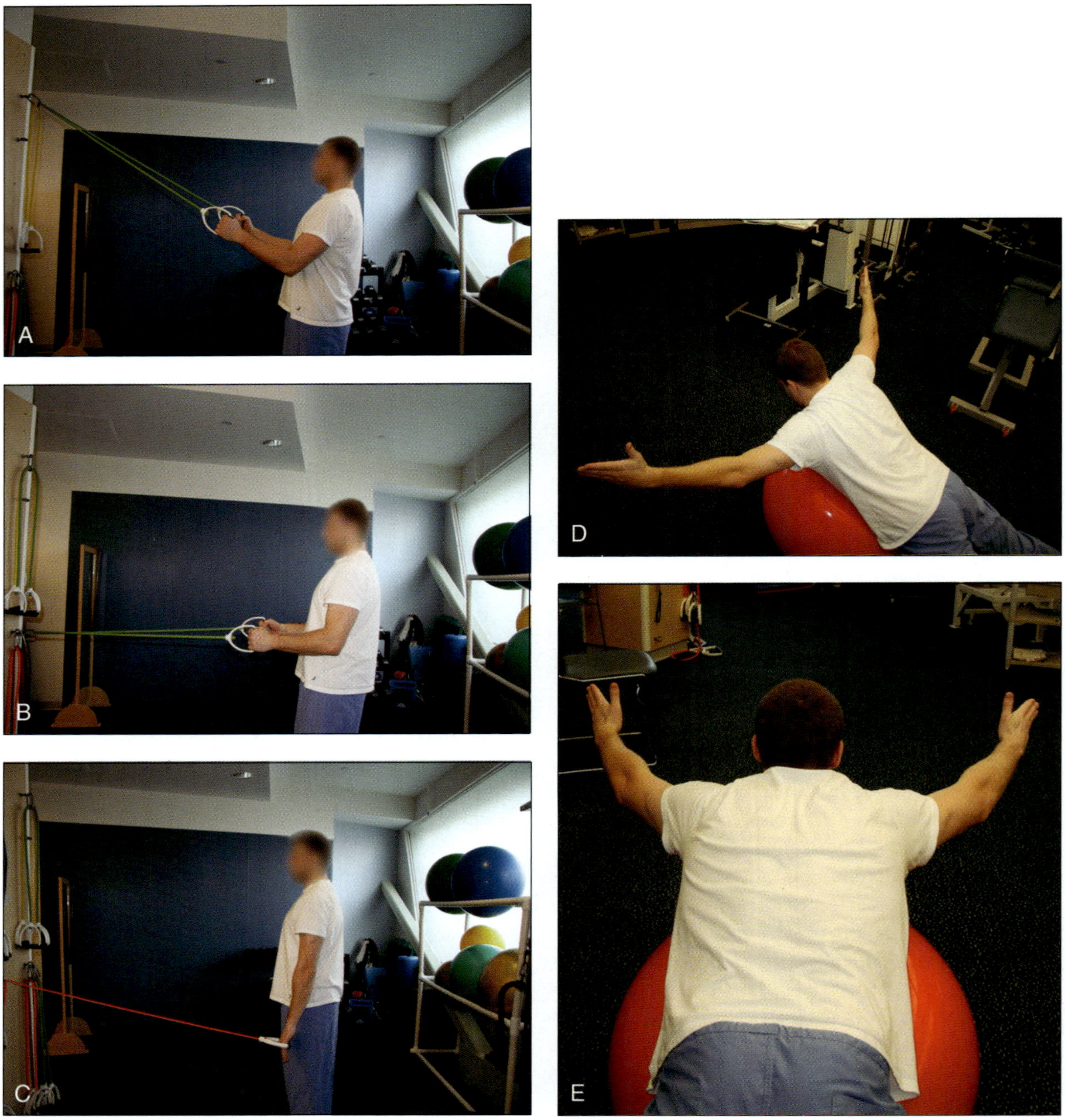

Photographs show isotonic exercises. Rowing exercises performed at upper (**A**), mid (**B**), and lower (**C**) levels. **D,** Horizontal abduction with external rotation (using a physiotherapy ball). **E,** Prone horizontal extension with the arm at 100°.

function and improve the patient's ability to exhibit and maintain scapular retraction (**Figure 5**). DeMay et al[50] demonstrated that contralateral single-limb stance during dynamic pulling exercises increased the activity of the lower trapezius, suggesting that position and motions of the lower extremity are capable of affecting shoulder muscle activation.

LHB Tendinopathy Associated With SLAP Lesions

A SLAP lesion is defined as injury to the superior labrum that extends anterior and posterior to the biceps anchor. By definition, the biceps tendon has been damaged; however, the extent to which the tendon displays signs of degeneration that may result in weakening of the attachment varies extensively. The incidence of SLAP lesions is higher among overhead athletes and military personnel.[51,52] Although several studies support surgical repair,[53-56] successful nonsurgical management has also been described.[30,57] Edwards et al[57] reported on a case series of 39 patients with a SLAP tear, 19 of whom were successfully treated nonsurgically. Scores on quality-of-life instruments and pain scales were markedly improved in the 19 patients who were treated nonsurgically. Return to sport was comparable with patients who underwent successful surgical treatment: 66% of patients returned to the same level of play in overhead sports.

The authors of this chapter offer a trial of nonsurgical treatment to patients with isolated SLAP lesions before surgical repair is attempted. In the case of acute injury, mobility exercises are initiated immediately in an effort to decrease associated morbidity. Active, assisted range of motion (ROM) is progressed as tolerated by the patient. Strengthening exercises are begun immediately and progressed as tolerated by the patient. Treating scapular dyskinesia and posterior shoulder tightness as described previously is often necessary in this group of patients.

Rehabilitation of the overhead athlete, including throwers and swimmers, can be particularly challenging because multiple shoulder structures are often involved. Many of these individuals exhibit anterior patholaxity, caused by his or her athletic performance.[58] When contracting, the LHB provides restraint to anterior humeral head translation, which increases in the presence of anterior patholaxity,[26] increasing strain on the LHB tendon. Nonsurgical management of the overhead athlete is beyond the scope of this chapter; however, impairments in this population often include posterior shoulder tightness, anterior patholaxity, SLAP lesions, and scapular dyskinesis.

FIGURE 5

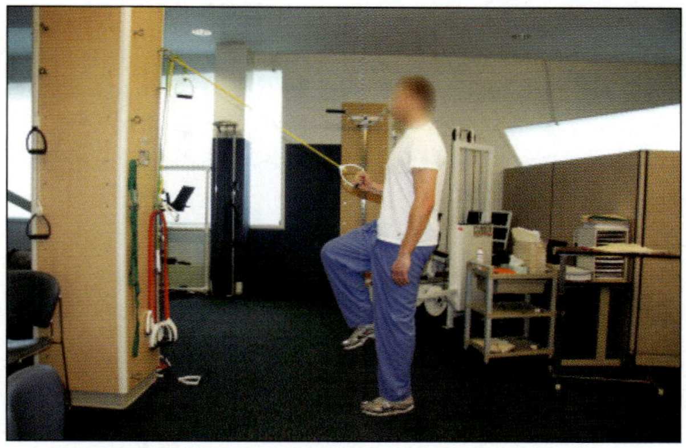

Photograph shows integration of the kinetic chain with scapular exercise. The patient performs a unilateral high-row exercise in contralateral single-leg stance to encourage scapular muscle activation.

LHB Tendinopathy Secondary to Tendon Instability

Biceps tendinopathy may result from instability of the tendon within the bicipital groove. Before entering the intertubercular groove, the LHB tendon is stabilized by several structures, including the superior glenohumeral ligament and the subscapularis tendon anteriorly and the coracohumeral ligament and the anterior fibers of supraspinatus tendon posterolaterally. The biceps pulley system provides stability to the LHB tendon by limiting movement while allowing the necessary gliding of the tendon in the groove to occur during arm movement.[59] Insult to these structures by means of traumatic injury or degeneration can create instability in the LHB tendon. Habermeyer et al[8] reported on 89 patients with arthroscopically diagnosed pulley lesions and found pathology of the LHB tendon, including synovitis, subluxation, dislocation, and partial or complete tears, in 80 patients (89.9%).

Nonsurgical management for LHB tendon instability is similar to that used for primary LHB tendinopathy in that treatment focuses on improving rotator cuff function and scapular mechanics. In the experience of this chapter's authors, it is important to be mindful of internal and external rotation exercises for the rotator cuff musculature. These exercises involve rotating the shoulder under load (for example, using exercise tubing and resistance cable) with the arm at the side and the elbow in 90° of flexion. This motion may be painful because of repetitive contact of the LHB tendon on the intertubercular groove as the humerus rotates. In these cases, rotator cuff exercises should be prescribed in a limited range and progressed carefully according to the patient's symptoms.

Postoperative Rehabilitation

Patients with persistent symptoms and functional limitations recalcitrant to nonsurgical rehabilitation are recommended for surgical intervention. Biceps tenodesis, biceps tenotomy, and SLAP repair are surgical procedures commonly performed to treat LHB tendon pathology. Despite the commonality, no evidence exists to support postoperative rehabilitation. Therefore, the authors of this chapter follow rehabilitation guidelines based on anatomy, pathoanatomy, and biologic healing for the progression of activities.

Biceps Tenodesis

Multiple biceps tenodesis procedures have been reported in the literature, including the bone tunnel, suture anchor, arthroscopic, and interference screw techniques.[16,60-64] Biceps tenodesis is often performed in conjunction with other procedures such as a rotator cuff repair. To develop a safe strategy for postoperative rehabilitation, it is critical to identify these procedures and recognize the healing times associated with these procedures.

Following biceps tenodesis, the arm is immobilized in a sling for 4 weeks to encourage healing of the biceps tendon in its new insertion site on the humerus. Shoulder motion in all planes and active, assisted elbow flexion are also performed. From weeks 4 to 12, active elbow ROM is permitted in all planes of motion. Rotator cuff and parascapular muscle strengthening exercises are also initiated. Direct strengthening of the biceps musculature is withheld until 12 weeks postoperatively.

Shoulder mobility exercises are initiated within the first week following surgery. The authors of this chapter prefer to initiate ROM exercises with limb-supported activities such as the table or wall slide (**Figure 6**). These closed chain exercises have been shown to elicit low levels of shoulder muscle activity.[65] The exercises can be started on a flat surface and gradually progressed to inclined surfaces, and finally, a vertical surface. The addition of supine flexion and pulley exercises also helps increase forward elevation. In the experience of the authors of this chapter, patients respond favorably to this progression because it allows the patient to gradually increase the level of muscle contribution with each exercise.

With concomitant rotator cuff repair, the arm is immobilized for 6 weeks in an abduction sling. Patients are allowed to perform supine external rotation to 30° and forward elevation as an active-assisted (patient-directed) or therapist-assisted exercise. These exercises should be performed passively to avoid placing stress on the repair as a result of excessive muscle activity of the rotator cuff musculature.

From weeks 6 through 12, intervention progresses with the goal of establishing full ROM at week 12. Exercises are selected based on the amount of strain that may be placed on the repaired rotator cuff as a result of the direction of motion (passive stretching) or contraction of the rotator cuff muscles (active or resistive motion). Exercises with minimal rotator cuff muscle activity and strain at the repair are performed early in the postoperative period whereas higher-demand, higher-strain exercises are reserved until the latter weeks following surgery. Rotator cuff-specific strengthening (resistance exercise) is delayed until after postoperative week 12 and progressed through week 18.

Biceps Tenotomy

Biceps tenotomy releases the LHB tendon from its attachment without any subsequent reattachment. Rehabilitation following biceps tenotomy is similar to that following biceps tenodesis in that attention is given to concomitant procedures. When biceps tenotomy is performed in isolation without concomitant procedures, the rate of rehabilitation may be accelerated and progressed as tolerated, because none of the healing tissues require protection. However, patients should be coun-

FIGURE 6

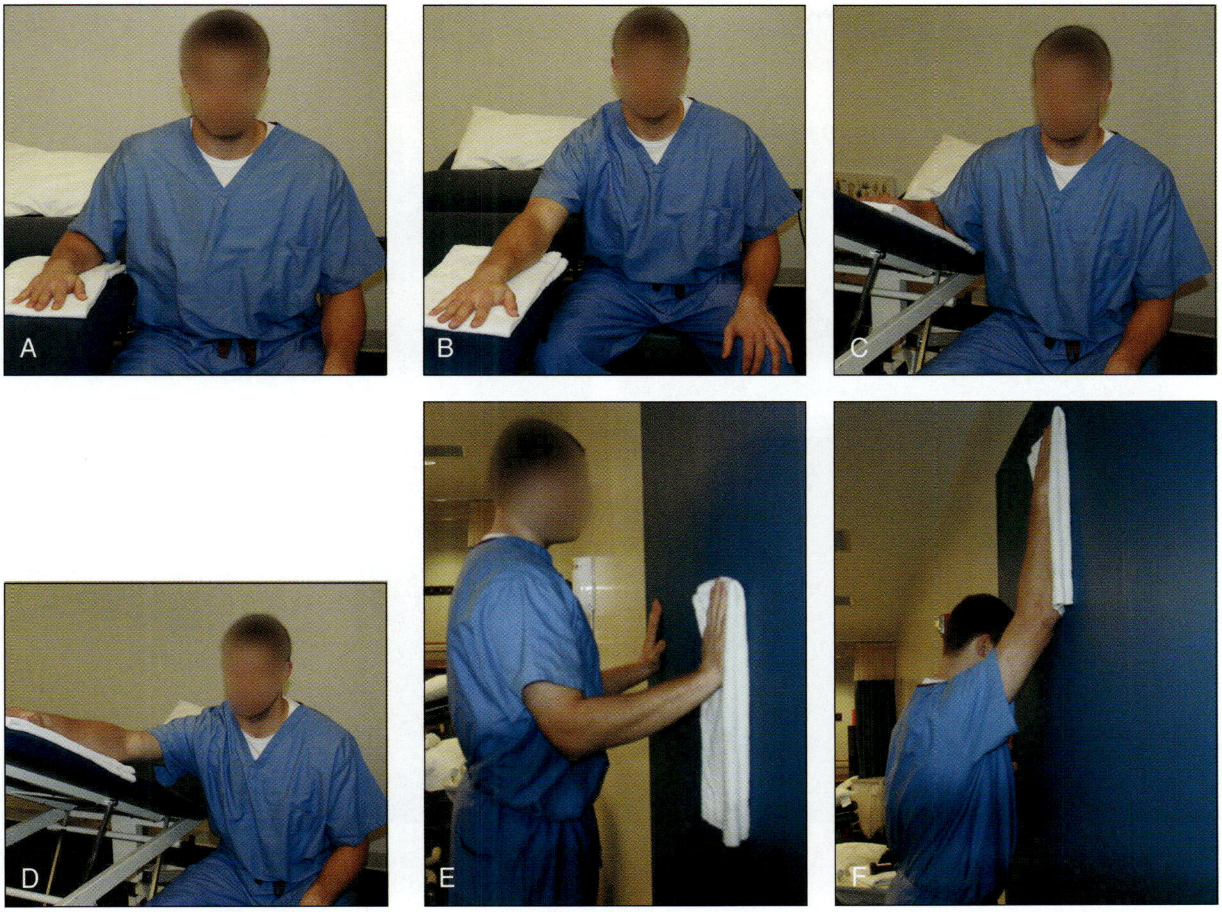

Photographs show limb-supported range of motion. With the hand placed on a flat surface (**A**) the patient slides his hand forward (**B**). The exercise is progressed by gradually inclining the surface (**C, D**), ending with a vertical surface (**E, F**).

seled about the potential for a Popeye (cosmetic) deformity.[66,67] Some authors suggest that this finding may be more likely to occur with an aggressive approach to rehabilitation, prompting slower initiation of movement.[31]

The authors of this chapter prefer to progress postoperative rehabilitation as tolerated by the patient. Although ROM following isolated biceps tenotomy is not expressly limited, progressing exercise too quickly can result in continued pain and dysfunction. If pain is persistent, ROM exercises can be adjusted to focus on high frequency (motion exercises performed three to four times per day), at low intensity (within a pain-free ROM or ROM to pain) for short durations (20 to 30 repetitions or for 2 to 3 minutes). This approach allows existing motion to be maintained and carefully increased while facilitating a reduction in pain and inflammation.

SLAP Repair

The postoperative guidelines for SLAP repair are similar to those for tenodesis in that the selection and progression of activities is based on anatomy, pathoanatomy, and biologic healing. Following SLAP repair, patients are immobilized for 4 weeks to protect the repair. The

FIGURE 7

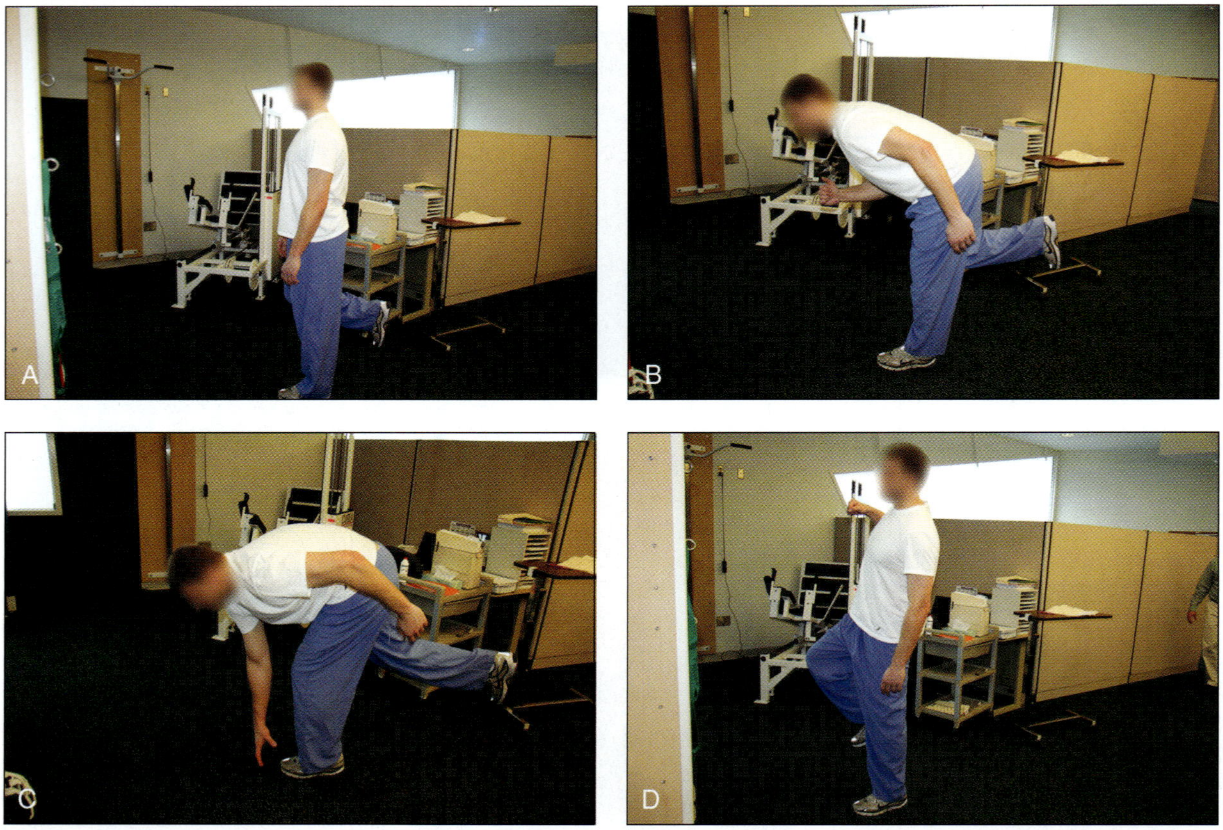

Photographs show kinetic chain exercises. **A, B,** The single-leg trunk bend. **C, D,** The lawnmower exercise.

selection and progression of rehabilitation activities is based largely on the potential stress placed on the repair site. To avoid placing stress on the repair via the peel-back mechanism, external rotation is limited during the first 6 weeks following repair. The peel-back mechanism occurs when the shoulder is in a position of abduction and end ROM in external rotation and can produce torsional force at the base of the biceps,[68] limiting external rotation to 30° for the first 6 weeks. As with biceps tenodesis, patients are progressed by means of prescribed exercises and techniques that decrease the assistance needed, with the goal of establishing full ROM at 12 weeks.

Closed chain scapular exercises can be initiated within the first 2 weeks of rehabilitation. These exercises unload the weight of the upper extremity, allowing the patient to focus on isolating the scapular motion. The low row (**Figure 3, A**) and scapular clock (**Figure 3, B**) exercises are useful during this period to facilitate scapular motion and control. At 6 weeks postoperatively, these exercises can be advanced to rowing with tubing or cable resistance, with integration of combined motions of the upper extremity.

Early integration of kinetic chain exercises is also recommended to enhance the recovery of shoulder function and improve the patient's ability to produce and maintain scapular retraction. Based on the kinetic link model, these exercises combine leg and trunk activity with shoulder motion to reinforce normally occurring movement patterns of the upper extremity.[69,70] Single-leg trunk bends and the lawnmower exercise are examples of commonly prescribed kinetic chain exercises (**Figure 7**). After week 6, rotator cuff strengthening is initiated but restricted to exercises with the arm at the side (0° of abduction) until 12 weeks. From week 12 through week 18, overhead exercises such as those in external rotation at 90° can be initiated and progressed.

Strengthening exercises for the biceps musculature should be progressed according to the type of repair. Dodson and Altchek[30] described the differences regarding the progression of biceps activity based on the extent of bicipital involvement. During SLAP repair, the LHB tendon may be resected or repaired. If the LHB tendon is repaired, resisted biceps activities (elbow flexion, forearm supination) is withheld for the first 12 weeks to allow healing to occur. Conversely, if the LHB tendon is resected, biceps activities can begin between 6 and 8 weeks following repair.[30]

Conclusion

Rehabilitation plays an important role in the treatment of patients with LHB tendinopathy. In nonsurgical management, identifying potential contributing factors of the musculoskeletal system that are amenable to therapy-based interventions is essential for the development of an effective plan of care. Postoperatively, biceps tenodesis and biceps tenotomy are often performed in conjunction with other procedures. Recognition of healing time frames associated with these procedures is necessary to develop a safe strategy for rehabilitation. A thorough evaluation of the integrity of soft-tissue structures and shoulder girdle mechanics is of paramount importance. Common findings associated with biceps tendinopathy include a tight posterior shoulder, rotator cuff dysfunction, and scapular dyskinesia. Interventions should target the identified impairments, with the principal goal of ultimately restoring optimal shoulder function.

References

1. Galasso O, Gasparini G, De Benedetto M, Familiari F, Castricini R: Tenotomy versus tenodesis in the treatment of the long head of biceps brachii tendon lesions. *BMC Musculoskelet Disord* 2012;13:205.
2. Delle Rose G, Borroni M, Silvestro A, et al: The long head of biceps as a source of pain in active population: tenotomy or tenodesis? A comparison of 2 case series with isolated lesions. *Musculoskelet Surg* 2012;96 (Suppl 1):S47-S52.
3. Favorito PJ, Harding WG III, Heidt RS Jr: Complete arthroscopic examination of the long head of the biceps tendon. *Arthroscopy* 2001;17(4):430-432.
4. Chen CH, Chen CH, Chang CH, et al: Classification and analysis of pathology of the long head of the biceps tendon in complete rotator cuff tears. *Chang Gung Med J* 2012;35(3):263-270.
5. Pill SG, Walch G, Hawkins RJ, Kissenberth MJ: The role of the biceps tendon in massive rotator cuff tears. *Instr Course Lect* 2012;61:113-120.
6. Ahrens PM, Boileau P: The long head of biceps and associated tendinopathy. *J Bone Joint Surg Br* 2007;89(8):1001-1009.
7. Bennett WF: Correlation of the SLAP lesion with lesions of the medial sheath of the biceps tendon and intra-articular subscapularis tendon. *Indian J Orthop* 2009;43(4):342-346.
8. Habermeyer P, Magosch P, Pritsch M, Scheibel MT, Lichtenberg S: Anterosuperior impingement of the shoulder as a result of pulley lesions: A prospective arthroscopic study. *J Shoulder Elbow Surg* 2004;13(1):5-12.
9. Zhao W, Zheng X, Liu Y, et al: An MRI study of symptomatic adhesive capsulitis. *PLoS One* 2012;7(10):e47277.
10. Curtis AS, Snyder SJ: Evaluation and treatment of biceps tendon pathology. *Orthop Clin North Am* 1993;24(1):33-43.
11. Hsu SH, Miller SL, Curtis AS: Long head of biceps tendon pathology: Management alternatives. *Clin Sports Med* 2008;27(4):747-762.
12. Krüger M, Bischof-Léger E: Frequency of biceps tendon tenosynovitis from crutches: A sonographical observation. *Z Rheumatol* 2008;67(1):62, 64-67.
13. Murthi AM, Vosburgh CL, Neviaser TJ: The incidence of pathologic changes of the long head of the biceps tendon. *J Shoulder Elbow Surg* 2000;9(5):382-385.
14. Patton WC, McCluskey GM III: Biceps tendinitis and subluxation. *Clin Sports Med* 2001;20(3):505-529.
15. Post M, Benca P: Primary tendinitis of the long head of the biceps. *Clin Orthop Relat Res* 1989;(246):117-125.
16. Depalma AF, Callery GE: Bicipital tenosynovitis. *Clin Orthop* 1954;3(3):69-85.
17. Longo UG, Loppini M, Marineo G, Khan WS, Maffulli N, Denaro V: Tendinopathy of the tendon of the long

head of the biceps. *Sports Med Arthrosc* 2011;19(4): 321-332.

18. Yamaguchi K, Keener JD, Galatz LM: Disorders of the biceps tendon, in Iannotti JP, Williams GR, eds: Disorders of the Shoulder: Diagnosis and Management, ed 2. Philadelphia, PA, Lippincott, Williams and Wilkins, 2007.
19. Khazzam M, George MS, Churchill RS, Kuhn JE: Disorders of the long head of biceps tendon. *J Shoulder Elbow Surg* 2012;21(1):136-145.
20. Arnoczky SP, Lavagnino M, Egerbacher M: The mechanobiological aetiopathogenesis of tendinopathy: Is it the over-stimulation or the under-stimulation of tendon cells? *Int J Exp Pathol* 2007;88(4):217-226.
21. Zhang J, Wang JH: Mechanobiological response of tendon stem cells: Implications of tendon homeostasis and pathogenesis of tendinopathy. *J Orthop Res* 2010;28(5):639-643.
22. Wang JH: Mechanobiology of tendon. *J Biomech* 2006;39(9):1563-1582.
23. Kannus P, Józsa L: Histopathological changes preceding spontaneous rupture of a tendon: A controlled study of 891 patients. *J Bone Joint Surg Am* 1991;73(10): 1507-1525.
24. Joseph M, Maresh CM, McCarthy MB, et al: Histological and molecular analysis of the biceps tendon long head post-tenotomy. *J Orthop Res* 2009;27(10): 1379-1385.
25. Snyder SJ, Banas MP, Karzel RP: An analysis of 140 injuries to the superior glenoid labrum. *J Shoulder Elbow Surg* 1995;4(4):243-248.
26. Rodosky MW, Harner CD, Fu FH: The role of the long head of the biceps muscle and superior glenoid labrum in anterior stability of the shoulder. *Am J Sports Med* 1994;22(1):121-130.
27. Youm T, ElAttrache NS, Tibone JE, McGarry MH, Lee TQ: The effect of the long head of the biceps on glenohumeral kinematics. *J Shoulder Elbow Surg* 2009;18(1):122-129.
28. Longo UG, Berton A, Marinozzi A, Maffulli N, Denaro V: Subscapularis tears. *Med Sport Sci* 2012;57:114-121.
29. Longo UG, Berton A, Papapietro N, Maffulli N, Denaro V: Biomechanics of the rotator cuff: European perspective. *Med Sport Sci* 2012;57:10-17.
30. Dodson CC, Altchek DW: SLAP lesions: An update on recognition and treatment. *J Orthop Sports Phys Ther* 2009;39(2):71-80.
31. Ryu JH, Pedowitz RA: Rehabilitation of biceps tendon disorders in athletes. *Clin Sports Med* 2010;29(2):229-246, vii-viii.
32. Pfahler M, Branner S, Refior HJ: The role of the bicipital groove in tendopathy of the long biceps tendon. *J Shoulder Elbow Surg* 1999;8(5):419-424.
33. De Mey K, Danneels L, Cagnie B, Cools AM: Scapular muscle rehabilitation exercises in overhead athletes with impingement symptoms: Effect of a 6-week training program on muscle recruitment and functional outcome. *Am J Sports Med* 2012;40(8):1906-1915.
34. Holmgren T, Björnsson Hallgren H, Öberg B, Adolfsson L, Johansson K: Effect of specific exercise strategy on need for surgery in patients with subacromial impingement syndrome: Randomised controlled study. *BMJ* 2012;344:e787.
35. Tate AR, McClure PW, Young IA, Salvatori R, Michener LA: Comprehensive impairment-based exercise and manual therapy intervention for patients with subacromial impingement syndrome: A case series. *J Orthop Sports Phys Ther* 2010;40(8):474-493.
36. Kibler WB, Uhl TL, Maddux JW, Brooks PV, Zeller B, McMullen J: Qualitative clinical evaluation of scapular dysfunction: A reliability study. *J Shoulder Elbow Surg* 2002;11(6):550-556.
37. Tate AR, McClure P, Kareha S, Irwin D, Barbe MF: A clinical method for identifying scapular dyskinesis, part 2: Validity. *J Athl Train* 2009;44(2):165-173.
38. McClure P, Tate AR, Kareha S, Irwin D, Zlupko E: A clinical method for identifying scapular dyskinesis, part 1: Reliability. *J Athl Train* 2009;44(2):160-164.
39. Borstad JD: Measurement of pectoralis minor muscle length: Validation and clinical application. *J Orthop Sports Phys Ther* 2008;38(4):169-174.
40. Borstad JD, Ludewig PM: Comparison of three stretches for the pectoralis minor muscle. *J Shoulder Elbow Surg* 2006;15(3):324-330.
41. Michener LA, McClure PW, Karduna AR: Anatomical and biomechanical mechanisms of subacromial impingement syndrome. *Clin Biomech (Bristol, Avon)* 2003;18(5):369-379.
42. Borstad JD, Mathiowetz KM, Minday LE, Prabhu B, Christopherson DE, Ludewig PM: Clinical measurement of posterior shoulder flexibility. *Man Ther* 2007;12(4):386-389.

43. Jari S, Sallay P: Quantification of posterior capsule tightness and motion loss in patients with shoulder impingement. *Am J Sports Med* 2001;29(4):534.
44. Tyler TF, Nicholas SJ, Roy T, Gleim GW: Quantification of posterior capsule tightness and motion loss in patients with shoulder impingement. *Am J Sports Med* 2000;28(5):668-673.
45. Tyler TF, Roy T, Nicholas SJ, Gleim GW: Reliability and validity of a new method of measuring posterior shoulder tightness. *J Orthop Sports Phys Ther* 1999;29(5): 262-274.
46. Myers JB, Oyama S, Wassinger CA, et al: Reliability, precision, accuracy, and validity of posterior shoulder tightness assessment in overhead athletes. *Am J Sports Med* 2007;35(11):1922-1930.
47. Burkhart SS, Morgan CD, Kibler WB: The disabled throwing shoulder: spectrum of pathology. Part III: The SICK scapula, scapular dyskinesis, the kinetic chain, and rehabilitation. *Arthroscopy* 2003;19(6):641-661.
48. Johansen RL, Callis M, Potts J, Shall LM: A modified internal rotation stretching technique for overhand and throwing athletes. *J Orthop Sports Phys Ther* 1995;21(4):216-219.
49. McClure P, Balaicuis J, Heiland D, Broersma ME, Thorndike CK, Wood A: A randomized controlled comparison of stretching procedures for posterior shoulder tightness. *J Orthop Sports Phys Ther* 2007;37(3):108-114.
50. De Mey K, Danneels L, Cagnie B, Van den Bosch L, Flier J, Cools AM: Kinetic chain influences on upper and lower trapezius muscle activation during eight variations of a scapular retraction exercise in overhead athletes. *J Sci Med Sport* 2013;16(1):65-70.
51. Sayde WM, Cohen SB, Ciccotti MG, Dodson CC: Return to play after Type II superior labral anterior-posterior lesion repairs in athletes: A systematic review. *Clin Orthop Relat Res* 2012;470(6):1595-1600.
52. Kampa RJ, Clasper J: Incidence of SLAP lesions in a military population. *J R Army Med Corps* 2005;151(3): 171-175.
53. Van Kleunen JP, Tucker SA, Field LD, Savoie FH III: Return to high-level throwing after combination infraspinatus repair, SLAP repair, and release of glenohumeral internal rotation deficit. *Am J Sports Med* 2012;40(11):2536-2541.
54. Neuman BJ, Boisvert CB, Reiter B, Lawson K, Ciccotti MG, Cohen SB: Results of arthroscopic repair of type II superior labral anterior posterior lesions in overhead athletes: Assessment of return to preinjury playing level and satisfaction. *Am J Sports Med* 2011;39(9):1883-1888.
55. Park JH, Lee YS, Wang JH, Noh HK, Kim JG: Outcome of the isolated SLAP lesions and analysis of the results according to the injury mechanisms. *Knee Surg Sports Traumatol Arthrosc* 2008;16(5):511-515.
56. Keener JD, Brophy RH: Superior labral tears of the shoulder: Pathogenesis, evaluation, and treatment. *J Am Acad Orthop Surg* 2009;17(10):627-637.
57. Edwards SL, Lee JA, Bell JE, et al: Nonoperative treatment of superior labrum anterior posterior tears: Improvements in pain, function, and quality of life. *Am J Sports Med* 2010;38(7):1456-1461.
58. Yiannakopoulos CK, Mataragas E, Antonogiannakis E: A comparison of the spectrum of intra-articular lesions in acute and chronic anterior shoulder instability. *Arthroscopy* 2007;23(9):985-990.
59. Werner A, Mueller T, Boehm D, Gohlke F: The stabilizing sling for the long head of the biceps tendon in the rotator cuff interval: A histoanatomic study. *Am J Sports Med* 2000;28(1):28-31.
60. Boileau P, Krishnan SG, Coste JS, Walch G: Arthroscopic biceps tenodesis: A new technique using bioabsorbable interference screw fixation. *Arthroscopy* 2002;18(9):1002-1012.
61. Froimson AI, O I: Keyhole tenodesis of biceps origin at the shoulder. *Clin Orthop Relat Res* 1975;112:245-249.
62. Gilcreest EL: Dislocation and elongation of the long head of the biceps brachii: An analysis of six cases. *Ann Surg* 1936;104(1):118-138.
63. Mazzocca AD, Bicos J, Santangelo S, Romeo AA, Arciero RA: The biomechanical evaluation of four fixation techniques for proximal biceps tenodesis. *Arthroscopy* 2005;21(11):1296-1306.
64. Mazzocca AD, Cote MP, Arciero CL, Romeo AA, Arciero RA: Clinical outcomes after subpectoral biceps tenodesis with an interference screw. *Am J Sports Med* 2008;36(10):1922-1929.
65. Wise MB, Uhl TL, Mattacola CG, Nitz AJ, Kibler WB: The effect of limb support on muscle activation during shoulder exercises. *J Shoulder Elbow Surg* 2004;13(6):614-620.

66. Bradbury T, Dunn WR, Kuhn JE: Preventing the popeye deformity after release of the long head of the biceps tendon: An alternative technique and biomechanical evaluation. *Arthroscopy* 2008;24(10):1099-1102.
67. Boileau P, Baqué F, Valerio L, Ahrens P, Chuinard C, Trojani C: Isolated arthroscopic biceps tenotomy or tenodesis improves symptoms in patients with massive irreparable rotator cuff tears. *J Bone Joint Surg Am* 2007;89(4):747-757.
68. Burkhart SS, Morgan CD: The peel-back mechanism: Its role in producing and extending posterior type II SLAP lesions and its effect on SLAP repair rehabilitation. *Arthroscopy* 1998;14(6):637-640.
69. McMullen J, Uhl TL: A kinetic chain approach for shoulder rehabilitation. *J Athl Train* 2000;35(3): 329-337.
70. Kibler WB, Livingston B: Closed-chain rehabilitation for upper and lower extremities. *J Am Acad Orthop Surg* 2001;9(6):412-421.

Index

Page numbers followed by *f* indicate figures, and page numbers followed by *t* indicate tables

C

D

E

G

H

I

J

K

L

M

N

O

P

R

S

T

Y